Advances in HIV/AIDS Research

Advances in HIV/AIDS Research

Edited by **Roger Mostafa**

hayle
medical

New York

Published by Hayle Medical,
30 West, 37th Street, Suite 612,
New York, NY 10018, USA
www.haylemedical.com

Advances in HIV/AIDS Research
Edited by Roger Mostafa

© 2015 Hayle Medical

International Standard Book Number: 978-1-63241-027-6 (Hardback)

Contents

	Preface	VII

Part 1	Special Clinical Cares	1

Chapter 1	HIV-1 Treatment-Experienced Patients: Treatment Options and Management Gail Reid and Richard M. Novak	3
Chapter 2	Special Considerations in the Management of HIV Infection in Pregnancy Chi Dola, Sean Kim and Juliet Tran	21
Chapter 3	InforMatrix Nucleoside/Nucleotide Reverse Transcriptase Inhibitors "Backbones" Gerrit Schreij and Rob Janknegt	39

Part 2	New Therapy Strategies	63

Chapter 4	Cell-Delivered Gene Therapy for HIV Scott Ledger, Borislav Savkovic, Michelle Millington, Helen Impey, Maureen Boyd, John M. Murray and Geoff Symonds	65
Chapter 5	Gene Therapy for HIV-1 Infection Lisa Egerer, Dorothee von Laer and Janine Kimpel	91
Chapter 6	Crippling of HIV at Multiple Stages with Recombinant Adeno-Associated Viral Mediated RNA Interference Ramesh B. Batchu, Oksana V. Gruzdyn, Aamer M. Qazi, Assaad Y. Semaan, Shelly M. Seward, Christopher P. Steffes, David L. Bouwman, Donald W. Weaver and Scott A. Gruber	117
Chapter 7	HIV-Screening Strategies for the Discovery of Novel HIV-Inhibitors María José Abad, Luis Miguel Bedoya and Paulina Bermejo	135

Part 3   Vaccine Development   147

Chapter 8   HIV Vaccine   149
Alexandre de Almeida, Telma Miyuki Oshiro,
Alessandra Pontillo and Alberto José da Silva Duarte

Chapter 9   Towards a Functional Cure for HIV Infection:
The Potential Contribution of Therapeutic Vaccination   171
Maja A. Sommerfelt

Part 4   Beyond Conventional   189

Chapter 10   Substance Abuse Treatment Utilizing Medication
Assisted Treatment as HIV Prevention   191
Thomas F Kresina, Robert Lubran and Laura W. Cheever

Chapter 11   Micronutrient Synergy
in the Control of HIV Infection and AIDS   213
Raxit J. Jariwalla, Aleksandra Niedzwiecki and Matthias Rath

Chapter 12   The Pertinence of Applying Qualitative
Investigation Strategies in the Design
and Evaluation of HIV Prevention Policies   227
Carmen Rodríguez, Teresa Blasco,
Antonio Vargas and Agustín Benito

Permissions

List of Contributors

Preface

Every book is a source of knowledge and this one is no exception. The idea that led to the conceptualization of this book was the fact that the world is advancing rapidly; which makes it crucial to document the progress in every field. I am aware that a lot of data is already available, yet, there is a lot more to learn. Hence, I accepted the responsibility of editing this book and contributing my knowledge to the community.

This book presents HIV/AIDS researches on treatment, new developments, pathogenesis and other related fields which offer a good foundation for development of clinical patient care. This book includes contributions of scientists and researchers who have extensively researched about HIV/AIDS. Translational model is one of the initial steps for progressing HIV/AIDS clinical research. Advanced researches should directly benefit HIV/AIDS patients when linked to the care of patients. The book discusses important topics under the sections: Special Clinical Cares; New Therapy Strategies; Vaccine Development and Beyond Conventional. It aims to assist interested individuals in the study of HIV/AIDS by providing informative and valuable data.

While editing this book, I had multiple visions for it. Then I finally narrowed down to make every chapter a sole standing text explaining a particular topic, so that they can be used independently. However, the umbrella subject sinews them into a common theme. This makes the book a unique platform of knowledge.

I would like to give the major credit of this book to the experts from every corner of the world, who took the time to share their expertise with us. Also, I owe the completion of this book to the never-ending support of my family, who supported me throughout the project.

Editor

Part 1

Special Clinical Cares

HIV-1 Treatment-Experienced Patients: Treatment Options and Management

Gail Reid and Richard M. Novak
University of Illinois, Chicago
U.S.A.

1. Introduction

Human immunodeficiency virus (HIV) and acquired immune deficiency syndrome (AIDS) are a global health crisis of unprecedented dimensions, causing over 25 million deaths worldwide since it was first recognized as a disease entity in the early 1980s.(Joint United Nations Program on HIV/AIDS 2008) In 2008 alone, there were approximately 2.7 million newly infected and over 33 million persons living with HIV globally, of whom between 1.8 and 2.3 million died.(Joint United Nations Program on HIV/AIDS 2011) In the 24 years since zidovudine was approved for the treatment of HIV infection, remarkable advances have been made in the understanding of disease pathogenesis and translating that knowledge into practical therapeutics. Most notably, the advent of highly active antiretroviral therapy (HAART) has transformed HIV from an inevitably fatal disease to one that, if managed appropriately, can be considered a chronic condition. As a result, the overall number of people living with HIV is increasing as these regimens extend life and as new infections outnumber AIDS deaths. (www.unaids.org; Joint United Nations Program on HIV/AIDS 2011)

The number of HIV treatment regimens has grown exponentially, particularly in the past decade. This, coupled with advances in the understanding of disease pathogenesis and progression, has made HIV disease management among the most dynamic fields in modern medicine. A number of guidelines have been developed to assist practitioners with often complex treatment decisions. These include the 2010 International AIDS Society (IAS/IAS-USA) guidelines and the 2011 US Department of Health and Human Services (DHHS) HIV treatment guidelines.(Thompson, et al., 2010; http//:www.aidsinfo.nih.gov; Thompson, et al., 2010; United States Department of Health and Human Services (US DHHS) Panel on Antiretroviral Guidelines for Adults and Adolescents 2011)

Close to 30 individual drugs and fixed-dose combinations are available to treat HIV. Despite the availability of a broad range of individual antiretroviral treatments and combinations, drug resistance remains a common phenomenon, and treatment failure is still frequently observed. Moreover, treatment advances—together with recent demographic shifts—have resulted in a dramatic expansion in the population of treatment-experienced patients. This group comprises an ever-increasing proportion of the patients whom HIV clinicians are called upon to treat. This review attempts to integrate guideline recommendations and evidence from recent clinical trials to identify best practices in the management of these patients.

2. The treatment-experienced patient

According to the IAS, the primary goal of antiretroviral therapy is to increase disease-free survival through the maximal suppression of viral replication and preservation of immunologic function.(Thompson, et al., 2010; Hammer, et al., 2008) Optimal therapy for patients with HIV depends on carefully balancing these benefits with the risks for drug toxicity, potential emergence of viral resistance, and the understanding that HIV infection is a chronic disease that requires continuous therapy – often for decades. These considerations are complicated in the treatment-experienced patient, as these patients often have accumulated resistance mutations to a number of drugs in existing antiretroviral drug classes. Modifications of treatment regimens may be forced by undue toxicity, drug-drug interactions, or outright virologic failure. While, theoretically, it is optimal for patients to remain on a single treatment until virologic failure, regimens may also be modified to improve convenience and/or ameliorate minor or cosmetic side effects, ultimately improving adherence and increasing time to virologic failure.(Thompson, et al., 2010; Hammer, et al. 2008)

3. Defining treatment failure

Treatment failure may be defined based on HIV RNA response to therapy (virologic failure), changes in CD4+ cell count (immunologic failure), and the occurrence or recurrence of HIV-related events after ≥ 3 months on an antiretroviral regimen (clinical progression). (US Department of Health and Human Services (DHHS) Panel on Antiretroviral treatment guidelines for adults and adolescents 2011, http://aidsinfor.nih.gov)

Virologic failure may be characterized as persistent HIV RNA viral load above 200 copies/mL. (US DHHS HIV treatment guidelines 2011) Occasional episodes of viral detection between 51 and 1000 copies/mL may occur due to laboratory variation or other transient viral illness. However, frequent and/or consistent viremia is a strong indicator of treatment failure and must be addressed to prevent selection of drug-resistant virus.

Immunologic failure is the failure to achieve and maintain an adequate CD4+ T-cell response despite virologic suppression. Although an absolute definition has not been agreed upon by experts, immunologic failure can generally be considered as failure to increase CD4+ cell counts above 350–500 cells/mm^3 over 4–7 years of treatment.(US DHHS HIV treatment guidelines 2011) Alternatively, it may be defined as failure to increase CD4+ cell count by 50–100 cells/mm^3 above baseline during the first year of a new therapy, or a decline in CD4+ cell count to below baseline while on therapy.(US DHHS HIV treatment guidelines 2011)

Clinical progression is the occurrence or recurrence of HIV-related conditions (a new AIDS defining illness or death) after ≥3 months of HAART, excluding immune reconstitution syndromes.(US DHHS HIV treatment guidelines 2011)

While virologic failure, immunologic failure, and clinical progression are closely related, all three may not occur simultaneously. In general, virologic failure precedes immunologic failure and clinical progression of disease; however, the period between overt virologic failure and detectable suppression of CD4+ cell count and/or HIV-related events can span from months to years.(US DHHS HIV treatment guidelines 2011; Deeks, et al., AIDS 2002)

4. Assessing treatment failure

In general, treatment failure cannot be attributed to any single cause. When assessing individual patients with treatment failure, it is important to recognize that multiple reasons for failure may occur in a single patient. These include:

1. patient-specific factors, such as earlier calendar year of starting therapy, high baseline HIV RNA level, lower nadir CD4+ cell count, prior AIDS diagnosis, the presence of comorbidities such as depression or active substance use, and infection with a drug-resistant virus;
2. medication noncompliance and/or missed clinic appointments;
3. medication side effects and toxicity, potentially leading to noncompliance;
4. suboptimal pharmacokinetics, including variable absorption, metabolism, penetration, food/fasting requirements, and drug and natural product interactions; and
5. suboptimal potency of the antiretroviral regimen.(http://aidsinfo.nih.gov)

Of these reasons, suboptimal adherence and toxicities account for the majority (26%−64%) of treatment failures and discontinuations.(d'Arminio Monforte, et al. AIDS 2000; Mocroft A, et al. AIDS 2001)

5. Addressing treatment failure

Careful assessment of the reasons for treatment failure is critical, as approaches to subsequent therapy differ based on the combination of risk factors in the individual patient. Of the potential reasons for failure summarized above, all except certain patient-specific risk factors can be addressed through appropriate attention to maintaining adherence (either to the current regimen or to a new regimen) and careful assessment of all of the patients' current medications, including but not limited to HAART, treatments for comorbid conditions, and natural health products.

5.1 Noncompliance

Unless the patient was infected with resistant virus, treatment failure implies inadequate adherence to antiretroviral therapy. The development of drug resistance requires concurrent antiretroviral drug exposure and ongoing viral replication. Thus, even intermediate adherence (e.g., 70%−90% compliance) is associated with considerable risk for the development of drug-resistant strains of HIV, as a result of ongoing low-level drug exposure and intermittent viral replication. (Lucas GM, et al., J Antimicrob Chemother 2005) For this reason, it is worthwhile to target 90%−100% compliance in patients with HIV.

The causes of nonadherence must be identified and addressed in cooperation with the patient to avoid future treatment failures and the accumulation of drug-resistance mutations. Numerous reasons for nonadherence to medication have been described in the literature. These include, but are not limited to, regimen complexity (a particular problem in HIV treatment), (Ammassari, et al., Neurology 2003) side effects, (Ammassari, et al., JAIDS 2001) failure to understand dosing directions, illiteracy,(Kalichman, et al., J Natl Med Assoc 1999) substance abuse, (Power , et al., AIDS Pt Care STDS 2003) psychological issues, (Gibbie, et al., Sex Health 2007) cost, missed appointments, and lack of social supports..

Routinely discussing adherence with patients at each visit may improve medication adherence. Pill boxes are helpful for patients who are busy or forgetful and have the additional benefit of being highly cost-effective. In one study, its use resulted in a significant

4% improvement in adherence that correlated with a significant reduction in viral load. (Petersen M, et al. CROI 2007)

5.2 Side effects and toxicities

When treatment fails, the patient should be carefully assessed for side effects and their duration and severity. In some cases, side effects are transiently associated with the initiation of a new regimen. However, ongoing side effects should first be managed, if possible, by using symptomatic treatment (e.g., antiemetics and antidiarrheals). Alternatively, substitution of one drug for another in the same therapeutic class may reduce symptoms. For example, tenofovir or abacavir may be used to replace zidovudine in patients with gastrointestinal symptoms or anemia.(US DHHS HIV treatment guidelines 2011) Changing drug classes altogether is also an option in patients who experience side effects with multiple alternative drugs within the same class.

5.3 Pharmacokinetic parameters

The risk for treatment failure is increased if the patient is not taking the medication correctly (e.g., with or without food and otherwise, as directed). Similarly, treatment may fail if the patient is taking other medications, prescription or over the counter, that may affect drug absorption or metabolism (e.g., proton pump inhibitors).

The effect of natural health products, such as herbs and vitamins, is underappreciated as a source of potentially detrimental interactions with antiretroviral treatment. Data suggest that more than two thirds of HIV patients take natural or alternative health products, (Rivera, et al., J Natl Med Assoc 2005) and that many physicians are not aware of their patients' use of "natural" or alternative health products. The complexities of accounting for interactions between these products and antiretroviral treatments are compounded by the fact that natural health products are not produced to a generally accepted standard, and there may be wide variability in potency between and within brands. Moreover, many natural health products are complex mixtures that may contain components that influence drug metabolizing enzymes and drug transporters.(Lee LS, et al. CID 2006) Table 1 presents some known interactions between antiretroviral drugs and natural health products.

5.4 Drug resistance

When noncompliance, side effects and toxicities, and potential pharmacokinetic interactions have been excluded, drug resistance should be considered. Resistance testing should be performed while the patient is still on the failing regimen or within 4 weeks of discontinuation, and before starting a new regimen. In general, changing therapy for virologic failure is warranted for detectable viremia >1000 copies/mL. Some authorities suggest a more aggressive approach, in which therapy is changed for any repeated, detectable viremia (e.g., two consecutive HIV RNA >50 copies/mL after suppression to <50 copies/mL in a patient receiving antiretroviral treatment), but this is not routine practice.(http://aidsinfo.nih.gov)

5.4.1 Drug resistance testing

Resistance testing may be accomplished through genotype or phenotype testing. Two types of resistance assays are available in clinical practice. Genotypic assays involve sequencing HIV-1 genes to detect mutations that confer HIV-1 drug resistance, whereas phenotypic assays use cell-culture based viral replication assays in the presence and absence of drugs.

	St. John's wort	Echinacea	Milk thistle	Garlic	Vitamin E
PIs	Should not be coadministered; may cause significant decrease in PI levels	Possible interaction; echinacea may interact with ARVs that are CYP 3A4 or CYP 2C9 substrates	Possible interaction, except for indinavir; milk thistle may inhibit CYP3A4	Possible interaction; garlic may inhibit CYP3A4 GI toxicity has been reported with coadministration of garlic and ritonavir	Should not be coadministered with tipranavir/ritonavir; may increase the risk of bleeding
NNRTIs	Should not be coadministered; may cause significant decrease in NNRTI levels (including etravirine)	Possible interaction; echinacea may interact with ARVs that are CYP 3A4 or CYP 2C9 substrates	Possible interaction; milk thistle may inhibit CYP 3A4	Possible interaction; garlic may inhibit CYP 3A4	Unknown
NRTIs	No evidence for interaction	No evidence for interaction	No evidence for interaction	No evidence for interaction	No evidence for interaction
Integrase inhibitor (raltegravir)	No evidence for interaction	No evidence for interaction	No evidence for interaction	No evidence for interaction	No evidence for interaction
CCR5 antagonist (maraviroc)	Coadministration not recommended; expected to decrease maraviroc concentrations	Possible interaction; echinacea may interact with ARVs that are CYP 3A4 and CYP 2C9 substrates	Possible interaction; milk thistle may inhibit CYP 3A4	Possible interaction; garlic may inhibit CYP 3A4	No evidence for interaction

Table 1. Known Interactions Between Antiretroviral (ARV) Therapies and Natural Health Products

CYP, cytochrome P; GI, gastrointestinal; NNRTI, non-nucleoside reverse transcriptase inhibitor; NRTI, nucleoside reverse transcriptase inhibitor; PI, protease inhibitor.

(Reyataz, Intelence, Aptivus, & Selzentry package inserts; Gorski, et al., 2004; Mills, et al., 2005; Venkataramanan, et al., 2000; Foster, et al., 2001; Laroche, et al., 1998; Lee, et al., 2006)

Both tests can accurately identify resistance only in the predominant virus in patients, so a substantial proportion of the circulating virus may be resistant even in patients with negative results.(Schuurman, et al., J Clin Microbiol 1999) Furthermore, drug resistance testing is limited, because it does not predict the activity of antiretroviral agents when used in combination and requires a viral load >1000. Also, it only reveals resistance based on drug pressure, so it is important to consider all prior genotype tests, as these mutations will remain, even if not currently detectable. In addition to these methods, "virtual phenotyping" utilizes genotype data to evaluate *in vitro* drug susceptibility of the virus; for most antiretroviral agents, this test predicts actual phenotypic resistance.(Perez-Elias, et al., Antivir Ther 2003) Despite limitations, the preponderance of evidence suggests an advantage for the use of genotypic testing over standard of care in the selection of regimens for patients with treatment failure.(Hirsch, et al., CID 2003) Compared with standard of care, the patients allocated to the genotyping arms of these studies had substantially greater decreases in plasma HIV RNA levels and were more likely to achieve undetectable HIV RNA levels. In contrast, trials of phenotypic testing versus standard of care have not produced such clear-cut results, with variable outcomes in different studies. (Hirsch, CID 2003; Melnick, et al., abstract #786 CROI 2000; Cohen, et al., AIDS 2002; Torti, et al., CID 2005; Dunn, et al., JAIDS, 2005; Vray, et al., 2003; Wegner, et al., CID 2004). A recent clinical study compared outcomes in patients randomly assigned to either genotypic testing or genotypic plus virtual phenotypic testing. (Hales, et al, PLoS Clin Trials 2006) After 48 weeks, no significant differences were observed between the two groups in terms of mean change from baseline plasma HIV RNA and mean change from baseline CD4+ cell count, suggesting that resistance testing with genotyping alone is sufficient for the management of HIV infection. Tables 2, 3, and 4 indicate resistance mutations for the three major classes of antiretrovirals.

6. 2011 Guidelines for the management of treatment-experienced patients

When selecting appropriate treatment, all resistance testing should be considered, as should the patient's treatment history, comorbidities, concomitant medications, and prior intolerance. Treatment should be individualized based on these factors.

In patients with limited prior treatment but with no resistance, the potential for nonadherence should be evaluated and strongly considered. Resumption of the same regimen or initiation of a new regimen should be considered, with genotypic testing within 4 - 6 weeks to determine whether a resistant viral strain emerges if viral suppression cannot be achieved. In patients with limited prior treatment who are receiving protease inhibitors (PIs), thought should be given to intensifying one drug or boosting. The primary goal of therapy is to resuppress HIV RNA levels to undetectable levels and to prevent further selection of resistance mutations. (http://aidsinfo.nih.gov)

In patients with limited prior treatment and recognized drug resistance, maximal HIV RNA suppression (e.g., to <50 copies/mL) is required to prevent the selection of additional resistance mutations. (Thompson, et al, 2010; http://aidsinfo.nih.gov) Changes in the treatment regimen should be considered to minimize selection of resistance mutations. New regimens should include ≥2 active agents. (Thompson, et al, 2010; http://aidsinfo.nih.gov) Resistance mutations for nucleoside analog reverse transcriptase inhibitors (NRTIs), non-NRTIs (NNRTIs), and PIs are noted in Tables 2, 3, and 4, respectively. Effects of Protease mutations are noted in Table 5.

In patients with extensive prior treatment and drug resistance, maximal viral suppression is warranted to prevent the accumulation of additional resistance mutations. Antiretroviral drugs from newer classes should be considered. If viral suppression is impossible to achieve, the primary goal is to preserve immunologic function and prevent clinical progression. When a new regimen with two fully active agents cannot be identified, it is reasonable to observe the patient on the same regimen rather than changing the regimen, depending on the stage of HIV disease. (Thompson, et al, 2010; http://aidsinfo.nih.gov)

Patients with significant treatment experience and drug-resistant virus can often still achieve undetectable viral loads and the goal is still to reestablish suppression of the virus.

NRTI	Resistance mutations (IAS-USA)	Mutations associated with reduced RC
All currently approved NRTIs	69 insertion complex: M41L, A62V, 69 insert, K70R, L210W, T215Y/F, K219Q/E	
All currently approved NRTIs except tenofovir	151 complex: A62V, V75I, F77L, F116Y, Q151M	Q151M
All currently approved NRTIs	Thymidine analogue-associated mutations (TAMs): M41L, D67N, K70R, L210W, T215Y/F, K219Q/E	
Abacavir	K65R, L74V, Y115F, M184V	K65R, M184V
Didanosine	K65R, L74V	K65R
Emtricitabine	K65R, M184V/I	K65R, M184V
Lamivudine	K65R, M184V/I	K65R, M184V
Stavudine	M41L, D67N, K70R, L210W, T215Y/F, K219O/E	
Tenofovir	K65R, K70E	K65R
Zidovudine	M41L, D67N, K70R, L10W, T215Y/F, K219Q/E	

Table 2. NRTI resistance mutations
AS, International Aids Society; NRTI, nucleoside reverse transcriptase inhibitor; RC, replicative capacity.
Johnson, et al., 2009; Garcia-Perez, et al., 2005; Girardet, et al., 2007; White, et al., 2002)

NNRTI	Resistance mutations (IAS-USA)	Mutations associated with reduced RC
Delavirdine	K103N, V106M, Y181C, Y188L, P236L	V106A, G190C/S/E/Q/V/T, P225H, M230L, and P236L
Efavirenz	L100I, K103N, V106M, V108I, Y181C/I, Y188L, G190S/A, P225H	V106A, G190C/S/E/Q/V/T, P225H, M230L, and P236L
Nevirapine	L100I, K103N, V106A/M, V108I, Y181C/I, Y188C/L/H, G190A	V106A, G190C/S/E/Q/V/T, P225H, M230L, and P236L

Table 3. NNRTI Resistance Mutations
NNRTI, non-nucleoside reverse transcriptase inhibitor; RC, replicative capacity.
(Johnson, et al., 2009; Archer, et al., 2000; Huang, et al., 2003; Wirden, et al., 2003)

(US DHHS HIV management guidelines) NRTIs, in particular, have been shown to retain antiviral activity in patients with drug-resistant virus. Moreover, continued use of both NRTIs and PIs can select for drug-resistance mutations that reduce viral fitness. (Deeks, et al., 2005) If complete viral suppression is not feasible, the goals of treatment should be maintenance or improvement of CD4+ cell count and preventing clinical progression. Discontinuation is not recommended unless the patient has a high CD4+ count. Data suggest that partial virologic suppression of >0.5 to 1.0 $\log_{10}$ copies/mL below baseline is associated with clinical benefit; larger and more sustained reductions in HIV RNA are directly correlated with lower risk for disease progression. (Murray, et al., 1999) In addition, a "holding regimen" will maintain poor viral fitness. For example, the M184V mutation, which increases resistance to lamivudine and emtricitabine, decreases viral fitness and increases the antiviral activity of zidovudine, stavudine, and tenofovir. (Whitcomb, et al., 2003) Therefore, maintaining this resistance mutation by continuing lamivudine or emtricitabine can enhance the effect of zidovudine, stavudine, and/or tenofovir. (Wegner, et al., CID 2004)

Protease inhibitor	Major resistance mutations (IAS-USA)	Mutations associated with reduced RC
Atazanavir +/- ritonavir	I50L, I84V, N88S	I50L
Fosamprenavir/ritonavir	I50V, I84V	I50V, I84V
Darunavir/ritonavir	I47V, I50V, I54M/L, L76V, I84V	
Indinavir/ritonavir	M46I/L, V82A/F/T, I84V	
Lopinavir/ritonavir	V32I, I47V/A, L76V, V82A/F/T/S	
Nelfinavir	D30N, L90M	D30N, N88S, L90M
Saquinavir/ritonavir	G48V, L90M	
Tipranavir/ritonavir	I47V, Q58E, T74P, V82L/T, I84V	

Table 4. Major Protease Inhibitor Resistance Mutations
IAS, International Aids Society; RC, replicative capacity.
(Johnson, et al., 2009; Archer, et al., 2000; Martinez-Picado, et al., 1999; Prado, et al., 2002; Resch, et al., 2002; Wirden, et al., 2003; Reyataz prescribing information)

In some highly treatment-experienced patients, the addition of enfuvirtide should also be considered. In the T-20 versus Optimized Regimen Only (TORO) studies, adding enfuvirtide to an optimized background regimen was associated with significant antiretroviral and immunologic benefit in patients with >6 months of previous treatment with agents in three classes of antiretroviral drugs and/or resistance to drugs in these classes.(Lalezari, et al., 2003) Notably, enfuvirtide is most effective when given with other active drugs. As shown in the TORO study, enfuvirtide monotherapy is associated with a high rate of emerging resistance. (Lalezari, et al., 2003)

DHHS guidelines indicate no consensus on how to define or treat immunologic failure in the setting of a virologic response. (US DHHS HIV management guidelines) Patients with discordant responses (e.g., undetectable HIV RNA but low CD4+ cell counts) should continue to receive their current treatment, unless they are taking zidovudine or didanosine, which have been shown to be myelosuppressive. However, time to immune response is variable and may even take years. In these cases, changing these drugs, if possible, is recommended. Additionally, changing trimethoprim-sulfamethoxazole prophylaxis to dapsone or aerosolized pentamidine may be warranted in this group in order to enhance immunologic response further. This should be considered prior to changing an antiretroviral regimen that is successfully suppressing viral load.

7. Beyond the guidelines: Investigational therapeutic approaches

Numerous permutations of various treatment strategies have been attempted. Below are several of the more commonly investigated therapeutic approaches.

7.1 Structured treatment interruptions

The CPCRA 064 study found that there was an increased risk of death, a long-term negative effect on CD4+ cell count, and no virologic or clinical benefit associated with a structured treatment interruption.(Lawrence, et al., 2006) Based on these, it is advised to not discontinue an ARV regimen in an adherent patient except for in the presence of drug resistance and when awaiting genotype results.

7.2 Double-boosted PIs

Double-boosted PIs (two PIs plus ritonavir) may be clinically effective by increasing blood levels to the point where resistance is overcome.(Staszewski, et al., 2006) This approach raises major issues, however, in terms of drug interactions and may be suitable only for patients who have exhausted all other options. This is not strongly advised or recommended and the patient should be referred to an HIV specialist.

7.3 Mega-HAART

Multiple-drug rescue therapy (e.g., >5 antiretrovirals) has the complication of severe drug interactions. Thus, this is a last resort in highly selected patients and should be managed by an HIV specialist.(Montaner, et al., 2001)

8. New treatment options

Over the past 3 years, a number of new treatment options have been approved by the US Food and Drug Administration, including drugs from entirely new classes: maraviroc, a CCR5 antagonist, and raltegravir, an integrase inhibitor. Drug interactions of these newly approved agents are summarized in Table 6.

Effect	TPV	LPV	ATV	DRV
Decreased virologic response	no firm data	6 or more mutations	Increasing number of mutations	I47V, I54M, T74P, I84V
High level resistance	no firm data	7 – 8 mutations; I47A, V32I; L76V+3 mutations	I50L, I84V, N88S	3+of: V11I, V32I, L33F, I47V, I50V I54M/L, G73S, L76V, I84V, L89V
Possible increased virologic response	L24I, I50L/V, F53Y/L/W, I54L, L76V		M46I + L76V without other mutations	V82A

Table 5. Impact of Protease Inhibitor Resistance Mutations: Effects of different PI mutations on different PIs

*ATV, atazanavir; DRV, darunavir; LPV, lopinavir; TPV, tipranavir. PI, Protease Inhibitor (Norton, et al., 2008; DeMeyer, et al., 2009; Descamps, et al., 2009; Mo, et al., 2005; Friend, et al., 2004; Kagan, et al., 2005; Rhee, et al., 2010; Schapiro, et al., 2010, and Marcelin, et al., 2008; all as cited by Johnson, et al., 2010)

8.1 Newer protease inhibitors

In the RESIST-1 and RESIST-2 trials (Randomized Evaluation of Strategic Intervention in Multidrug Resistant Patients with Tipranavir), tipranavir-ritonavir plus optimized best regimen provided superior virologic and immunologic responses over 48 weeks compared with patients who received an investigator-selected ritonavir-boosted comparator PI plus optimized background regimen. (Hicks, et al., 2006) Gastrointestinal disorders transaminitis, and hyperlipidemia were more frequent in patients who received tipranavir ritonavir compared with the control group. Tipranavir carries black-box warnings regarding the risk for hepatitis and hepatic decompensation as well as fatal and non-fatal intracranial hemorrhage. (Aptivus package insert, Boehringer Ingelheim Pharmaceuticals 2008) Tipranavir's unique resistance profile makes it valuable in patients who have failed prior PI-containing regimens. (Marcelin, et al., 2008) Tipranavir is approved for highly treatment-experienced HIV patients or those with multiple PI resistance mutations.

Ritonavir-boosted darunavir has shown superiority to boosted comparator PIs in treatment-experienced patients, including those with PI mutations. (Clotet, et al., 2007) The POWER 1, POWER 2, and POWER 3 (Performance Of TMC114/r When evaluated in treatment-Experienced patients with PI Resistance) studies found 40%–44% attained viral suppression among treatment-experienced patients who had previously failed other PI-based regimens. Thus, darunavir is also valuable in patients with significant resistance. (Lefebvre, et al., Abstract H-1387, ICAAC 2006) Darunavir is approved for both treatment-experienced and treatment-naïve patients. Table 5 shows the impact of protease mutations on resistance to various PIs.

8.2 New non-NRTI

The DUET 1 and 2 (TMC125-0216: a phase 3 study to investigate the efficacy, tolerability, and safety of TMC125(etravirine) as part of an antiretroviral regimen, with optimized background regimen in HIV-1 infected patients with limited to no treatment options) trials examined the efficacy of etravirine, a second-generation NNRTI, in treatment-experienced adult patients with virological failure on stable antiretroviral therapy and documented genotypic evidence of NNRTI resistance, viral load >5000 copies/mL, and ≥3 primary PI mutations.(Lazzarin, et al., 2007; Madruga, et al., 2007) Etravirine was associated with superior virologic suppression compared with placebo, with up to 62% of patients in the etravirine group achieving undetectable viral loads, compared with 44% in the placebo group. (Lazzarin, et al., 2007; Madruga, et al., 2007) Etravirine exhibits retained activity despite multiple NNRTI mutations, with high rates of sustained efficacy at 48 weeks in heavily treatment-experienced patients. (Haubrich, et al, Abstract #790, CROI 2008; Johnson M, et al., Abstract #792, CROI, 2008) The tolerability profile is comparable to placebo, with the exception of a rash. It is associated with significant drug interactions and should not be used with unboosted PIs, boosted atazanavir, fosamprenavir, tipranavir, or other NNRTIs.[49](Intelence package insert, Tibotech Therapeutics 2008) The mutation Y181 decreases susceptibility to etravirine, but does not eliminate efficacy altogether. (Johnson, et al, 2010; http://aidsinfo.nih.gov)

8.3 New class: CCR5 antagonist

Maraviroc, the first drug in this class to be licensed, is active against chemokine receptor R5- but not X4-tropic viruses in vitro. In the MOTIVATE 1 and MOTIVATE 2 (Maraviroc versus Optimized Therapy in Viremic Antiretroviral Treatment-Experienced Patients) trials, patients who had R5-tropic virus and had been treated with or had resistance to three antiretroviral drug classes, and had HIV RNA >5000 copies/mL, demonstrated increased CD4+ counts and more sustained viral suppression at 48 weeks following treatment with maraviroc compared with placebo, and with comparable adverse event outcomes. (Gulick, et al., 2008) Maraviroc is not effective in patients with mixed-tropic virus infection; it is indicated for the treatment of patients infected with only CCR5-tropic HIV who are either treatment naïve, or who have evidence of viral replication and HIV strains resistant to multiple antiretroviral agents.(Selzentry package insert, Pfizer, Inc.) Patients that may benefit from having a regimen including maraviroc can be identified via any of several assays available to assess the presence of the CCR5 tropic virus and the minority CXCR4 (X4) strains. (Reeves, et al., Abstract H-1026, ICAAC, 2007)

8.4 New class: Integrase inhibitor

Raltegravir, the first-in-class integrase inhibitor, was examined in combination with optimized background regimen in two identical, placebo-controlled trials in patients infected with triple-class drug-resistant HIV-1 in whom antiretroviral therapy had failed. (Steigbigel, et al., 2008) At 48 weeks of therapy, 62.1% and 32.9% of raltegravir and placebo patients, respectively, had suppressed HIV RNA viral load. Raltegravir is approved in combination with other antiretroviral agents for the treatment of HIV infection in treatment-naïve or treatment-experienced adult patients who have evidence of viral replication and HIV-1 strains resistant to multiple antiretroviral agents. (Isentress package insert, Merck & Co)

9. Drugs under investigation

A new integrase inhibitor, Dolutegravir (Glaxo Smith Kline) is in phase 2 clinical trials and is active against raltegravir-resistant strains, revealing a higher genetic barrier to resistance (Seki, et al., abstract #555, CROI 2010; Eron, et al., abstract #151LB, CROI 2011).
GSK2248761 is a once daily NNRTI currently in phase 2b studies with activity against virus with many NNRTI mutations, including efavirenz resistant strains. (Kim, et al., abstract #628, CROI 2011; Kim, et al., abstract #631, CROI 2011) In addition, this drug appears to have an additive to synergistic antiviral effect when coadministered with other antiretrovirals. (Vavro, et al. abstract #520, CROI 2011)
BI-C is a non-catalytic site integrase inhibitor that may have activity against virus resistant to other integrase inhibitors. It has shown very good biological and pharmacological profiles and is now in Phase 1 clinical trials. (Fenwick, et al., abstract #523, CROI 2011)

9.1 New classes(future)

These are not currently approved and have yet to start Phase 3 clinical trials, however, they show promise as potential future new drug classes. Their possible addition to the current arsenal of antiretrovirals is particularly important for the treatment experienced patient.

9.1.1 Attachment inhibitors

Currently in very early trials, this class shows the possibility for potent antiretroviral activity against HIV-1 infection. (Nettles, et al., abstract #49, CROI 2011). New targets include the gp 120 glycoprotein, which allows attachment of virus to CD4+ cells. (Nowicka-Sans, et al., abstract #518, CROI 2011)

9.1.2 Gag inhibitors

Another potentially new class of antiviral drugs being investigated are gag inhibitors. This drug targets the HIV-1 capsid and exhibited inhibition of the early phase of its life cycle. (Urano, et al., abstract #525, CROI 2011)

	Interactions with other ARVs	Selected interactions with non-ARV drugs
Etravirine	Should not be coadministered with: • Tipranavir/ritonavir • Fosamprenavir/ritonavir • Atazanavir/ritonavir • Unboosted PIs • NNRTIs Dose adjustment not established with Saquinavir, consider Saquinavir 1000mg bid + Ritonavir 100mg bid If with Maraviroc: MVC 600mg bid MVC 150mg bid (if with Ritonavir boosted darunavir)	Drug concentration monitoring recommended when used with antiarrythmics INR monitoring recommended when used with warfarin; clopidogrel should not be coadministered Certain anticonvulsants, including carabamazepine, phenobarbital, and phenytoin, can cause significant decreases in etravirine plasma concentrations Dose adjustments may be necessary for coadministration with itraconazole, ketoconazole, voriconazole; coadminister with caution and follow drug levels Clarithromycin alternatives should be considered Rifampin, rifapentine, and rifabutin may cause significant decreases in etravirine plasma concentrations Etravirine may increase plasma concentrations of diazepam , dose adjustment may be necessary Dexamethasone should be used with caution, as etravirine levels may decrease. Interaction with certain statins has been detected Etravirine may be coadministered with methadone; however, clinical monitoring for withdrawal symptoms is recommended, as methadone maintenance therapy may need to be adjusted Administer with immunosuppressants with caution; levels of cyclosporine, tacrolimus, and sirolimus may be decreased
Raltegravir	No effect expected on the following drug classes: PIs, NNRTIs that would	No effect expected on methadone, opioid analgesics, statins, azole antifungals,

	require dose adjustments	proton pump inhibitors, oral contraceptives, anti-erectile dysfunction agents
	No clinically meaningful effect on lamivudine, tenofovir	
	Recommended dose of raltegravir may be coadministered with efavirenz, nevirapine	Caution recommended when coadministering with rifampin; reduces plasma concentrations of raltegravir
	Recommended dose of raltegravir may be coadministered with boosted tipranavir or atazanavir	Recommended dose of raltegravir may be coadministered with rifabutin ; recommend 800 mg twice daily with coadministered rifampin
Maraviroc	Dose reduction to 150 mg twice daily with PIs (except tipranavir/ritonavir), delaviridine	Dose reduction to 150 mg twice daily with ketoconazole, itraconazole, clarithromycin, other strong CYP 3A inhibitors (e.g., nefazadone, telithromycin)
	No dose adjustment (300 mg twice daily) with tipranavir/ritonavir, nevirapine, NRTIs	Dose increase to 600 mg twice daily with CYP 3A inducers including rifampin, carbamazepine, phenobarbital, phenytoin
	Dose increase to 600 mg twice daily with CYP 3A inducers including efavirenz	No clinically relevant effect on midazolam, oral contraceptives (ethinylestradiol and levonorgestrel)
	No effect on zidovudine, lamivudine	

Table 6. Drug Interactions of Newly Approved Antiretroviral Therapies
ARV, antiretroviral; INR, International Normalized Ratio; CYP, cytochrome; NNRTI, non-nucleoside reverse transcriptase inhibitor; NRTI, nucleoside reverse transcriptase inhibitor; PI, protease inhibitor.
(Aptivus, Invirase, Isentress, Kaletra, Lexiva, Prezista, Reyataz, Selzentry, Sustiva, Viracept, and Viramune prescribing information)

10. Conclusion

Managing treatment-experienced patients poses considerable challenges, not the least of which includes selecting appropriate therapy to maximize clinical benefit, minimize toxicities, and avoid drug-drug interactions. The best approach to these patients is preventative. As noted above, with appropriate attention to medication adherence and addressing the side effects and toxicities of antiretroviral medications proactively, many patients can remain on the first regimen for many years. In the real world, however, a substantial proportion of patients fail to adhere to their medication. Many suffer from overt toxicities and/or minor/cosmetic side effects that affect compliance with treatment and eventually necessitate a switch in regimen. Given the broad spectrum of available agents—including the recent advent of two entirely new classes of antiretroviral agents—the majority of patients have reasonably well-tolerated therapeutic options that, with appropriate attention to all aspects of the clinical and patient experience, can provide sufficient long-term efficacy which has transformed HIV from an inevitably fatal disease to one that can truly be considered a chronic condition.

11. Author disclosure statement

Gail Reid has no competing financial interests.
Richard Novak has been the Recipient of Research Grants from Merck, GlaxoSmithKline, and Abbott Laboratories.

12. References

Ammassari, A., R. Murri, et al. (2001). "Self-reported symptoms and medication side effects influence adherence to highly active antiretroviral therapy in persons with HIV infection." J Acquir Immune Defic Syndr 28(5): 445-9.

Ammassari, A. A., F. Starace, et al. (2003). "Medication adherence among HIV+ adults: effects of cognitive dysfunction and regimen complexity." Neurology 61(5): 723-4; author reply 724.

Boehringer Ingelheim Pharmaceuticals (2008). "Aptivus Prescribing Information."

Bristol-Meyers Squibb Inc (2008). "Reyataz Prescribing Information."

Clotet, B., N. Bellos, et al. (2007). "Efficacy and safety of darunavir-ritonavir at week 48 in treatment-experienced patients with HIV-1 infection in POWER 1 and 2: a pooled subgroup analysis of data from two randomised trials." Lancet 369(9568): 1169-78.

Cohen, C. J., S. Hunt, et al. (2002). "A randomized trial assessing the impact of phenotypic resistance testing on antiretroviral therapy." Aids 16(4): 579-88.

d'Arminio Monforte, A., A. C. Lepri, et al. (2000). "Insights into the reasons for discontinuation of the first highly active antiretroviral therapy (HAART) regimen in a cohort of antiretroviral naive patients. I.CO.N.A. Study Group. Italian Cohort of Antiretroviral-Naive Patients." Aids 14(5): 499-507.

Deeks, S. G., J. D. Barbour, et al. (2002). "Duration and predictors of CD4 T-cell gains in patients who continue combination therapy despite detectable plasma viremia." Aids 16(2): 201-7.

Deeks, S. G., R. Hoh, et al. (2005). "Interruption of treatment with individual therapeutic drug classes in adults with multidrug-resistant HIV-1 infection." J Infect Dis 192(9): 1537-44.

Archer RH, Dykes C, Gerondelis P, et al. Mutants of human immunodeficiency virus type 1 (HIV-1) reverse transcriptase resistant to nonnucleoside reverse transcriptase inhibitors demonstrate altered rates of RNase H cleavage that correlate with HIV-1 replication fitness in cell culture. J Virol. 2000 Sep;74(18):8390-401.

Dunn DT, Green H, et al. (2005). "A randomized controlled trial of the value of phenotypic testing in addition to genotypic testing for HIV drug resistance: evaluation of resistance assays (ERA) trial invetigators."Journal of Acquired Immune Deficiency Syndrome. 38:553-9.

Eron, J., Kumar, P., Lazzarin, A., Richmond, G., Soriano, V., Huang, J., Vavro., C., Ait-Khaled, M., Min, S., and Yeo., J. "DTG in Subjects with HIV Exhibiting RAL Resistance: Functional Monotherapy Results of VIKING Study Cohort II" Abstract #151LB, CROI 2011.

Fenwick, C, Bethel, R, Bonneau, P., et al., "Identification of BI-C, a Novel HIV-1 Non-catalytic Site Integrase Inhibitor." abstract #523, CROI 2011, Boston.

Foster, B. C., M. S. Foster, et al. (2001). "An in vitro evaluation of human cytochrome P450 3A4 and P-glycoprotein inhibition by garlic." J Pharm Pharm Sci 4(2): 176-84.

Garcia-Perez J, Sanchez-Palomino S, Perez-Olmeda M, Fernandez B, Alcami J. (2007). A new strategy based on recombinant viruses as a tool for assessing drug susceptibility of human immunodeficiency virus type 1.J Med Virol. 79:127-37.

Gibbie, T., M. Hay, et al. (2007). "Depression, social support and adherence to highly active antiretroviral therapy in people living with HIV/AIDS." Sex Health 4(4): 227-32.

Gorski, J. C., S. M. Huang, et al. (2004). "The effect of echinacea (Echinacea purpurea root) on cytochrome P450 activity in vivo." Clin Pharmacol Ther 75(1): 89-100.

Gulick, R. M., J. Lalezari, et al. (2008). "Maraviroc for previously treated patients with R5 HIV-1 infection." N Engl J Med 359(14): 1429-41.

Hales, G., C. Birch, et al. (2006). "A randomised trial comparing genotypic and virtual phenotypic interpretation of HIV drug resistance: the CREST study." PLoS Clin Trials 1(3): e18.

Hammer, S. M., J. J. Eron, Jr., et al. (2008). "Antiretroviral treatment of adult HIV infection: 2008 recommendations of the International AIDS Society-USA panel." JAMA 300(5): 555-70.

Haubrich, R, Cahn, P, Grinsztejn, B., et al., "DUET-1: Week 48 Results of a pase III Randomized double blind trial to evaluate the efficacy and safety of TMC125 vs placebo in 612 treatment experienced HIV-1 infected patients." abstract #790, CROI, 2008, Boston.

Hicks, CB, Cahn, P, cooper, DA, et al. (2006) "Durable efficacy of tipranavir-ritonavir in combination with an optimised background regimen of antiretroviral drugs for treatment-experienced HIV-1 infected patients at 48 weeks in the Randomized Evaluation of Strategic Intervention in multi-drug reSistant patients with Tipranavir (RESIST) studies: an analysis of combined data from two randomised open-label trials. Lancet 368:466-475.

Hirsch, M. S., F. Brun-Vezinet, et al. (2003). "Antiretroviral drug resistance testing in adults infected with human immunodeficiency virus type 1: 2003 recommendations of an International AIDS Society-USA Panel." Clin Infect Dis 37(1): 113-28.

Johnson, M, Campbell, T, Clotet, B., et al. "DUET-2: Week 48 Results of a Phase III Randomized double blind Trial to Evaluate the Efficacy and Safety of TMC125 vs Placebo in 591 Treatment experienced HIV-1 infected patients . Abstract #792. CROI, 2008, Boston.

Johnson VA, Brun-Vézinet F, Clotet B, et al. (2010) Update of the Drug Resistance Mutations in HIV-1: December 2010. Top HIV Med. 18;5: 156-163

Joint United Nations Program on HIV/AIDS (2008). "Report on the global AIDS epidemic. Available at: http://www.unaids.org/en/KnowledgeCentre/HIVData/GlobalReport/2008/200 8_Global_report.asp. Accessed 6 December 2008."

Kalichman, S. C., S. Catz, et al. (1999). "Barriers to HIV/AIDS treatment and treatment adherence among African-American adults with disadvantaged education." J Natl Med Assoc 91(8): 439-46.

Kim, J, Wire, MB, Lovern, M.. "Dose seclection for Phase IIb studies of GSK2248761, a next generation NNRTI, using PK/PD/VD Model and Trial Simulation." abstract #628, CROI, 2011, Boston.

Kim, J, Gould, E, Lou, Y, Piscitelli, S. "Lack of drug-drug interaction between the NRRTI GSK2248761 and RAL." abstract #631, CROI, 2011, Boston.

Lalezari, J. P., K. Henry, et al. (2003). "Enfuvirtide, an HIV-1 fusion inhibitor, for drug-resistant HIV infection in North and South America." N Engl J Med 348(22): 2175-85.

Laroche, M. and S. Choudhri (1998). "Severe gastrointestinal toxicity with concomitant ingestion of ritonavir and garlic." Can J Infect Dis 9(Suppl A): 76A.

Lawrence, J., K. H. Hullsiek, et al. (2006). "Disadvantages of structured treatment interruption persist in patients with multidrug-resistant HIV-1: final results of the CPCRA 064 study." J Acquir Immune Defic Syndr 43(2): 169-78.

Lazzarin, A., T. Campbell, et al. (2007). "Efficacy and safety of TMC125 (etravirine) in treatment-experienced HIV-1-infected patients in DUET-2: 24-week results from a randomised, double-blind, placebo-controlled trial." Lancet 370(9581): 39-48.

Lee, L. S., A. S. Andrade, et al. (2006). "Interactions between natural health products and antiretroviral drugs: pharmacokinetic and pharmacodynamic effects." Clin Infect Dis 43(8): 1052-9.

Lefebvre, E., M. De Bethune, et al. (2006). "Impact of use of TPV, LPV & (f)APV at screening on TMC114/r virologic response in treatment-experienced patients in POWER 1,2, & 3. Interscience Conference on Antimicrobial Agents and Chemotherapy 2006. Abstract no. H-1387."

Lucas, G. M. (2005). "Antiretroviral adherence, drug resistance, viral fitness and HIV disease progression: a tangled web is woven." J Antimicrob Chemother 55(4): 413-6.

Madruga, J. V., P. Cahn, et al. (2007). "Efficacy and safety of TMC125 (etravirine) in treatment-experienced HIV-1-infected patients in DUET-1: 24-week results from a randomised, double-blind, placebo-controlled trial." Lancet 370(9581): 29-38.

Marcelin, A. G., B. Masquelier, et al. (2008). "Tipranavir-ritonavir genotypic resistance score in protease inhibitor-experienced patients." Antimicrob Agents Chemother 52(9): 3237-43.

Melnick, D. A., J. Rosenthal, et al. "Impact of phenotypic antiretroviral drug resistance testing on the response to salvage antiretroviral therapy (ART) in heavily experienced patients. In: Program and abstracts of the 7th Conference on Retroviruses and Opportunistic Infections (San Francisco). Alexandria, VA: Foundation for Retrovirology and Human Health, 2000:222. Abstract no. 786."

Merck & Co (2008). "Isentress prescribing information."

Mills, E., K. Wilson, et al. (2005). "Milk thistle and indinavir: a randomized controlled pharmacokinetics study and meta-analysis." Eur J Clin Pharmacol 61(1): 1-7.

Mocroft, A., M. Youle, et al. (2001). "Reasons for modification and discontinuation of antiretrovirals: results from a single treatment centre." Aids 15(2): 185-94.

Montaner, J. S., P. R. Harrigan, et al. (2001). "Multiple drug rescue therapy for HIV-infected individuals with prior virologic failure to multiple regimens." Aids 15(1): 61-9.

Murray, J. S., M. R. Elashoff, et al. (1999). "The use of plasma HIV RNA as a study endpoint in efficacy trials of antiretroviral drugs." Aids 13(7): 797-804.

Nettles, R, Schurmann, D, Zhu, L, et al. "Pharmacodynamics, Safety, and Pharmacokinetics of BMS-663068: A Potentially First-in-class oral HIV Attachment Inhibitor." Abstract #49, CROI, 2011, Boston.

Nowicka-Sans, B, Gong, Y-F, Ho, H-T, et al., "Antiviral Activity of a New SMall Molecule HIV-1 Attachment Inhibitor, BMS-626529, the Parent of BMS-663068." abstract #518, CROI 2011, Boston.

Perez-Elias, M. J., I. Garcia-Arata, et al. (2003). "Agreement degree between simultaneous real phenotype and virtual phenotype in patients from the REALVIRFEN study. Abstract no 808." Antivir Ther 8(Suppl 1).

Petersen, M., Y. Wang, et al. (2007). "Pill-box organizers are associated with improved ARV adherence, and viral suppression and are cost effective. Conference on Retroviruses and Opportunistic Infections CROI 2007. Abstract no. 524."

Pfizer Inc (2007). "Selzentry Prescribing Information."

Piliero, PJ, Parkin, N, Mayers, D. "Impact of protease (PR) mutations L33F/I, V82A, I84V, and L90M on ritonavir (RTV)-boosted protease inhibitor susceptibility. abstract H-998, ICAAC, 2006, San Francisco.

Power, R., C. Koopman, et al. (2003). "Social support, substance use, and denial in relationship to antiretroviral treatment adherence among HIV-infected persons." AIDS Patient Care STDS 17(5): 245-52.

Reeves, JD, Han, D, Liu, Y, et al. "Enhancements to the Trofile HIV Coreceptor Tropism Assay Enable Reliable Detection of CXCR4-using subpopulations at less than 1%. " abstract #H-1026, ICAAC, 2007, Chicago.

Resch W, Ziermann R, Parkin N, Gamarnik A, Swanstrom R. (2002) Nelfinavir-resistant, amprenavir-hypersusceptible strains of human immunodeficiency virus type 1 carrying an N88S mutation in protease have reduced infectivity, reduced replication capacity, and reduced fitness and process the Gag polyprotein precursor aberrantly. J Virol. Sep;76(17):8659-66.

Rivera, J. O., A. Gonzalez-Stuart, et al. (2005). "Herbal product use in non-HIV and HIV-positive Hispanic patients." J Natl Med Assoc 97(12): 1686-91.

Schuurman, R., L. Demeter, et al. (1999). "Worldwide evaluation of DNA sequencing approaches for identification of drug resistance mutations in the human immunodeficiency virus type 1 reverse transcriptase." J Clin Microbiol 37(7): 2291-6.

Seki, T, Kobayashi, M, Wakasa-Morimoto, C., et al. "S/GSK1349572 Is a Potent Next Generation HIV Integrase Inhibitor and Demonstrates a Superior Resistance Profile Substantiated with 60 Integrase Mutant Molecular Clones." abstract #555, CROI, 2010, San Francisco.

Staszewski, S., E. Babacan, et al. (2006). "The LOPSAQ study: 48 week analysis of a boosted double protease inhibitor regimen containing lopinavir/ritonavir plus saquinavir without additional antiretroviral therapy." J Antimicrob Chemother 58(5): 1024-30.

Steigbigel, R. T., D. A. Cooper, et al. (2008). "Raltegravir with optimized background therapy for resistant HIV-1 infection." N Engl J Med 359(4): 339-54.

Thompson MA, Aberg JA, Cahn P, et al; International AIDS Society-USA. (2010) "Antiretroviral treatment of adult HIV infection: 2010 recommendations of the International AIDS Society-USA panel." JAMA 304;3:321–333.

Tibotech Therapeutics (2008). "Intellence prescribing information."

Torti C, Quiros-Roldan E, Regazzi M, et al. (2005) "A randomized controlled trial to evaluate antiretroviral salvage therapy guided by rules-based or phenotype-driven HIV-1 genotypic drug-resistance interpretation with or without concentration-controlled intervention: the Resistance and Dosage Adapted Regimens (RADAR) Study." Clinical Infectious Disease, 40: 1828-36

United States Department of Health and Human Services (US DHHS) Panel on Antiretroviral Guidelines for Adults and Adolescents (2008). "Guidelines for the use of antiretroviral agents in HIV-1-infected adults and adolescents. Available at http://aidsinfo.nih.gov/contentfiles/AdultandAdolescentGL.pdf. Accessed 13 December 2008."

Urano, Emiko, Kuramochi, N, et al., "A Novel HIV-1 Inhibitor Targeting Gag Screened by Yeast Membrane-associated 2-hybrid System." abstract #525, CROI 2011, Boston.

Vavro, Cindy, Ferris, R, Edelstein M, Standring D, and StClair M. "GSK2248761 Retains potency against many NNRTI resiance mutants and is additive to synergistc in combination with other ART." abstract #520, CROI 2011, Boston.

Venkataramanan, R., V. Ramachandran, et al. (2000). "Milk thistle, a herbal supplement, decreases the activity of CYP3A4 and uridine diphosphoglucuronosyl transferase in human hepatocyte cultures." Drug Metab Dispos 28(11): 1270-3.

Vray M, Meynard JL, Dalban C, et al. (2003) "Predictors of the virological response to a change in the antiretroviral treatment regimen in HIV-1 infected patients enrolled in a randomized trial comparing genotyping, phenotyping and standard of care (Narval trial)". Antiviral Therapy. 8:427-34.

Wegner, S, Wallace, MR, Aronson, NE, et al. (2004) "Long-term efficacy of routine access to antiretroviral-resistance testing in HIV type I infected patients: results of the clinical efficacy of resistance testing trial." CID, 38:723-30.

Whitcomb, J. M., N. T. Parkin, et al. (2003). "Broad nucleoside reverse-transcriptase inhibitor cross-resistance in human immunodeficiency virus type 1 clinical isolates." J Infect Dis 188(7): 992-1000.

White KL, Margot NA, Wrin T, Petropoulos CJ, Miller MD, Naeger LK. (2002) "Molecular mechanisms of resistance to human immunodeficiency virus type 1 with reverse transcriptase mutations K65R and K65R+M184V and their effects on enzyme function and viral replication capacity. Antimicrob Agents Chemother. Nov;46(11):3437-46.

Wirden M, Simon A, Schneider L, et al. (2003) "Interruption of nonnucleoside reverse transcriptase inhibitor (NNRTI) therapy for 2 months has no effect on levels of human immunodeficiency virus type 1 in plasma of patients harboring viruses with mutations associated with resistance to NNRTIs." J Clin Microbiol. Jun;41(6):2713-5.

2

Special Considerations in the Management of HIV Infection in Pregnancy

Chi Dola, Sean Kim and Juliet Tran

Department of Obstetrics and Gynecology, Tulane University School of Medicine
New Orleans, Louisiana
USA

1. Introduction

In the industrialized world, significant development and interventions were made since the HIV epidemic and they contributed to improved maternal health and low perinatal transmission rates. However, not all questions about this infection in pregnancy were answered. At times, obstetric health care providers for HIV-infected pregnant women were faced with certain clinical situations where there was limited available data to help direct treatment planning. This chapter will discuss recent data on various special considerations encountered in the management of HIV infection in pregnancy.

2. Apparent lack of prenatal care and the lack of knowledge of available treatment to decrease perinatal transmission among HIV-infected women

Vertical transmission of HIV infection was significantly reduced by offering HIV testing to pregnant women and implementing the Pediatrics AIDS Clinical Trials Group (PACTG) protocol 076 (Connor et al., 1994). The success of this protocol was dependent on women seeking prenatal care, where they were offered HIV screening and appropriate treatment for affected pregnancies and their newborns. However, HIV-infected women often do not obtain prenatal care. As a whole, 5–10% of women in the United States receive inadequate or no prenatal care (Kogan et al., 1998). HIV-infected women are even less likely to seek prenatal care. According to a study by Minkoff et al., 50% of HIV-infected women who gave birth at a municipal hospital in New York City did not have prenatal care (Minkoff et al., 1990). In a survey of HIV-infected women in Philadelphia, only a third of these pregnant women reported adequate prenatal care and 20% had no prenatal care (Turner et al., 1996). Additionally, these women often failed to disclose their HIV infectious status when they presented for labor and delivery. Fifty percent of the women with inadequate prenatal care were actually aware of their HIV infection but did not choose to disclose to their caretaker when they presented for delivery at the Medical Center of LA in New Orleans (Centers for Disease Control and Prevention [CDC], 2004). This troubling data implies that many HIV-infected women unknowingly, as a consequence of a lack of knowledge, infect their unborn children despite the availability of treatments to reduce vertical transmission (Dola et al., 2010). These findings stress the importance of educating the public on the currently available interventions to reduce vertical transmission of HIV infection.

One of the barriers to decreasing perinatal transmission is that HIV-infected women do not obtain early prenatal care and thus exclude themselves from available interventions. Heath care providers must understand why HIV infected women are less likely to utilize prenatal services. Lancioni et al. reported that issues normally encountered in women without prenatal care - such as transportation, lack of child care, lack of insurance, and scheduling of appointments - were not found to be the reason why HIV infected women do not seek prenatal care. Rather, these women opted out of prenatal services because they feared the risk of disclosure and the anticipated anger from health care providers because they chose to continue their pregnancy (Lancioni et al., 1999). Eliminating the social stigma about HIV infection and educating health care providers about these women's fears and concerns could help reduce the barriers in seeking prenatal care (Dola et al., 2010).

3. Limitations of benefits of rapid HIV testing in labor and delivery

In the United States, approximately 144 – 226 infants are infected annually with HIV (CDC, 2007). Many of these infants were born of mothers who were not tested early in pregnancy or did not receive the appropriate prophylaxis treatment (CDC, 2007). Approximately a quarter of all people currently infected with HIV are not aware of their infectious status (Marks et al, 2006). Therefore, HIV screening during prenatal care is a necessity for the success of PACTG protocol 076. In addition, there is a high rate of HIV infection amongst women without prenatal care (Lindsay et al., 1991). Thus, those who most need it are excluded from the benefits of the PACTG protocol 076 and other obstetrical interventions to decrease perinatal transmission.

Rapid HIV testing is now available to allow undiagnosed HIV-infected women one last vital opportunity to be tested for the infection and to decrease the risk of transmitting the disease to their newborns. By virtue of the fast availability of the rapid HIV test result, it is hoped that interventions can be instituted to decrease perinatal transmission. If a woman tested reactive on the rapid HIV test, she will be counseled appropriately and if agreed, she will be administered zidovudine prophylaxis during labor along with obstetrical interventions, and her neonate will receive prophylactic zidovudine after birth. This abbreviated regimen of zidovudine has been shown to be cost-effective (Stringer et al., 1999) and can decrease vertical transmission (Wade et al., 1998). Studies by Wade et al. show a reduction of vertical HIV transmission to 10% when zidovudine prophylaxis begins intrapartum compared to 27% in those without any treatment (Wade et al., 1998).

Rapid HIV testing is an excellent concept to allow undiagnosed HIV-infected women one last chance to decrease the risk of infecting their newborn, however, the benefits of rapid HIV tests may not be fully appreciated due to a large percentage of these women presenting in advanced labor, after rupture of membranes, or when they deliver shortly after arrival to the labor unit. Dola et al. retrospectively analyzed 350 parturients without prior prenatal care at their institution who presented to the labor unit with unknown HIV serostatus (Dola et al., 2010). These women often presented in active labor with cervical dilation of ≥ 5 cm (48.6%); another 15.2% presented at complete cervical dilation of 10 centimeters, and 43% presented after ruptured membranes. The benefit of early detection of HIV infection via rapid testing may be less obvious in these women as perinatal transmission might already have occurred. Another 5.5% of these women even missed the benefits of rapid HIV testing by delivering their baby prior to their arrival to the hospital. It could be postulated that no benefit can be gained from a rapid HIV test result to direct effective management of these patients during their labor and delivery (Dola et al., 2010). However, early oral zidovudine treatment for the newborn can be facilitated by early detection of the infection by rapid HIV testing on admission. Even so, recent studies reported conflicting data regarding the effectiveness of administering only zidovudine prophylaxis to neonates after delivery (Wade et al., 1998; Fiscus et al., 1999).

Although results from rapid HIV testing is readily available - the median turn-around time is 66 minutes based on the CDC-sponsored MIRIAD Study (Bulterys et al.,2004), or 45 minutes with the OraQuick Rapid HIV-1 Antibody Test at point-of-care hospitals (Cohen et al., 2003), Dola et al. reported that 22% of their study patients delivered within one hour after arrival to the labor and delivery unit, 31.6% within 2 hours, 38.4% within 3 hours, and 47.2% within 4 hours. Therefore, in order for any rapid HIV test to be of use, the test result turnaround time, the time for counseling, and the time to availability of the zidovudine treatment must be constricted to within a few hours after admission (Dola et al., 2010).

As a consequence, the full benefit of the rapid HIV tests may not be realized in patients who typically present without prenatal care - mostly in advanced labor and with rupture membranes (Dola et al., 2010). Due to the high prevalence of HIV infection in women without prenatal care (Lindsay et al., 1991), and until the rapid HIV testing results become available, obstetricians should consider these unregistered parturients as infected with HIV when they present for labor and delivery - refraining from certain common obstetrics practices (i.e. artificial rupture of membranes and the placement of an invasive fetal scalp electrode) to avoid inadvertly increasing the risk of perinatal transmission (Dola et al., 2010).

4. HIV rescreening in late pregnancy – should all women be rescreened?

A case report from Steele (Steele, 2010) describes three cases of infants whose mothers were screened negative for HIV infection in their first trimester of pregnancy. Since their mothers were not considered at high risk for HIV infection, they were not retested in the later stage of pregnancy according to the revised Centers for Disease Control and Prevention (CDC) guidelines (CDC, 2006; Branson et al., 2006). These mothers must have been infected with HIV later in their pregnancy as they were diagnosed with HIV infection shortly after delivery. Of these 3 infants, 2 developed an HIV infection (Steele, 2010).

The revised CDC guidelines (Branson et al., 2006) recommended repeat testing for HIV infection in late pregnancy but before 36 weeks of gestation for women at high risk for acquiring the infection. Women requiring repeat testing would include: those with high risk behaviors, those living in 20 states with high incidence of HIV infection, those receiving care at facilities with incidence of HIV infection of at least 1 per 1,000 women screened, and those with signs and symptoms consistent with acute HIV infection (Branson et al., 2006). These guidelines were placed as beneficial interventions to reduce mother-to-child transmission (MTCT) of HIV could have been implemented in mothers not identified as HIV infected until late in pregnancy or until the onset of labor (Wade et al., 1998).

Sansom et al, further supports the necessity of rescreening for HIV in the third trimester as it could prove to be cost-effective in preventing MTCT in a community with an HIV incidence of 1 per 1,000 person-years or higher. They argue that primary HIV infection may go undetected in women who continue to practice high-risk behaviors during pregnancy and in those with initial tests performed before HIV antibody development (Sansom et al., 2003). According to one study of 407 HIV-positive mothers, eight seroconversions happened after a negative test result during or just before pregnancy. Three of the 8 seroconversions resulted in perinatal HIV transmissions (Fiscus et al., 1999).

In an effort to further reduce perinatal transmission, Patterson et al. recommended that repeat HIV testing should be done in late pregnancy and again at time of labor and delivery along with the use of reflex RNA testing for women with negative antibody to detect acute HIV infection (Patterson et al, 2007). Furthermore, Gray et al reported that the risk of acquisition of HIV infection increased by 2-fold in pregnancy after adjustment for behaviors risk factors (Gray et al., 2005). Although the evidence is inconclusive, this increased risk could be due to the hormonal changes in pregnancy, which could affect genital tract mucosa (Jacobson et al., 2000; Michael et al., 1997) or immune responses (Brahin, 2002; Beagley & Gockel, 2003), resulting in susceptibility to HIV infectivity.

This above case report presented by Steele and the above arguments on cost-effectiveness of rescreening in late pregnancy support a recommendation for late pregnancy HIV screening - possibly including RNA reflex testing for those with negative antibody to the virus- of all women instead of only women known to have risk factors. However, a barrier to putting this into practice is that not all insurance companies will cover the cost of a repeat HIV screening in late pregnancy for all pregnant women unless the CDC revises its guidelines (Steele, 2010).

5. Cesarean section in HIV-infected women – Are there any maternal or neonatal morbidities?

Scheduled cesarean section prior to labor is recommended at 38 weeks gestation for women with a viral load above 1,000 copies/ml to further prevent vertical transmission of HIV infection (American College of Obstetricians and Gynecologists [ACOG], 2004). The combination of cesarean delivery and antiretroviral medications have been demonstrated to effectively reduce mother-to-child transmission of HIV disease (The International Perinatal HIV Group, 1999; The European Mode of Delivery Collaboration, 1999;Mofenson, 2002; Burdge et al., 2003; Mandelbrot et al., 1998; Kind et al., 1998). Cesarean deliveries are not without significant complications even for HIV-negative women (Allen et al., 2003; Makoha et al., 2004). Therefore, HIV-positive women could theoretically be at greater risk for post-operative complications due to a relatively weakened immune system or immunodeficient status. However, there are conflicting reports from the currently available data with regard to post-cesarean morbidities incurred by HIV-infected women (The European Mode of Delivery Collaboration, 1999; Maiques-Montesinos et al., 1999; Grubert et al., 2002; Rodriguez et al., 2001; Marcollet et al., 2002; Watts et al., 2000). Most studies report an increased risk of post-operative morbidity, mostly infectious, in HIV-positive women compared with HIV-negative control subjects (Coll et al., 2002; Grubert el al., 1999; Vimercati et al., 2000). Additionally, the risk of complications is correlated with the degree of immunosuppression (Jamieson et al., 2007). Thus, those who most benefit from scheduled cesarean delivery to decrease vertical transmission would sustain the highest risk of complication from the procedure.

A Cochrane review (Read & Newell; 2005) summarizes six studies (European Mode of Delivery Collaboration, 1999; Marcollet et al., 2002; Watts et al., 2000; Read et al., 2001; Faucher et al., 2001; Fior et al., 2004) which compare the complication rates in women receiving scheduled cesarean delivery, non-elective cesarean delivery, and vaginal delivery. Post-operative morbidity was highest in women who underwent a non-elective cesarean delivery.

Vaginal delivery resulted in the lowest post-partum morbidity. Of note, most of these morbidities were post-operative fever, anemia, endometritis, and wound infection (Jamieson et al., 2007). Maternal deaths are rare, and these studies did not have adequate sample sizes to assess any potential differences in maternal mortality rate (Jamieson et al., 2007). Given that these HIV-infected women are at high risk for post-operative infectious morbidities, prophylactic antibiotics should be given according to ACOG guidelines for all women who undergo cesarean delivery (American College of Obstetricians and Gynecologists [ACOG], 2003). However, most of these studies were performed prior to the recommendation to give prophylactic antibiotics at least 30 minutes prior to cesarean delivery instead of after cord clamping, which has been shown to decrease the risk of post-operative infection. It would be interesting to determine whether this newly recommended practice would reduce the risk of post-operative infection in these HIV-infected women.

Current ACOG guidelines recommends scheduled cesarean delivery in HIV infected women, emphasizing the importance of performing the surgery prior to the onset of labor or rupture of membranes to reduce the risk of vertical transmission (ACOG, 2004) and that cesarean delivery performed after the onset of labor or after rupture of membranes is of unclear benefit with regard to decreasing vertical transmission. Based on the previously mentioned data, these cesarean deliveries after onset of labor or after rupture of membrane could be associated with an increase in maternal infectious morbidity (Rodriguez et al., 2001; Marcollet et al., 2002; Read et al., 2001; Duarte et al., 2006). Therefore, when an HIV-infected woman attempts vaginal delivery, she should be counseled for the increased risk of post-operative morbidity should she require an emergent cesarean delivery (Cavasin et al., 2009). Marcollet et al. recommends that HIV-infected women with a low probability of having a successful vaginal delivery should consider a scheduled cesarean delivery (Marcollet et al., 2002).

Overall, as the cost for treating postpartum morbidity is relatively low in comparison to the cost incurred by pediatric HIV infection, it appears that scheduled cesarean delivery is cost-effective (Halpern et al., 2000; Mrus et al., 2000; Ratcliffe et al., 1998).

ACOG recommends that scheduled cesarean delivery in the absence of medical or obstetrical indications should not be performed at less than 39 weeks of gestation, due to increased risk of neonatal respiratory morbidity (ACOG, 2001). This risk of respiratory morbidity for neonates born via cesarean section would closely approximate that of neonates born via the vaginal route at 39 weeks of gestation (Tita et al., 2009). In HIV-infected women with viral load greater than 1,000 copies/ml, both ACOG and the U.S. Public Health Service recommend scheduled cesarean delivery at 38 weeks for prevention of vertical transmission of the HIV infection (ACOG, 2001; Public Health Service Task Force, 2010). The gestational age of 38 weeks instead of 39 weeks was chosen as the timing for scheduled cesarean delivery with the intent to avoid spontaneous labor and rupture of membranes. Recent data reaffirmed an increased risk of neonatal morbidity even for those neonates born just a few days before 39 weeks of gestation (Tita et al., 2011). To address this valid clinical concern of a potential increase in neonatal respiratory distress syndrome in deliveries at 38 weeks in an effort to prevent mother-to-child transmission of HIV disease, Livingston et al and the IMPACT Protocol 1025 Study group (Livingston et al., 2010) performed a prospective cohort study. They concluded that after adjustment for gestational age and birth weight, the mode of delivery was not significantly associated with respiratory distress syndrome (p=.10), although a trend toward an increased risk for respiratory distress syndrome was noted among neonates delivered by cesarean section (either elective and non-elective) when compared to those delivered via the vaginal route. The overall rate of neonatal respiratory distress syndrome among those born beyond 37 weeks by all modes of delivery is low: 3.4% for 37 weeks, 1.0% for 38 weeks, and 1.1% at 39 weeks. Among those neonates born via elective cesarean delivery at 38 weeks of gestation, there were only 2 out of 227 neonates who had respiratory distress syndrome. This is reassuring data and it appears that respiratory distress syndrome at this late gestational age could be readily managed, although, an admission to the intensive care nursery for treatment might invoke significant parental distress. In the counseling of patients on scheduled cesarean section at 38 weeks to prevent vertical transmission, one must include the small potential risk of neonatal respiratory distress syndrome. This small risk from iatrogenic premature delivery must then be balanced against the risk of less effective prevention of vertical transmission with the onset of labor or rupture of membranes if expectant management is continued until 39 weeks of gestation. The results from this study are the first available data and are reassuring with regard to the low rate of neonatal morbidity associated with current guidelines recommending scheduled cesarean delivery at 38 weeks, therefore further research in this area is needed to provide more robust data regarding this intervention for decreasing vertical transmission.

6. The challenge of prenatal diagnosis in HIV infected - women

The current standard of care offers prenatal diagnosis to the general obstetrics population. In pregnancies complicated by HIV infection, there is a suspicion of a higher rate of false-positive results when these women are screened with the maternal serum multiple marker test (Yudin et al., 2003). This may lead to a higher risk for HIV infected women to require definitive testing with genetic amniocentesis. Therefore it is important to review the current data on the usefulness of biochemical marker screening test in pregnant HIV-infected women.

Variations in beta-hCG and AFP levels have been shown in HIV-infected pregnancies (Yudin et al., 2003; Einstein et al., 2004). This may make calculating the risk for Down syndrome difficult and might result in further diagnostic procedures. Additionally, a patient's immune status (CD4+ count) and viral load may be associated with abnormal screening test results (Neale et al., 2001; Gross et al., 2003). However, the mechanism for these alterations of the tested biochemical markers is unclear. It has been postulated to be due to the altered maternal immune status or the impact of highly active antiretroviral therapy on feto-maternal transfer of these markers, their metabolism or their excretion by the mother (Yudin et al., 2003).

In contrast to the above findings, Brossard et al (Brossard et al., 2008) concluded that these tests were still useful in a HIV-infected population composed of 214 women for first trimester screening tests and 209 women for risk assessment for neural tube defects. Although, they also found a lower median of the MoM of beta-human chorionic gonadotrophin and pregnancy-associated plasma protein-A in HIV-infected women when compared to controls, they did not believe that such differences impacted the risk estimation for Down syndrome or neural tube defects (Brossard et al., 2008).

Similarly, Le Meaux et al. studied a cohort of HIV-infected women in France and noted that untreated HIV-infection was associated with lower maternal alpha fetoprotein levels but there was no increase in false-positive rates in their double marker screening test (which included serum AFP and total beta-hCG levels) (Le Meaux et al., 2008). Therefore, future esearch - with larger sample sizes - is needed to further investigate the plausible nechanisms for the alterations in these biochemical markers in HIV-infected women. f indeed HIV-infected women had a higher rate of false-positive maternal serum multiple narker screening test results it may warrant that they are more likely to require definitive liagnostic testing, which includes invasive procedures such as amniocentesis. Caution is equired for HIV infected pregnant women who need amniocentesis because there is a *otentially iatrogenic risk for perinatal transmission which might be related to elevated naternal viral load (Bucceri et al., 2001). Such invasive procedures might result in infected naternal blood leaking into the amniotic cavity as the needle is traversing the uterine wall *r an anterior placenta (Giorlandino et al., 1996).

)ata regarding the safety of prenatal diagnostic procedures - in pregnancies complicated by IIV infection - are scant and based on a very small number of participants. Older studies onducted prior to the widespread use of zidovudine suggest an increased risk of infecting he unborn child through invasive diagnostic tests - such as amniocentesis, amnioscopies nd other needle puncture procedures (Mandelbrot et al., 1996). With the use of zidovudine nd HAART, the risk of perinatal transmission from invasive diagnostic tests may be greatly educed (Shapiro et al., 1999; Maiques et al., 2003). Other studies with small numbers of tudy patients (ranging from 6-11 women) reported no perinatal transmission in newborns Bucceri et al., 2001; Ekoukou et al., 2008; Coll et al., 2006). In total, of the data collected from *ublished studies, amongst the women who underwent invasive procedures there were 28 nfected newborns from 82 women who did not receive antiretroviral treatment, 2 infected *ewborns from 24 women who received zidovudine treatment only, and no infected *ewborns from 78 women who received HAART treatment, (p = 0.0001) (Ekoukou et al., !008). Thus, it appears that the significant decline in the rate of perinatal transmission after *nvasive procedures performed during pregnancy could possibly reflect the beneficial *mpact of anti-retroviral therapy (Ekoukou et al., 2008). Additionally, the potential risk of *erinatal transmission might not be as great as it was once thought to be with the *mplementation of HAART. However, we must consider that the above studies are limited *y their small number of study participants.

\ policy to guide physicians to provide adequate counseling to HIV-infected women *egarding the potential risks of early invasive prenatal diagnostic tests, and the optimal *pproach to such procedures is much needed. We venture to offer the following conclusions *egarding prenatal diagnosis in HIV-infected women based on the above limited data. HIV-nfected pregnant women should be offered biochemical marker testing for prenatal liagnosis since it is unclear whether the variations in these marker levels are significant. If nvasive sampling of the amniotic fluid is warranted, then careful judgment must be used to :onsider the patient's risk factors for vertical transmission. Patient should be counseled that *ased on studies with small sample sizes, the risk of iatrogenic transmission of the HIV *irus to the fetus is much lower than previously thought in the setting of optimal viral *uppression and HAART. Ideally, patients undergoing invasive testing should be on *ntiretroviral therapy and have undetectable viral loads (Watts, 2002). Additionally, care *hould be taken to avoid penetrating the placenta during the procedure as this could :heoretically increase maternal and fetal blood mixing, or directly inoculate the fetal blood Giorlandino et al., 1996). Prenatal diagnosis should not be performed in women whose HIV *erology is unknown, given the above concern of iatrogenic risk and the need for *ppropriate therapy prior to the procedure. There is a great need for continued *nvestigations on which to establish future policy and protocol on this topic.

7. Management of PPROM in women infected with HIV

The duration of rupture of membrane plays an important role in vertical transmission of HIV infection in term pregnancies. Minkoff et al. described a significantly increased rate of perinatal transmission of HIV infection in term women with low CD 4 count if they have ruptured their membranes for more than 4 hours (Minkoff et al., 1995). Other studies confirmed Minkoff's work and found an increase of perinatal transmission from 14% to 25% in the setting of rupture of membranes for greater than 4 hours (Landesman et al., 1996). Furthermore, there is a significant rise in transmission – from 8% to 31% – among women with AIDS if delivery is postponed past 24 hours after rupture of membranes (International Perinatal HIV Group, 2001).

These data reporting an increase in vertical transmission of the HIV infection after prolonged period of ruptured membranes pose a significant obstetrical dilemma for the management of women infected with HIV who had preterm premature rupture of the membranes (PPROM). The question is should all these HIV-infected women with PPROM be delivered at the time of first diagnosis with PPROM to avoid prolonged rupture of membranes, which potentially can lead to an increase in perinatal transmission of the disease? Does current data suggest that we should commit these HIV-infected pregnancies with PPROM to extreme prematurity with immediate delivery to avoid the risk of perinatal transmission of HIV? Available data on expectant management of PPROM in HIV infected women are limited. Currently available are two studies on PPROM in HIV infected women. The first study by Aagaard-Tillery et al. (Aagaard-Tillery et al. 2006) in 2006 evaluated the management and outcomes of 7 HIV pregnancies complicated by PPROM. They were diagnosed with PPROM, were expectantly management, and subsequently delivered between 25 to 32 weeks gestation. The mean latency for these patients was 17.1 days with a median of 5 days; one woman had a latency of 92 days. Two of 6 infants became infected with HIV through vertical transmission. The mothers of these two HIV-infected infants either did not receive antepartum or intrapartum antiretroviral therapy or only received treatment in the antepartum period with zidovudine monotherapy. Based on their results, the authors questioned whether expectant management is possible in the setting of PPROM in HIV-infected women, provided that they receive prophylactic combination antiretroviral therapy.

A second study in 2007 by Alvarez et al. (Alvarez et al., 2007) reported data on 18 cases of HIV infected women with PPROM at ≤ 34 weeks of gestation from a single center, delivering at an average gestational age of 31 weeks. The latency period before delivery ranged from 4 to 336 hours. Of those cases, 10 patients had been managed with antenatal antiretroviral therapy and did not have mother-to-child-transmission of HIV regardless of the duration of ruptured membranes, viral load, or maternal CD4 count. The remaining 8 cases did not receive antenatal antiretroviral therapy and received only intrapartum nevirapine. Two of these eight neonates sustained perinatal transmission of HIV; their mothers did not have prenatal care and did not receive antenatal antiretroviral therapy. In this study, the perinatal transmission rate for HIV was 11.1% (2/18).

Although these two studies show encouraging outcomes and are very thought provoking, safety of expectant management of PPROM could not be ascertained based on the small number of study participants. From the above data, we concluded that for HIV-infected women with PPROM at a very young gestational age who has suppressed viral load and on antenatal HAART, expectant management to allow in-utero lung maturation might be considered. However, as risk of morbidity from preterm birth is decreased at tertiary care center beyond 30-32 weeks, there might be more advantageous for expedite delivery. The benefits of expectant management are still uncertain in patients not receiving antiretroviral treatment. Future studies on HIV infected women with PPROM prior to 34 weeks gestation are necessary to arrive at the optimal care plan.

8. Could viral load in genital tract secretions have a role in perinatal transmission?

Maternal viral load was determined to be the most important risk factor in perinatal transmission of HIV infection (The European Collaborative Study, 1999). Efforts in reduction of MTCT of HIV involve optimal suppression of viral load with the implementation of HAART. However, perinatal transmission was reported among women with undetectable maternal serum viral load (Cao et al., 1997; Sperling et al., 1996). Provocative data was gathered by the European Collaborative study. The investigators reported a 2% risk of vertical transmission among women with low viral load who delivered after 37 weeks by elective cesarean section and 11% among those delivered via the vaginal route (The European Collaborative Study, 1999). This might imply that other factors play an important role in the perinatal transmission besides maternal serum viral load. One explanation for the perinatal transmission in the setting of low plasma viral load and the protective effect from cesarean section could be that viral shedding in the female genital tract could have a role in perinatal transmission and that there might be a discordance between HIV-1 RNA levels in blood and cervicovaginal secretions (Garcia-Bujalance et al., 2004). HIV-1 RNA has been detected from the female cervicovaginal tract (Cu Uvin & Caliendoa, 1997) and treatment with HAART can suppress HIV-1 RNA to below detectable levels in both the genital tract and plasma of non-pregnant women (Cu Uvin et al., 2000).

Several studies noted a strong correlation between the level of HIV-1 viral load in the genital tract and the plasma (Hart et al., 1999; Kovacs et al., 1999). However, in non-pregnant women with undetectable plasma viral load, HIV-1 RNA load can be found in their genital tract (Debiaggi et al., 2001). Conversely, some studies reported no correlation between the viral load in the plasma and genital shedding of non-pregnant women (Rasheed et al., 1996). One study from Kovacs et al. (Kovacs et al., 2001) reports that although there was a positive correlation between RNA concentrations in the plasma and the genital tract, 4% (9 of 252 women) of their population had higher RNA concentrations in the genital secretions and two women had at least 10-fold higher RNA levels in genital tract secretions than in plasma. Different genotypic variants of HIV-1 were found in the blood and cervicovaginal lavage according to another study (Shaheen et al., 1999). Garcia-Bujalance et al. reported 2 cases in 38 HIV-1 infected pregnant women with a low plasma viral load of <50 copies/mL but with detectable viral load in their vaginal secretions (Garcia-Bujalance et al., 2004).

Another factor in reducing MTCT of HIV infection can perhaps be determined by viral shedding in the female genital tract. The lack of correlation between the viral load in blood plasma and genital tract secretions might suggest that there is still risk for perinatal transmission in women with undetectable viral load in the plasma (Iribarren et al., 2001). More studies are needed to investigate on the roles of genital tract viral shedding in perinatal transmission and the possible benefit of using both plasma and cervicovaginal secretion viral loads despite undetectable viral plasma load in choosing the vaginal route of delivery.

9. Should assisted reproductive technology be available for HIV-infected men and women?

Currently, about 80% of women infected with HIV are of reproductive age (CDC, 2001). With the current advent and widespread use of HAART in industrialized countries, HIV infection has become a chronic disease and those who are affected with the disease can now live longer and with a better quality of life (Kambin & Batzer, 2004). Furthermore, with current interventions, the risk of MTCT of HIV infection is now significantly declined to approximately 2% (The Ethics Committee of the American Society for Reproductive Medicine [ASRM], 2010). As a result, HIV-infected men and women may elect to have children. However, for discordant couple, reproduction may result in the risk of horizontal transmission to the uninfected partner.

The Ethics Committee of the American Society for Reproductive Medicine (ASRM) established guidelines in 1994 for patients infected with HIV who might request or require assisted reproductive technologies (Ethics Committee of the American Fertility Society, 1994). The committee made the following recommendations due to their concern about potential horizontal transmission to the uninfected partner and vertical transmission to the couple's child and the potential problem to the offspring as the infected parent might succumb to the disease. Their recommendations are as follows: couples seeking support are encouraged to test for HIV infection, development of written policies on infertility treatment for HIV-infected people by each institution, counseling of consequences of using infected sperm, and advising couples on the alternative options of donor sperm, adoption, or not having children (Ethics Committee of the American Fertility Society, 1994).

Since then, better understanding of the disease has been achieved, and the beneficial impact of HAART significantly improved survival and quality of life for HIV-infected persons, along with improved technique to provide virus-free sperm for reproductive assistance. Thus, in 2006, ASRM published its revision of the original guidelines. Obstetric health care providers should be aware of these revisions so that they can appropriately counsel their patients.

Approximately 1 in 500 – 1,000 episodes of unprotected intercourse is estimated to result in horizontal transmission of the HIV infection to an uninfected partner (Mandelbrot et al., 1997). Therefore, in discordant couples where the woman is infected with HIV and her partner is negative, ASRM discussed the use of homologous insemination with the uninfected male partner's sperm to achieve pregnancy and to avoid the risk of transmission (ASRM, 2010).

In discordant couples (with the male partner being infected), intercourse without condom use at the time of ovulation to attempt conception could reduce but does not eliminate the risk of infecting the partner. According to one study, the reported seroconversion rate was 4.3% for couples that employed timed intercourse to attempt conception (Sauer et al., 2009). Couples should be counseled against this unsafe method as they could still infect their partner. For these instances of male-infected sero-discordant couples, specific methods for sperm preparation and testing (density gradient and swim-up technique to obtain sperm and PCR virus detection assay) have been described (Kambin et al., 2004; Sauer et al., 2009; Semprini et al., 1998). The final sperm sample was used only if it tested negative on these assays (Semprini et al., 1998). These techniques resulted in less than 1% of the samples testing positive for the virus and thus was discarded (Semprini et al., 1998). These techniques can markedly reduce the chance of HIV transmission to the female partner and child. Specifically, Semprini et al. reported data on almost 1,600 inseminations of 513 HIV-uninfected women in which there were 228 pregnancies. At a follow-up rate of 97.5% at 3 months, and 92% at one year, all mothers and children were uninfected (Semprini et al., 1998). Similarly, there was no report of transmitted HIV infection to the mother or child with intrauterine insemination (Kambin et al., 2004) or intracytoplasmic sperm injection (Sauer et al., 2009) technique. For these male-positive discordant couples, extensive counseling should be performed regarding transmission risk-reduction techniques (ASRM, 2000). Health care providers should not overlook HIV-infected men and women's desire to have children. They should make every effort to encourage these men and women to obtain care at the institutions with most effective methods to provide appropriate treatment and to reduce the chance of infecting their partner and child.

10. Conclusion

Significant progress was made in understanding HIV virology and important interventions were developed to reduce mother-to-child-transmission of this disease since the epidemic of this disease. Most obstetricians caring for HIV-infected women are familiar with these commonly employed interventions. However, there are still many difficult clinical situations where only scant data is available to direct management, in part due to the fortunately low prevalence of the disease in industrialized countries. We hope readers of this chapter would continue to report their challenging clinical encounters and thus, would contribute to the better care of these pregnant HIV-infected women. The review of these special considerations, hopefully, will aid obstetricians in their plan of care, raise valid questions, and suggest areas of future research directions.

11. References

Aagaard-Tillery, K., Lin, M.G., Lupo, V., Buchbinder, A., & Ramsey, P.S. (2006). Clinical Study – Preterm Premature Rupture of Membranes in Human Immunodeficiency Virus Infected Women: A Novel Case Series. Infectious Diseases in Obstetrics and Gynecology; 2006:53234.

ACOG Committee on Obstetric Practice.(2004) Scheduled Cesarean Delivery and the Prevention of Vertical Transmission of HIV Infection. ACOG Committee Opinion No 234, May 2004.

Allen, V.M., O'Connell, C.M., Liston, R.M., & Baskett, T.F. (2003). Maternal morbidity Associated with cesarean delivery without labor compared with spontaneous onset of labor at term. Obstet Gynecol 2003; 102:477-82.

Alvarez, J.R., Bardeguez, A, Iffy, L., & Apuzzio, J.J.(2007). Preterm premature rupture of membranes in pregnancies complicated by human immunodeficiency virus infection: A single center's five-year experience. The Journal of Maternal-Fetal and Neonatal Medicine, 2007; 20(12):853-857.

American College of Obstetricians and Gynecologists. (2001). Scheduled cesarean delivery and the prevention of vertical transmission of HIV infection. ACOG Committee Opinion 234. Int J Gynaecol Obstet. 2001;73:279–81.

American College of Obstetricians and Gynecologists. (2003). Prophylactic antibiotics in labor and delivery: ACOG practice bulletin no. :47. Obstet Gynecol 2003;102:875-82.

Beagley, K.W., & Gockel, C.M. (2003). Regulation of innate and adaptive immunity by female sex hormones oestradiol and progesterone. FEMS Immunol Med Microbiol, 2003;39:13-22.

Brabin L. (2002). Interactions of the female hormonal environment, susceptibility to viral infections, and disease progression. AIDS Patient Care STDS 2002; 16: 211-21.

Branson, B.M., Handsfield, H.H., Lampe, M.A., Janssen, R.S., Taylor, A.W., Lyss, S.B., et al. (2006). Revised recommendations for HIV testing of adults, adolescents, and pregnant women in health-care settings. MMWR Recomm Rep 2006;55(RR-14): 1-17.

Brossard, P., Boulvain, M., Coll, O., Barlow, P., Aebi-Popp, K., Bischof, P., Martinez de Teja, B. (2008). Swiss HIV Cohort Study; Swiss HIV Mother and Child Cohort Study. Is screening for fetal anomalies reliable in HIV-infected pregnant women? A multicentre study. AIDS, 2008;22(15):2013-7.

Bucceri, A.M., Somigliana, E., Vignali, M. (2001). Early invasive diagnostic techniques During pregnancy in HIV-infected women. Acta Obstet Gynecol Scand, 2001;80(1):82-3.

Bulterys, M., Jamieson, D.J., O'Sullivan, M.J., & et al. (2004). Rapid HIV-1 Testing During Labor. A Multicenter Study. JAMA.2004;292:219-223.

Burdge, D.R., Money, D.M., Forbes, J.C., Walmsley, S.L., Smaill, F.M., Boucher, M., & et al. (2003). Canadian consensus guidelines for the management of pregnancy, labour and delivery and for postpartum care in HIV-positive pregnant women and their offspring. CMAJ 2003; 168.

Cao, Y., Krogstad, P., Korber, B.T., et al. (1997). Maternal HIV-1 viral load and vertical transmission of infection: the Ariel Project for the prevention of HIV transmission from mother to infant. Nat Med, 1997;3:549-552.

Cavasin, H., Dola, T., Uribe, O., & et al. (2009). Postoperative infectious morbidities of cesarean delivery in Human Immunodeficiency Virus-Infected Women. Infect Dis Obstet Gynecol. 2009;2009:827405. Epub 2009 May 25

Centers for Disease Control and Prevention (CDC). (2004). Rapid HIV Antibody Testing During Labor and Delivery for Women of Unknown HIV Status. A Practical Guide and Model Protocol. January 2004.

CDC. (2006). Sexually transmitted diseases treatment guidelines. Morb Mortal Wkly Rep, 2006;55(RR-11):14.

CDC. (2007). HIV/AIDS Fact sheet. Mother-to-Child (Perinatal) HIV transmission and prevention. October 2007.

CDC. (2001). HIV/ADIS Surveillance Report. 2001;13.

Cohen, M.H., Olszewski, Y., Brandon, B., & et al. (2003) Using point-of-care testing to make rapid HIV-1 tests in labor really rapid. AIDS. 2003;17:2121-2123.

Coll, O., Fiore, S., Floridia, M., & et al. (2002). Pregnancy and HIV infection: a European consensus on management. AIDS, 2002; 16(suppl):S1-18.

Coll, .O, Suy, A., Hernandez, S., Pisa, S., Lonca, M., Thorne, C., & Borrell, A. (2006). Prenatal diagnosis in human immunodeficiency virus-infected women: a new screening program for chromosomal anomalies. Am J Obstet Gynecol, 2006;194(1):192-8.

Connor, E.M., Sperling, R.S., Gelber, R., & et al. (1994). Reduction of maternal-infant transmission of human immunodeficiency virus type 1 with zidovudine treatment. N. Engl J Med. 1994;331:1173-1180.

u Uvin, S. & Caliendoa, A.M. (1997). Cervicovaginal human immunodeficiency virus secretion and plasma viral load in human immunodeficiency virus-seropositive women. Obstetrics & Gynecology, 1997;90(3): 739-743.

u Uvin, S., Caliendoa, A.M., Reinert, S., Chang, A., Juliano-Remollino, C., Flanigan, T.P., Mayer, K.H., & Carpenter, C.C.J. (2000). Effect of highly active antiretroviral therapy on cervicovaginal HIV-1 RNA. AIDS, 2000;14:415-421.

)ebiaggi, M., Zara, F., Spinillo, A., De Santolo ,A., Maserati, R., Bruno, R., Sacchi, P., Achilli, G., Pistorio, A., Romero, E., & Filice, G. (2001). Viral excretion in cervicovaginal secretions of HIV-1 infected women receiving antiretroviral therapy. Eur J Clin, 2001; 20:91-96.

)ola, C.P., Tran, T., Duong, C., Federico, C., DeNicola, N., & Maupin, R. (2010). Rapid HIV testing and obstetrical characteristics of women with unkown HIV serostatus at time of labor and delivery. J Natl Med Assoc. 2010; 102(12):1158-64.

)uarte, G., Read, J., Gonin, R., & et al. (2006). Mode of delivery and postpartum morbidity in Latin American and Caribbean countries among women who are infected with human immunodeficiency virus-1: The NICHD International Site Development Initiative (NISDI) Perinatal Study. Am J Obstet Gynecol (2006) 195: 215-29.

instein, F.H., Wright, R.L., Trentacoste, S., Gross, S., Merkatz, I.R., & Bernstein, P.S. (2004). The impact of protease inhibitors on maternal serum screening analyte levels in pregnant women who are HIV positive. Am J Obstet Gynecol, 2004;191(3):1004-8.

koukou, D., Khuong-Josses, M.A., Ghibaudo, N., Mechali, D., & Rotten, D. (2008). Amniocentesis in pregnant HIV-infected patients. Absence of mother-to-child viral transmission in a series of selected patients. Eur J Obstet Gynecol Reprod Biol, 2008;140(2):212-7. Epub 2008 Jun 27.

ithics Committee of the American Fertility Society. (1994). Ethical considerations of assisted reproductive technologies. Fertil Steril 1994;62 (Suppl1):85s.

ithics Committee of the American Society for Reproductive Medicine. (2010). Human immunodeficiency virus and infertility treatment. Fertility and Sterility, 2010;94(1): 11-15.

aucher, P., Batallan, A., Bastian, H., & et al. (2001). Management of pregnant women infected with HIV at Bichat Hospital between 1990 and 1998: analysis of 202 pregnancies. Gynecol Obstet Fertil 2001;29:211-25.

iore S, Newell ML, Thorne C. Higher rates of post-partum complications in HIV-infected than in uninfected women irresptive of mode of delivery. AIDS 2004;18:933-8

iscus SA, Adimora AA, Schoenbach VJ, McKinney R, Lim W, Rupar D, et al. Trends in human immunodeficiency virus (HIV) counseling, testing, and antiretroviral treatment of HIV-positive women and perinatal transmission in North Carolina. J Infect Dis 1999;180:99–105.

iscus SA, Schoenbach VJ, Wilfert C. Short courses of zidovudine and perinatal transmission of HIV. N Engl J Med. 1999 Apr 1; 340 (13): 1040 - 1.

García-Bujalance S, Ruiz G, De Guevara CL, Peña JM, Bates I, Vázquez JJ, Gutiérrez A. Quantitation of human immunodeficiency virus type 1 RNA loads in cervicovaginal secretions in pregnant women and relationship between viral loads in the genital tract and blood. Eur J Clin Microbiol Infect Dis.,2004;23(2):111-5. Epub 2004 Jan 20.

Giorlandino C, Gambuzza G, D'Alessio P, Santoro ML, Gentili P, Vizzone A. Blood contamination of amniotic fluid after amniocentesis in relation to placental location. Prenat Diag, 1996;16:180-2

Gray R, Li X, Kigozi G, Serwadda D, Brahmbhatt H, Wabwire-Mangen F, et al. Increased risk of incident HIV during pregnancy in Rakai, Uganda: a prospective study. Lancet 2005; 366:1182–1188.

Gross S, Castillo W, Crane M, Espinosa B, Carter S, DeVeaux R, Salafia C. Maternal serum alpha-fetoprotein and human chorionic gonadotropin levels in women with human immunodeficiency virus. Am J Obstet Gynecol, 2003;188(4):1052-6.

Grubert TA, Reindell D, Belohradsky BH, Gurtler L, Stauber M, Dathe O. Rates of postoperative complication among human immunodeficiency virus-infected women who have undergone obstetric and gynecologic surgical procedures. CID 2002; 34:822-30.

Grubert TA, Reindell D, Kastner R, Lutz-Friedrich R, Belohradsky BH, Datha O. Complications after caesarean section in HIV-1 infected women not taking antiretroviral treatment. Lancet, 1999;354:1612-3.

Halpern MT, Read JS, Ganoczy DA, Harris Dr. Cost-effectiveness of cesarean section delivery to prevent mother-to-child transmission of HIV-1. AIDS 2000;14:691-700.

Hart CE, Lennox JL, Pratt-Palmore M, Wright TC, Schinazi RF, Evans-Strickfaden TE, Bush TJ, Schenell C, Conley LJ, Clancy KA, Ellerbrock TV. Correlation of human immunodeficiency virus type 1 RNA levels in blood and the female genital tract. J Infect Dis, 1999;179:871-882.

International Perinatal HIV Group. Duration of ruptured membranes and vertical transmission of HIV-1: A metaanalysis ßfrom 15 prospective cohort studies. AIDS 2001;15:357-368.

Iribarren JA, Ramos JR, Guerra L, Coll O, De Jose MI, Domingo P, Fortuny C, Miralles P, Parras F, Pena JM, Rodrigo C, Vidal R. Prevencion de la transmison vertical y tratamiento de la infeccion por el virus de la immunodeficiencia humana en la mujer embarazada. Enferm Infec Microbiol Clin, 2001;19:314-335.

Jacobson DL, Peralta L, Farmer M, Graham NMH, Gaydos C, Zenilman J. Relationship of hormonal contraception and cervical ectopy as measured by computerized planimetry to chlamydial infection in adolescents. Sex Transm Dis 2000; 27: 313–19.

Jamieson DJ, Read JS, Kourtis AP, Durant TM, Lampe MA, Dominguez KL. Cesarean delivery for HIV-infected women: recommendations and controversies. Am J Obstet Gynecol. 2007 Sep;197(3 Suppl):S96-100.

Kambin S, Batzer F. Assisted reproductive technology in HIV serodiscordant couples. Sex Reprod Menopause 2004;2:92–100.

Kind C, Rudin C, Siegrist C, Wyler C, Biedermann K, Lauper U. Prevention of vertical HIV transmission: additive protective effect of elective Cesarean section and zidovudine prophylaxis. AIDS 1998; 12:205–10.

Kogan, MD, Martin JA, Alexander GR, Kotelchuck M, Ventura SJ, Frigoletto FD. The changing pattern of prenatal care utilization in the US, 1981 – 1995, using different prenatal care indices. JAMA 1998; 279: 1623 – 8.

Kovacs, A., Chan, L.S., Chen, Z.C., Meyer, W., Muderspach, L., Young, M., Anastos, K., & Levine, A.M. (1999). HIV-1 RNA in plasma and genital tract secretions in women infected with HIV-1. J Acquir Immune Defic Syndr, 1999;22:124-131.

Covacs, A., Wasserman, S., Burns, D., Wright, D., Cohn, J., Landay, A., Weber, K., Cohen, M., Levine, A., Minkoff, H., Miotti, P., Palefsky, J., Young, M., Reichelderfer, P., & the DATRI and WIHS Study Groups. (2001). Determinants of HIV-1 shedding in the genital tract of women. The Lancet, 2001;358(9293): 1593-1601.

Lancioni, C., Harwell, T., & Rutstein, R.M. (1999). Prenatal care and HIV infection. AIDS Patient Care STDS. 1999 Feb; 13 (2); 97 – 102.

Landesman, S.H., Kalisha, L.A., Burns, D.N,. Minkoff, H,. Fox, H.E., Zorrilla, C., Garcia, P., Fowler, M.G., Mofenson, L., & Tuomala, R. (1996). Obstetrical factors and the transmission of human immunodeficiency virus type 1 from mother to child. The Women and Infants Transmission Study. N Engl J Med, 1996;334:1617–1623.

Le Meaux, J.P., Tsatsaris, V., Schmitz, T., Fulla, Y., Launay, O., Goffinet, F., & Azria, E. (2008). Maternal biochemical serum screening for Down syndrome in pregnancy with human immunodeficiency virus infection. Obstet Gynecol, 2008;112(2 Pt 1):223-30.

Lindsay, M.K., Feng, T.I., Peterson, H.B., & et al. (1991). Routine human immunodeficiency infection screening in unregistered and registered inner-city parturients. Obstet Gynecol. 1991; 77: 599 – 603.

Livingston, E., Huo, Y., Patel, K., Brogly, S.B., Tuomala, R., Scott, G.B., Bardeguez, A., Stek, A., & Read, J.S. (2010). For the International Maternal Pediatric Adolescent AIDS Clinical Trials Group (IMPAACT) Protocol 1025 Study. Mode of Delivery and Infant Respiratory Morbidity Among Infants Born to HIV-1 infected Women. Obstet Gynecol, 2010; 116(2 Pt 1): 335–343.

Maiques, V., García-Tejedor, A., Perales, A., Córdoba, J., & Esteban, R.J. (2003). HIV detection in amniotic fluid samples. Amniocentesis can be performed in HIV pregnant women? Eur J Obstet Gynecol Reprod Biol, 2003;108(2):137-41.

Maiques-Montesinos, V., Cervera-Sanchez, J., Bellver-Pradas, J., Abad-Carrascosa, A., & Serra, V. (1999). Post-cesarean section morbidity in HIV-positive women. Acta Obstet Gynecol Scand 1999; 78:789-92.

Makoha, F.W., Felimban, H.M., Fathuddien, M.A., Roomi, F., & Ghabra, T. (2004). Multiple cesarean section morbidity. Int J Gynaecol Obstet 2004; 87:227-32.

Mandelbrot, L., Heard, I., Henrion-Geant, E., & Henrion, R. (1997). Natural conception in HIV-negative women with HIV-infected partners. Lancet 1997;349:850–1.

Mandelbrot, L., Le Chenadec, J., Berrebi, A., Bongain, A., Bénifla, J.L., Delfraissy, J.F., & et al. (1998). Perinatal HIV-1 transmission: interaction between zidovudine prophylaxis and mode of delivery in the French Perinatal Cohort. JAMA 1998; 280:55-60.

Mandelbrot, L., Mayaux, M.J., Bongain, A., Berrebi, A., Moudoub-Jeanpetit, Y., Bénifla, J.L., Ciraru Vigneron, N., Le Chenadec, J., Blanche, S., & Delfraissy, J.F. (1996). Obstetric factors and mother-to-child transmission of human immunodeficiency virus type 1: the French perinatal cohorts. SEROGEST French Pediatric HIV Infection Study Group. Am J Obstet Gynecol, 1996;175(3 Pt 1):661-7.

Marcollet, A., Goffinet, F., Firtion, G., Pannier, E., Le Bret, T., Brival, M., & et al. (2002). Differences in postpartum morbidity in women who are infected with the human immunodeficiency virus after elective cesarean delivery, emergency cesarean delivery, or vaginal delivery. Am J Obstet Gynecol 2002; 186:784-9.

Marks, G., Crepaz, N., & Janssen, R.S. (2006). Estimating sexual transmission of HIV from persons aware and unaware that they are infected with the virus in the USA. AIDS 2006;20(10):1447-1450.

Michael, C.W. & Esfahani, F.M. (1997). Pregnancy-related changes: a retrospective review of 278 cervical smears. Diagn Cytopathol 1997; 17: 99-107.

Minkoff, H., Burns, D.N., Landesman, S., Youchah, J., Goedert, J.J., Nugent, R.P., Muenz, L.R., & Willoughby, A.D. (1995). The relationship of the duration of ruptured membranes to vertical transmission of human immunodeficiency virus. American Journal of Obstetrics and Gynecology, 1995;173:585-589.

Minkoff, H., McCalla, S., & Feldman, J. (1990). The relationship of cocaine use to syphilis and HIV infection among inner city parturient women. Am J Obstet Gynecol. 1990;163:521-526.

Mofenson, L.M. (2002). U.S. Public Health Service Task Force Recommendations for use of antiretroviral drugs in pregnant HIV-1 -infected women for maternal health and interventions to reduce perinatal HIV-a transmission in the United States. MMWR Recomm Rep 2002; 51(RR-18):1-58.

Mrus, J.M., Goldi, S.J., Weinstein, M.C., & Tsevat, J. (2000). The cost-effectiveness of elective cesarean delivery for HIV-infected women with detectable HIV RNA during pregnancy. AIDS, 2000;14:2543-52.

Neale, D., Magriples, U., Simpson, J., & Copel, J. (2001). HIV and biochemical screening: Is there a higher false-positive rate in the HIV population? Am J Obstet Gynecol, 2001;185(suppl):S189.

Patterson, K.B., Leone, P.A., Fiscus, S.A., Kurue, J., McCoy, S.I., Wolf, L., Foust, E., Williams, D., Eron, J.J., & Pilcher, C.D. (2007). Frequent detection of acute HIV infection in pregnant women. AIDS, 2007;21(17): 2303-2308.

Public Health Service Task Force. (2010). Recommendations for use of antiretroviral drugs In pregnant HIV-1-infected women for maternal health and interventions to reduce perinatal HIV-1 transmission in the United States. 2010. Available at: http://aidsinfo.nih.gov/contentfiles/PerinatalGL.pdf Retrieved April 13, 2011.

Rasheed, S., Li, Z., Xu, D., & Kovacs, A. (1996). Presence of cell-free human immunodeficiency virus in cervicovaginal secretions is independent of viral load in the blood of human immunodeficiency virus-infected women. Am J Obstet Gynecol, 1996;175:122- 130.

Ratcliffe, J., Ades, A.E., Gibb, D., Sculpher, M.J., & Briggs, A.H. (1998). Prevention of mother-to-child transmission of HIV-1 infection: alternative strategies and their cost-effectiveness. AIDS 1998;12:1381-8.

Read, J.S. & Newell, M.K. (2005). Efficacy and safety of cesarean delivery for prevention of mother-to-child transmission of HIV-1. Cochrane Database Syste Rev 2005;4:CD005479.

Read, J.S., Tuomala, R., Kpamegan, E., & et al. (2001). Mode of Delivery and postpartum morbidity among HIV infected women: The Women and Infants Transmission Study. JAIDS March, 2001 26(3): 236-45.

Rodriguez, E.J., Spann, C., Jamieson, D., & Lindsay, M. (2001). Postoperative morbidity associated with cesarean delivery among human immunodeficiency virus-positive women. Am J Obstet Gynecol 2001; 184:1108-11.

ansom, S., Jamieson, D., Farnham, P.G., Bulterys, M., & Fowler, M.G. (2003). Humman Immunodeficiency Virus Retesting During Pregnancy: Costs and Effectiveness in Preventing Perinatal Transmission. Obstetrics & Gynecology, 2003;102(4): 782-790.

auer, M.V., Wang, J.G., Douglas, N.C., Nakhuda, G.S., Vardhana, P., Jovanovic, V., & Guarnaccia, M.M. (2009). Providing fertility care to men seropositive for human immunodeficiency virus: reviewing 10 years of experience and 420 consecutive cycles of in vitro fertilization and intracytoplasmic sperminjection. Fertil Steril 2009;91:2455–60.

emprini, A.E., Levi-Setti, P., Ravizza, M., & Pardi, G. (1998). Assisted conception to reduce the risk of male-to female sexual transfer of HIV in serodiscordant couples: an update [abstract]. Presented at the 1998 Symposium on AIDS in Women, Sao Paulo, Brazil, September 14–15, 1998.

haheen, F., Sison, A.V., McIntosh, L., Mukhart, M., & Pomerantz, R.J. (1999). Analysis of HIV-1 in the cervicovaginal secretions and blood of pregnant and nonpregnant women. J Hum Virol, 1999;2:154-166.

hapiro, D.E., Sperling, R.S., Mandelbrot, L., Britto, P., & Cunningham, B.E. (1999). Risk factors for perinatal human immunodeficiency virus transmission in patients receiving zidovudine prophylaxis. Pediatric AIDS Clinical Trials Group protocol 076 Study Group. Obstet Gynecol, 1999;94(6):897-908.

perling, R.S., Shapiro, D.E., Cooms, R.W., & et al. (1996). Maternal viral load, zidovuidine treatment, and the risk of transmission of human immunodeficiency virus type 1 from mother to infant. N Engl J Med, 1996;355:1621-1629.

teele, R.W. (2010). Late Pregnancy Screening for Human Immunodeficiency Virus. The Pediatric Infectious Disease Journal, 2010: 72-73. E-pub ahead of print.

tringer, J.S. & Rouse, D.J. (1999). Rapid Testing and Zidovudine Treatment to Prevent Vertical Transmission of Human Immunodeficiency Virus in Unregistered Parturients: A Cost-Effectiveness Analysis. Obstetric & Gynecology. 1999; 94:34-40.

he European Collaborative study. (1999). Maternal viral load and vertical transmission of HIV-1: an important factor but not the only one. AIDS, 1999;13(11): 1377-1385).

he European Mode of Delivery Collaboration. (1999). Elective caesarean-section versus Vaginal delivery in prevention of vertical HIV-1 transmission: A randomized clinical trial. Lancet 1999; 353:1035-9.

he International Perinatal HIV Group. (1999). The mode of delivery and the risk of vertical transmission of human immunodeficiency virus type 1: a meta-analysis of 15 prospective cohort studies. N Engl J Med 1999; 340:977-87.

Tita, A.T., Lai, Y., Landon, M.B., Spong, C.Y., Leveno, K.J., Varner, M.W., Caritis, S.N., Meis, P.J., Wapner, R.J., Sorokin, Y., Peaceman, A.M., O'Sullivan, M.J., Sibai, B.M., Thorp, J.M., Ramin, S.M., & Mercer, B.M. (2011). Eunice Kennedy Shriver National Institute of Child Health and Human Development (NICHD) Maternal-Fetal Medicine Units Network (MFMU). Timing of elective repeat cesarean delivery at term and maternal perioperative outcomes. Obstet Gynecol, 2011;117(2 Pt 1):280-6

Tita, A.T., Landon, M.B., Spong, C.Y., Lai, Y., Leveno, K.J., Varner, M.W., Moawad, A.H., Caritis, S.N., Meis, P.J., Wapner, R.J., Sorokin, Y., Miodovnik, M., Carpenter, M., Peaceman, A.M., O'Sullivan, M.J., Sibai, B.M., Langer, O., Thorp, J.M., Ramin, S.M., Mercer, B.M.; Eunice Kennedy Shriver NICHD Maternal-Fetal Medicine Units

Network. Timing of elective repeat cesarean delivery at term and neonatal outcomes. N Engl J Med, 2009;360(2):111-20.

Turner, B.J., McKee, L.J., Siverman, N.S., &et al. (1996). Prenatal care and birth outcomes of a cohort of HIV-infected women. J Acquir Immune Defic Syndr 1996; 12:259 – 67.

Vimercati, A., Greco, P., Loverro, G., Lopalco, P.L., Pansini, V., & Selvaggi, L. (2000). Maternal complications after caesarean section in HIV infected women. Eur J Obstet Gynecol Reprod Biol, 2000;90:73-76.

Wade, N.A., Birkhead, G.S., Warren, B.L., & et al. (1998). Abbreviated regimens of zidovudine prophylaxis and perinatal transmission of the human immunodeficiency virus. N Engl J Med 1998; 339:1409-14.

Watts, D. (2002). Management of human immunodeficiency virus infection in pregnancy. N Engl J Med, 2002;346:1879-91.

Watts, D.H., Lambert, J.S., Stiehm, R., & et al. (2000). Complications according to mode of delivery among human immunodeficiency virus-infected women with CDS lymphocyte counts of ≤500/µL. Am J Obstet Gynecol July, 2000; 183 (1): 100-7.

Yudin, M.H., Prosen. T.L., & Landers. D.V. (2003). Multiple-marker screening in human Immunodeficiency virus-positive pregnant women: Screen positivity rates with the triple and quad screens. Am J Obstet Gynecol, 2003;189(4):973-6.

3

InforMatrix Nucleoside/Nucleotide Reverse Transcriptase Inhibitors "Backbones"

Gerrit Schreij[1] and Rob Janknegt[2]

[1]*Maastricht University Medical Centre, Maastricht*
[2]*Orbis Medical Centre, Sittard-Geleen*
The Netherlands

1. Introduction

InforMatrix is an interactive matrix model, in which pharmacotherapeutic strategies are supported in a rational manner by means of a transparent selection methodology. This is achieved through the use of an independent reporting made by interactive workshops in the field, in which participants are facilitated in the determination of their own preference.

The treatment of AIDS is directed by guidelines and continually being modified as a result of ongoing research and the arrival of new treatment options. The goal of this InforMatrix program on backbones of nucleoside/nucleotide reverse transcriptase inhibitors is to make a rational selection of a first choice medication possible. It is important in this to describe the selection process and to make this process transparent. The InforMatrix methodology is a tool in this, in which selection criteria are described; tested against the available literature and the various therapeutic alternatives evaluated as to their clinical value.

Below follows a short description of the InforMatrix methodology, of the subject, and a description of the various selection criteria.

1.1 InforMatrix methodology

InforMatrix is a so-called decision matrix technique, with which a group of experts in the subject determine, on the basis of criteria, an order of merit within various treatment options which have similar objectives. In this order of merit, the criteria are weighed against each other. After all, they do not all carry the same weight. Next, the various options per criterion are compared to each other. Data is necessary for this, both from literature as well as from own practice experience. The literature is tested by an independent ethisor for clinical value and evaluated per criterion.

The InforMatrix technique has six set criteria. These criteria are:

- *Effectiveness* (the actualization of positive outcomes and treatment goas)
- *Safety* (the avoidance of negative outcomes, such as hazardous side effects)
- *Tolerance* (the interruption of the care process due to less hazardous, generally transitory, but disturbing side effects)
- *Users' ease* (ease for the patient, for example, dosing frequency)
- *Usability* (what is the scope of the treatment freedom (interactions and such) and the ease for the caregiver)
- *Costs* (price per month)

These criteria are specifically described per selection subject ("operationalized").
The InforMatrix technique takes place in the following steps:
- Operationalization of the six criteria
- Literature synthesis
- Relative weighing of the six criteria
- Evaluation of the various treatment options on the basis of the literature and own knowledge and experience
- Synthesis of the weightings and evaluations in the selection matrix: calculation of order of merit

A group of experts in the field are requested to test the operationalization of the above six selection criteria in the framework of the treatment of HIV/AIDS in the care process for relevance. Following on to these selection aspects, the authors execute a literature synthesis. This results in a report, in which these means are evaluated on the basis of these selection criteria by a group of experts in the field. In this, the report is tested as far as its applicability in making a rational consideration of the treatment options possible.

The choice of nucleoside/nuclotide reverse transcriptase inhibitors and the assessment criteria

After the introduction of nucleoside/nuclotide reverse transcriptase inhibitors (NRTIs), the first antiretroviral drugs approved for the treatment of HIV, patients were initially treated with one drug (monotherapy) and later with two NRTIs (duotherapy). After the introduction of protease inhibitors effective treatment of the HIV infection was possible. This so called HAART (highly active antiretroviral therapy) initially consisted of a combination of 2NRTIs with a proteaseinhibitor (PI).

New classes of antiretrovirals have been developed and nowadays many more combinations of antiretrovirals are possible. A backbone therapy consisting of 2NRTIs in combination with a third drugs like a PI, a non-nucleoside reverse transcriptase inhibitor (NNRTI) or an integrase inhibitor is still chosen as an initial combination antiretroviral therapy (cART).

The treatment goal of cART is to attain an undetectable plasma viral HIV-1 load (VL), after which a recovery of immunity usually follows.

In a meta-analysis covering 64 clinical trials with in total 10,559 naive patients HAART consisting of 2NRTI/PI/ritonavir or 2NRTI/NNRTI both produce significantly higher percentages of patients with undetectable VL and a significantly higher increase of CD4 positive T-lymphocytescount (CD4 cell count) than cART consisting of 2NRTI/PI or 3NRTI **(1)**.

Although stavudine (d4T) is a effective anti-retroviral drug, especially in combination with didanosine, its use is no longer recommended because of the increased change for the development of lipoatrophy during treatment and high rates of mitochondrial toxicity **(2)**.

Combining ddI with tenofovir leads to a specific renal interaction causing high drug levels of didanosine and ddI toxicity resulting in decrease of CD4 cell count **(3)**. Lowering of ddI dosing leads to an increased change of developing virological failure **(4)**.

The following combinations are compared in this InforMatrix because they are recommended in the three major guidelines, the American DHHS Panel (December, 2009) **(5)**, the European AIDS Clinical Society (November, 2009) **(6)** and the International AIDS Society-USA Panel **(7)**

    a. Abacavir/lamivudine (fixed dose combination Kivexa® or Epzicom®) abbreviated as ABC/3TC b.　Didanosine/lamivudine or emtricitabine abbreviated as ddI/3TC or FTC

   c.　Tenofovir/emtricitabine (fixed dose combination Truvada®) abbreviated as TDF/FTC

   d.　Zidovudine/eamivudine (fixed dose combination Combivir®) abbreviated as ZVD/3TC

The following criteria and subcriteria were used:

.　Efficacy of anti-retroviral backbones
   1.1　Parameters of efficacy of anti-retroviral backbones
   1.2　Compliance, quality of life and durability of anti-retroviral backbones
   1.3　Development of resistance during treatment with anti-retroviral backbones

.　Safety of anti-retroviral backbones
   1.4　Grade 3 and 4, serious adverse events
   1.5　Documentation

.　Tolerability of anti-retroviral backbones
   1.6　Grade 1 and 2, mild to moderate adverse events

.　Easy of use
   1.7　Dosage frequency, number of tablets per day

.　Applicability
   1.8　Available strengths
   1.9　Drug interactions
   1.10 Approved indications
   1.11 Contra-indications
   1.12 Use in children and elderly
   1.13 Use in renal and hepatic disease
   1.14 Use in pregancy and lactation
   1.15 Special precautions

.　Cost

2. Efficacy of anti-retroviral backbones

2.1 Parameters of efficacy of anti-retroviral backbones

The efficacy of a cART, usually consisting of 2NRTIs in combination with a PI or NNRTI is judged by the results of its anti-retroviral efficacy, increase of CD4 cell count and change of developing resistance.

The combination of 3 NRTIs as initial therapy is no longer used since the availability of the results of the ACTG 5095 study (8). Limited data are available on combinations of one NRTI + NNRTI+PI the so called NUC-sparing regimen or other combinations. In has been shown in meta-analyses that HAART consisting of 2NRTIs + PI, not combined with ritonavir (as a booster) is virologically and immunologically less effective than 2NRTIs+NNRTI or 2NRTIs + PI combined with ritonavir (1).

The anti-retroviral efficacy of cART must lead to undetectable VL, less than 50 copies/mL (VL<50 c/mL), in older studies a pVL < 400 c/mL is used as measure of undetectability. If the VL does not become undetectable this almost always leads to the development of resistance and to antiviral inefficacy of a certain drug or a whole class of drugs resulting in a decrease of the CD4 cells. This ongoing decrease in the number of CD4 cells leads to HIV related diseases, AIDS and death. The antiviral efficacy is one of the most important parameter for the efficacy of a certain regimen. Te so called "regimen failure" which is a broader measure effectivity of an antiretroviral regimen includes not only virological failure but all other reaons for stopping a regimen such as adverse effects or death and indicates its clinical efficacy.

Studies in patients who are not pretreated (naive patients) and harbouring no significant resistant mutations provide the best indication of the antiviral and clinical efficacy.

The percentage of naive patients in a certain study after 48 weeks, but preferably longer, in the intent to treat analysis (ITT) showing a VL<50 c/mL, is regarded as the best parameter for clinical efficacy. Often missing data on participants (M) are considered as virologic failures (F) (ITT analysis M=F) (5).

Increase of CD4 cell count is of less importance as a parameter of efficacy, because an undetectable VL almost always leads to recovery of CD4 cell count and the mean increase in CD4 cell count is probably similar in the different strata of CD4 cell count when starting cART. For instance in the Athena Dutch cohort study the average increase in CD4 cell count after initiation of therapy was around 70 cells/mm^3 per year during seven years of continuous cART with an undetectable VL. In the first six months after start of cART the increase was on average around 140 cells/mm^3 . Patients starting cART when the CD4 cell count was above 500 cells/mm^3 had on average a lower increase CD4 cell of around 40 cells/mm^3 per year (9).

There are seven major randomized studies (10-17) comparing backbones combined with a similar third drug. The results of these comparative studies are summarised in Table 1.

In the three above mentioned guidelines two (3,5) recommend to start with TDF/FTC and ABC/3TC as an alternative to start with.

-In the HEAT (10) and ACTG 5202 (11,12) these two fixed dose combinations were compared with each other. In the HEAT study the third drug was a PI, lopinavir/ritonavir and in the ACTG 5202 it was a NNRTI, efavirenz or a PI, atazanavir/ritonavir. The HEAT study is an industry sponsored study.

ABC is known for its hypersensitivity reaction usually appearing in the first six week after starting ABC therapy. This hypersensitivity can lead to serious complications and death if not recognized. The presence of HLA-B5701 antigen is highly predictive for the chance of developing this hypersensitivity reaction (18).

In boths studies no determination for the presence of HLA-B5701 antigen was done.

In the HEAT study (10) the effectivity and CD4 cell count increase of both regimens after 48 weeks of treatment and safety after 96 weeks of treatmet was similar. In both treatment arms 2% of the participants had a grade 3-4 (19) decrease in renal function.

Of importance in this study is the fact that there was no difference in anti-vial efficacy between both treatment arms for participants with a high screening VL greater than 100,000 copies/ml (high VL). In the ACTG 5202 the anti-viral efficacy of the regimens were similar for participants with a screening VL less than 100,000 copies/ml (12) but not for those participants with a high screening VL. In the ACTG 5202, 43% of the participants had a high screening VL (11). At a median follow-up of 60 weeks, among the 797 patients with high VL, the time to virologic failure was significantly shorter in the ABC/3TC group than in the TDF/FTC group. There were 57 virologic failures (14%) in the ABC/3TC group versus 26 (7%) in the TDF/FTC group. The time to the first adverse event was also significantly shorter in the ABC/3TC arm. The increase in CD4 cells from baseline at week 48 was similar.

In an analysis of five pharmaceutical company sponsored trials with 872 paticipants with high sreening VL treated with   ABC/3TC and using the same criteria for virological failure as in the ACTG 5202 study there was no inceased chance for virological failure in this group **(20)**.

But in a meta-analysis of 12 trials with 4896 participants and also using the same criteria for virological failure as in the ACTG 5202 study TDF/FTC showed to be virological more effective than ABC/3TC **(21)**.

-In a number of trials **(13-17)** (see table 1) combination regimens with ZVD or combination regimens with d4T are less effective or result in a lower increase of CD4 cell count than in the comparative study arm.

For instance in two trials comparing ABC/3TC with ZVD/3TC **(14)** and TDF/FTC with ZVD/3TC **(13)** a significant lower increase in CD4 count is seen in both ZVD/3TC study arms than in the comparative study arms. In the 934 study **(13)** significant differences were seen in the proportion of patients with VL less than 50 copies/ml (80% versus 70%). Significant more patients in de ZVD/3TC arm had virologic failure, 4% versus <1% in the TDF arm.

More patients in theZVD/3TC group than in the TDF/FTC group had adverse events resulting in discontinuation of the study drugs **(13)**. These adverse events were mainly anemia, nausea, vomiting and fatigue. The authors concluded that through week 48, TDF/FTC proved to be superior in terms of virologic suppression, CD4 response and adverse events resulting in discontinuation of the study drugs.

Also in other studies, serious adverse events like anemia and leukopenia are seen in patients taking ZVD and are often a reason for stopping ZVD **(14, 15)**.

2.2 Compliance, quality of life and durability of anti-retroviral backbones

Good compliance is the cornerstone for succes of anti-retroviral therapy. Stress reduction, a good sociaal network and adequate information play an important role **(22)**. Irregular intake of medication by inadequate compliance leads to suboptimal plasma levels of the medication, thereby increasing development of resistance **(23, 24)** Compliance which leads to actual intake of > 95% of the prescribed medication is a predictor of efficacy of a regimen **(23,24)**.

Adverse events, the number of pills and dosage frequency determine compliance.

In different meta-analyses of 64 **(25)** and 20 **(26)** clinical trials it was shown that the number of tablets per day, dosage fequency and diet restrictions (with food or on an empty stomach) are important determinants of success of antiretroviral therapy. In the meta-analysis of 64 clinical trials **(25)** the number of tablets per day was the most important factor for success of cART.

A meta-analysis of 11 randomized trials revealed that the adherence rate was better with once-daily regimens than twice-daily regimens and this effect was more pronounced at the time of treatment initiation **(27)**.

No studies on quality of life (QoL) and compliance have been done linked to the seven major randomized studies mentioned above.

In a meta analysis, initial ART regimens, regimens containing TDF are equivalent to those containing AZT concerning serious adverse events. However, TDF showed to be superior to AZT in terms of immunologic response and adherence and less frequent emergence of resistance **(28)**.

In a review of twenty-two randomized controlled trials including all above mentioned backbones, including 8,184 HIV-treatment-naïve patients, the combination ddI/3TC was anti-virologic more effective and less toxic for discontinuation due to adverse events and more tolerable than its comparators. The combination TDF/3TC or FTC was more effective and less toxic only in the 144-week follow-up data (two trials, 1,119 patients). ABC/3TC had similar efficacy to its comparators, but more AIDS-defining events (29). In the Swiss cohort study, including 1318 naïve patients, between 2005 and 2008 drug toxicity remained a frequent reason for treatment modification. Initial treatment with ZVD/3TC was associated with a high rate of drug toxicity. (30) In general QoL is beter with a higher CD4 cell count and QoL is decreased in patients with a high VL. The effects of adverse events on QoL are independent of CD4 cell count and VL (31).

Acronime of study	Set up of study	Treatment arms Number of patients in each treatment arm ()	Third drug	ITT analysis: % patients with VL< 50 cop/mL	% patients with screening VL >100.000 copies/mL with VL< 50 copies/mL	CD4 increase cells/mm³	% patients stopping study drugs due to adverse events
HEAT Sudy #(10)	randomised dubble blind placebo controlled	ABC/3TC (343) versus TDF/FTC (345)	lopinavir/r	68% vs 67%	63% vs 65%	214 vs 193	up to week 96: 6% vs 6%
ACTG 5202# (11,12)	randomised blinded for backbone	ABC/3TC (388) versus TDF/FTC (393)	atazanavir/r or efavirenz	similar	75% vs 80%	194 vs 199	up to week 112: 5% vs 4%
Gilead 934 Study (13)	randomised open label	TDF/FTC(258) versus ZVD/3TC (259)	efavirenz	77% vs 68%**	not available	190 vs 158*	up to week 48: 5% vs 19%* up to week 144: 13% vs 34%*
CNA30024# (14)	randomised dubble blind	ABC/3TC (327) versus ZVD/3TC (327)	efavirenz	70% vs 69%	67% vs 67%	209 vs 155**	up to week 48: 14% vs 18%
GESIDA (15)	randomised open label	ddI/3TC (189) versus ZVD/3TC (187)	efavirenz	67% vs 63%	67% vs 63%	158 vs 163	up to week 48: 14% vs 26%
FTC 301 (16)	randomised dubble blind	ddI/FTC (286) versus d4T/ddI (285)	efavirenz	78% vs 59%***	67% vs 50%***	168 vs 134	up to week 60: 7% vs 15%
Gilead 903 Study(17)	randomised dubble blind placebo controlled	TDF/FTC (299) versus d4T/3TC (303)	efavirenz	82% vs 81%	not available	169 vs 167	up to week 48: 9% vs 9% up to week 96: 14% vs 15%

Table 1. Major characteristics and parameters of effectiviness of the seven important clinical trials comparing different backbones of during 48 to 96 weeks of treatment
HLA-B57 screening test not done at inclusion
Degree of significance between treatment arms * p< 0,05 ** p<0,005 ***p<0.001

2.3 Resistance development during treatment with anti-retroviral backbones

Inadequate compliance is the most important cause of virologic failure and resistance development (23,24). Repeated virologic failure with cumulation of resistances will lead to a decrease of the number of CD4 cells (immunologic failure), leading to HIV-related diseases, AIDS and death (clinical failure).

Development of resistance varies per class of anti-retroviral drugs and also within a class of antiretrovirals. For NRTIs, the development of resistance after initiation of cART is stongly associated with adherence. Resistance to antiretrovirals from the start of cART will develop

first and during follow-up in highest frequency to lamivudine, followed by development of resistance to NNRTIs, NRTIs and PIs (32).
A distinction between the different mutations to NRTI's is made between thymidine analoge mutations (TAMs), TAMs-associated mutations, evolving mainly during virologic failure when on therapy with thymidine analogues ZVD and d4T and the discriminatory mutations and the Q151M pathway mutations conferring for multiresistance. Mutations, an acumulation of mutations or the occurrence of multi-resistant mutations limit the number of effective combinations of NRTIs in the backbone for a second or third regimen.
For instance the K65R mutation (discriminatory mutation) can develop during failing therapy with TDF and will make ABC and ddI ineffective.
These drug-resistant viruses can be tranmitted and may limit the treatment options in treatment naïve patients.
The prevalence of transmitted drug resistance viruses since 2004 is similar in different Eropean countries and the Netherlands. In the Netherlands the prevalence of NRTI drug resistance in recent infection (naïve patients) is found to be around 5-6% and for intermediate or high level of resistance is around 2% (33)
Since2003 treatment guidelines recommend onbtaining a genotypic sequence at the start of cART.

3. Safety of anti-retroviral backbones

3.1 Grade 3 and 4, serious adverse events
The prevalence and incidence of grade 3 (severe adverse event) and grade 4 (potentially life threatening adverse event) adverse events (table according to NIAID, Division of AIDS) (19) provide information on the safety of anti-retrovirals. It is not always possible to determine which adverse events are caused by an individual drug or by the combination of drugs in a regimen. Grade 3-4 adverse events have major consequences for the patient and may lead to significant morbidity, hospitalisation and mortality. The medication must almost always be stopped, leading to an increased risk of resistant mutations, decrease in CD4 cell count and resulting impairment of physical condition and a lower quality of life (22,23,24,31).
Adverse events in the studies with mainly naive patients show highly variable incidences of grade 3 and 4 adverse events, ranging from 0-57%. On the basis of these studies, it is not possible to determine a certain pattern of side-effects. It is not clear which side-effects can be linked to the individual NRTI, to the backbone or other drugs. In some studies all grade 2-4 side-effects are summarised without full details (10,14,16). In other studies report only a selection of grade 3 and 4 clinical and or only laboratory adverse events are reported (11,12). The percentage of patients stopping study drugs because of adverse events ranged up to 34% (see table1). Several adverse events with changing severity have been associated with NRTIs (34).
Anemia, neutropenia and thrombocytopenia
Anemia and neutropenia (granulocytopenia) occur are 1.1-9.7% of the patients treated with ZVD. Higher percentages is seen in patients with AIDS, 15-61% (35). Serious grade 3 of 4 anemia and neutropenia are relatively rare with earlier initiation of treatment. Hematologic toxicity is more often seen with ZVD and rarely to never in treatment with other NRTIs. Combinations of NRTIs with other hemato-toxic medication may increase the incidence of serious anemia and neutropenia (35). Serious grade 3 of 4 thrombocytopenia due to cART, necessitating thrombocytes transfusions have been reported (35).

Pancreatitis:

In the older studies pancreatitis was seen in 4-7% of patients treated with ddI and d4T. In 6% of these patients pancreatis was fatal (35). Combinations of ddI/d4T double the risk and ddI/TDF also increase the risk of development of pancreatitis (36).

In the ACTG studies from October 1989 through July 1999 the overall pancreatitis rates were 0.61 per 100 person-years clinical and 2.23 per 100 person-years clinical/laboratory (36). The incidence of pancreatitis in the EuroSida cohort decreased over the years with earlier start of therapy and with higher CD4 cell counts. The incidence was 0.127 per 100 person-years over the years 2001-2006 (38).

Lactate acidosis (mitochondrial toxicity):

Lactate acidosis is a serious complication of the treatment with NRTIs, which occurs in around 0.9 times per 1000 years of treatment and often leads to serious morbidity and mortality (35).

In vitro studies have shown that inhibition of DNA polymerase gamma and other mitochondrial enzymes by NRTIs may lead to mitochondrial disfunction and cellular toxicity.

The clinical symptomatology of NRTI-induced mitochondrial toxicity consists of steatosis, hepatitis, lactate acidosis, myopathy, nephrotoxicity, peripheral neuropathy and pancreatitis. Studies with NRTIs in enzym assays and in cell cultures have shown that the following NRTIs are responsible for this mitochondrial toxicity, to a decreasing extent: ddI > d4T > ZVD (39). DNA polymerase gamma inhibition is not found in normal concentrations of ABC, 3TC and TDF (39).

Lipodystrophy:

Three forms of lipodystrophy are distinguished: lipoatrophy caused by loss of subcutaneous fat, fat accumulation or lipohypertrophy and mixed forms. It was described with cART in 1997 and may occur in all combinations of cART medication with a prevalence between 2-84%. Lipo-accumumulation like buffelo-hump and "crix belli" may be caused by PIs, lipoatrophy by NRTIs. Lipoatrophy may occur shortly after initiation of cART. In a large observational cohort, 62% of the patients who developed lipoatrophy has symptoms within one year. In this cohort a highly significant correlation was found between lipoatrophy and the use of d4T (40). It has been shown in observational cohort studies, clinical trials and in pathologic studies that lipoatrophy is specifically related to the use of NRTI especially d4T and in to a lesser extent to ZVD. Host factors have a modulating effect on the risk and the severity of lipoatrophy (2).

The development of lipoatrophy is a serious complication which often leads to a marked decrease of the quality of life. In clinical studies is was shown that lipoatrophy improved by the replacement of ZVD or d4T by ABC (41) or TDF (42).

Peripheral neuropathy

The occurrence of peripheral neuropathy is a well known complication of HIV-infection itself or due to a toxic effect on mitochondria induced by some NRTIs. Its incidence increases with the extent of immunodeficiency and older age. Patients who develop peripheral neuropathy tend to do so shortly after exposure to antiretroviral therapy and certain subgroup of patients are found to be more susceptible than others (43).

With ddI use the incidence of medication related sensoric neuropathy was 6.8 cases per 100 person years. In one study the relatieve risk is 1.4 fold higher in d4T use and 3.5 times higher in the combination of ddI/d4T compared to other NRTIs (44). In an other study peripheral neuropathy was reported in 3.0 cases per 100 person-years for ZVD monotherapy and in 2.2 cases per 100 person-years for ZVD/ddl **(43)**. Sensoric neuropathy has not been associated with the use of ABC,3TC, FTC and TDF.

Rash (hypersensitivity reaction) and muscle disorders

Drug hypersensitivity reactions are an important cause of morbidity in HIV-infected patients. The hypersensitivity reactions can be caused by each of the antiretroviral drugs in the cART regimen or by other concomitend prescribed drugs.

ABC is known for its hypersensitivity reaction usually appearing in the first six week after starting ABC therapy. Symptoms of this ABC related hypersensitivity reaction are nonspecific and can be difficult to distinguish from reactions to other drugs or conditions and can lead to serious complications and death if not recognized. The presence of HLA-B5701 antigen is highly predictive for the chance of developing this hypersensitivity reaction. ABC hypersensitivity reaction affects 5-8% of patients during the first six weeks of treatment **(18)**.

Hypersensitivity reactions to 3TC, FTC, ddI, TDF have been reported but occur very rarely **(45)**. Other forms of hypersensitivity reactions and rashes are related to the use of NNRTIs and PIs and are usually mild and self-limiting **(46)**.

Other serious adverse events like rhabdomyolysis, myopathy and cardiomyopathy are very rare complications, which are not clearly related to NRTIs. **(46)**.

Renal failure

Chronic kidney disease in HIV-positive persons can be caused by both HIV and traditional or non-HIV-related factors and antiretroviral drugs. Tenofovir has been associated with decline in renal funtion **(47,48,49)**.

Tenofovir is mainly cleared by glomerular filtration and active tubular secretion through tubular transport proteins. Interactions and competition of different anti-retrovirals with these transport proteins can lead to renal toxicity and increased blood levels. The combination of TDF/ddI leads to ~ 30% increased ddI levels and ddI related toxicity.

Up to February 2006, 27 individual cases of renal failure with or without proteinuria or Fanconi syndrome (renal tubular acidosis) have been described with the use of TDF **(47)**.

During a follow-up of 144 weeks of 600 patients in the 903 Study **(17,50)** comparing d4T/3TC/EFV with TDF/3TC/EFV no significant increases in mean creatinine level were seen in the 299 patients treated with tenofovir. In the Heat study **(10)** comparing ABC/3TC and TDF/FTC and in Study 934 **(13)** comparing ZVD/3TC and TDF/FTC during an obserervation period of respectively 96 weeks and 48 weeks no significant difference in renal function could be shown.

In the Swiss HIV Cohort Study **(48)** 363 treatment-naive patients or patients with treatment interruptions of more than 12 months starting either a TDF-based cART and 715 patients on a TDF-sparing regime were compared for the time to reach a 10 ml/min reduction in calculated GFR (cGFR). Apart from diabetes mellitus, higher baseline cGFR (by 10 ml/min), TDF use and boosted PI use were significantly associated with an increased risk for reaching a 10 ml/min reduction in cGFR during an observation time of two years.

During a median follow-up of 3.7 years in the EuroSida Study Group **(49)** 225 (3.3%) persons progressed to chronic kidney disease during 21.482 person-years follow-up, an incidence of 1.05 per 100 person-years follow-up. After adjustment for traditional factors associated with chronic kidney disease, increasing cumulative exposure to TDF and the PIs, indinavir, atazanavir and lopinavir/ritonavir were associated with a significantly increased rate of decline in renal function. No other antiretroviral drugs were associated with increased incidence of chronic kidney disease.

In a prospective observational cohort study at Johns Hopkins **(51)** patients taking both TDF and NRTIs experienced an initial decline in cGFR during the first 180 days of therapy, but cGFR stabilized between 180 and 720 days. In this study there was no difference between TDF and NRTI use in more than 25% or 50% decline in cGFR at 1 or 2 years or in change in cGFR at 6, 12, or 24 months. Those taking TDF and a PI/ritonavir had a greater median decline in cGFR than those taking TDF and a NNRTI at 6 months. There was no difference in median cGFR decline between those on an NRTI/PI/ritonavir versus those on an NRTI/NNRTI regimen.

The reversibility of TDF-related nephrotoxicity in 24 male patients who ceased TDF for renal impairment by retrospective assessment were determined **(52)**. Median eGFR pre-TDF was 74 mL/min/1.73 m^2 (using the Modified Diet in Renal Disease equation) and fell to 51 mL/min/1.73 m^2 at TDF cessation and increased to 58 mL/min/1.73 m^2 in a median of 13 months after TDF cessation. This decline in cGFR, most recent versus pre-TDF is significant. Results were similar using the Cockcroft-Gault equation for cGFR. Only 10 patients reached their pre-TDF cGFR.

Many patients on antiretroviral therapy have multiple medical problems and may take other potentially nephrotoxic drugs. It has been clearly shown that taking TDF in combination with PI may increase a decline in renal function.

In a systematic review **(53)** of a total of 17 studies (including 9 randomized, controlled trials) a significantly greater loss of kidney function was seen among patients using TDF, compared with control subjects (mean difference in eGFR was 3.92 mL/min, as well as a greater risk of acute renal failure. There was no evidence that TDF use led to increased risk of severe proteinuria, hypophosphatemia, or fractures.

Thus in some well designed randomized prospective trials **(10,17,50)** no decline in renal function during treatment with TDF has been noted. Some observational stusies have found evidence of mild decrease in kidney function in TDF treated patients and when TDF related renal toxicity was present it was not always fully reversible.

Cardiovascular risk and lipids

The risk of cardio vascular disease (CVD) and other non-AIDS conditions increases with age, but prevalence of these diseases by age is greater in HIV-positive populations. In a case-control study of HIV-infected patients and healthy HIV-negative individuals from an observational database comparing rates of 6 comorbidities,CVD, hypertension, renal failure, osteoporosis, diabetes, and hypothyroidism to be higher in HIV-infected patients **(54)**.

Numerous large observational cohort studies in Europe and the USA have found higher rates of acute myocardial infarction (MI) or coronary heart disease (CHD) in patients with HIV. (5-10) In a cross-sectional study of HIV-infected participants and controls without pre-existing CVD preclinical atherosclerosis assessed by carotid intima-medial thickness measurements in the internal/bulb and common carotid regions in HIV-infected participants and controls after adjusting for traditional CVD risk factors showed that HIV infection was accompanied by more extensive atherosclerosis **(61)**.

The higher risk among patients with HIV-infected patients held true for every age group analyzed and in multivariate analysis adjusting for demographics and common cardiovascular risk factors confirm that HIV infection is an independent predictor of acute MI, conferring nearly a two-fold risk. The risk of myocardial infarcion is found to be associated with the cumulative use of PIs in these studies **(55,56,59,60)**.

In the D.A.D cohort, a lage observational prospective cohort study with more than 30,000 HIV-infected patients in 212 clinics since 1999, it was found that ABC and ddI were associated with a higher risk of acute MI within each CVD risk category defined by the Framingham Risk Score **(62)**. Exposure to ABC within the most recent 6 months was associated with a 1.90 relative risk of acute MI. Subsequent analysis suggested cumulative use of ABC may also been associated with increased MI risk, although to a lesser extent than recent use **(63)**. Since that first publication, several reports on MI risk associated with ABC have appeared, and some of these analyses have not implicated ABC as an MI risk factor. Several studies have focused on possible mechanisms that may explain the increased risk on MI in patients taking ABC. In the largest analysis, SMART study investigators found higher levels of hsCRP and IL-6 in patients taking ABC than in patients not taking ABC **(64)** However, a study of 13 biomarkers in virologically suppressed patients taking ABC/3TC vs TDF/FTC found no significant change in either group after 48 weeks **(65)**. The results of the DAD study **(62)** could have been confounded by te so-called allocation biases such as high cardiovascular risk and renal function. In the Veterans Affairs Study a weak correlation between ABC use and MI was found, disappearing entirely after statistical adjustment for renal disease **(66)**.

In November 2008, DHHS guidelines reclassified abacavir from a preferred first-line agent to an alternate agent, partly because of these data on cardiovascular risk.

In the DAD study correcting the increased relative risk for antiretroviral-associated CVD for lipds attenuated this CVD risk by around 10% **(55)**. In the ACTG 5202 study **(11,12)** fasting lipids at week 48 had increased more in the ABC/3TC arm than in the TDF/FTC arm (respectively; total cholesterol 0,87 mmol/L versus 0,67 mmol/L and triglycerides 0.28 mmol/L versus 0.03 mmol/L) with no significant difference between groups in the change in the ratio of total cholesterol to HDL cholesterol. In a systemic review of 7 clinical trials with a total of 3,807 paticipants, studying initial treatment in naïve subjects receiving 2NRTIs/efavirenz regimens the mean change in total cholesterol from baseline to 48 weeks was significantly greater in patients taking a non-TDF containing regimen **(67)**.

Bone mineral density loss associated with HIV infection and cART

Many studies have documented an increased prevalence of osteopenia in HIV-infected individuals with dual x-ray absorptiometry bone densitometry (DEXA) scans. This finding is important since bone mineral density (BMD) predicts fracture risk **(68)**. A higher fracture rate has been demonstrated among HIV-infected subjects compared with controls in a large healthcare system.**(69)**. Many factors may play a role in the increased prevalence of osteopenia like vitamine D deficiency, low body mass, aging, corticosteroid use, alcoholism and HIV-infection.

Decreased BMD has been found in both treatment-naive and treated HIV-infected patients. Ongoing BMD loss over time has been observed in some treatment studies, although it is uncertain whether it is due to drug toxicity since it is difficult to differentiate between effects associated with antiretrovirals and other factors. In addition the presence and strength of antiviral-related factors is difficult to ascertain as combinations of classes of antiretroviral drugs are used.

In the GS 903 study comparing d4T/3TC and TDF/3TC, each combined with efavirenz in treatment-naive patients, after an an initial decrease in BMD was found in both study arms but stabilized after 24 weeks. By week 144, the mean decrease in BMD of the spine was significantly different 0.9% in the d4T/3TC arm and 2.2% in the TDF/3TC arm. At baseline there was a relatively high incidence of both osteopenia and osteoporosis in both study arms, but there was no significant difference in rates of new-onset osteopenia or progression to osteoporosis through week 144 **(70)**.

In the STEAL study, 360 virologically suppressed patients were randomized to switch their current NRTIs to either ABC/3TC or TDF/FTC. No significant change in spine or hip T scores were observed in the ABC/3TC arm, but BMD at spine and hip decreased in the TDF/FTC arm, and the difference between the regimens was statistically significant at weeks 48 and 96 (71).

In a study comparing the effect of TDF versus ABC based regimens on BMD, BMD decreased early during therapy in both arms before stabilizing. The mean loss of BMD was statistically greater with TDF and the loss correlated with biomarkers of bone turnover (72). Similar results were obtained in an other study comparing the safety aspects of ABC/3TC and TDF/FTC in 385 treatment-naive patients (73).

In the ACTG 5202 metabolic substudy, there was an initial reduction in BMD in all stady arms, which stabilized after 48 weeks. A significantly greater loss of BMD was seen at week 96 with TDF/FTC versus ABC/3TC. This included a significant 2% greater reduction in lumbar spine BMD and a significant 1.5% greater reduction in hip BMD. No difference was found in fracture rates between study arms at week 48 (74).

In the bone substudy of this trial, the initiation of antiretroviral therapy was associated with a decrease in bone mass of 2% to 4% that was independent of the regimen selected and stabilized by week 48; this decrease was greatest in patients who started a regimen that contained TDF (75).

Thus overall, BMD appears to decline to some degree during the first several months after initiation of cART, regardless of regimen, but the decline may be slightly greater with TDF containing regimens. However, there are no conclusive data showing that therapy-associated reductions in bone mineral density are also associated with an increased rate of fractures.

3.2 Documentation

The clinical documentation of the combinations is summarised in Table 2

	Number of clinical trials*	Years since registration
Zidovudine/Lamivudine or emtricitabine	532/23	>10 Emt: 8
Didanosine/Lamivudine or emtricitabine	165/10	>10 Emt: 8
Abacavir/Lamivudine or emtricitabine	160/15	> 10 Emt: 8
Tenofovir/emtricitabine or Lamivudine	78/115	>10 >10

Table 2. Documentation
* according to the definition of National Institute of Health/PubMed (www.ncbi.nih.gov)

4. Tolerability of anti-retroviral backbones

4.1 Grade 1 and 2, mild to moderate side-effects

The tolerability of a cART regimens is an important predictor of durability and long-term succes. Grade 1(mild adverse event) and grade 2 (moderate adverse event) (19) may have a

significant influence on compliance and quality of life (22,26) and on the durability of a certain combination. It is not always evident which drug in a cART regimen is responsible for which side-effect. The HIV-infection as such or complications of opportunistic infections may lead to symptoms marked as adverse events of anti-retroviral medication. General symptoms as fatigue, pain, anorexia, sleep and concentration disturbances occur frequently (46).
It is difficult to give a reliable estimation of the relative incidence of different grade of adverse events, based on the EMEA and FDA data (76), because of the relative lack of randomised comparative studies with extended follow-up and asufficient number of participants. Cohort studies yield better insight as to why patients switch or stop certain antiretroviral drugs and how long they keep using the same regimen, in comparison with randomised studies which usually have a limited follow-up time.
In the older cohort studies high rates of toxicity driven changes in antiretroviral drugs were common. For instance in the Swiss HIV Cohort Study, with 2,674 patients, 35% stopped treatment with at least one drug during the observation period of 3.2 years because of adverse events and/or intolerability and 41% stopped the combination of anti-retroviral drugs at least once or completely changed to another combination (77).
In the Italian ICONA-cohort (78), 36% of the 862 patients stopped because of side-effects during study period of 45 weeks and only 5% because of virologic failure.
Earlier initiation of cART, lower pill burden and dosing schemes of once or twice daily, together with declining toxicity, have improved tolerability.
In the Athena-cohort the incidence per 100 patient years of toxicity driven changes of cART during the first 3 years after the start of therapy decreased from 29% in 1996 to 15% in 2008. Significant decline in toxicity driven changes of cART started to be apparent after calendar year 2000. The incidence of toxicity driven changes of cART is highest in the first 3 month after initiation.

5. Easy of use

5.1 Ease of use (dosage frequency, number of tablets per day)
The combinations of ABC/3TC, TDF/FTC and ddI/FTC or 3TC can be given once daily. ZVD/3TC (Combivir®)has to be given twice daily. The other combinations are given once or twice daily. The combinations of ABCbacavir/Lamivudine (Kivexa®, Epzicom®) and TDT/FTC (Truvada ®) can be given as one tablet per day. TDT/FTC in combination with efavirenz can be given in one tablet (Atripla ®)
DdI is given 2 hours before or after food. The rest of the drugs can be taken irrespective of food.

6. Applicability

6.1 Availability of different formulations
Liquid or dispersible formulations are available for ddI.

6.2 Drug interactions
Abacavir
Abacavir is not significantly metabolised by CYP450, which makes serious reactions regarding inhibition or induction of CYP450 enzymes unlikely (80). No interactions were seen with adefovir, amprenavir, indinavir, ZVD and 3TC (50).

Enzymeinducers like rifampicin, phenobarbital and phenytoin may decrease the plasma concentrations of abacavir to a minor extent through an effect on UDP-glucuronyltransferases [72].
Alcohol may decrease the AUC of abacavir by 40% (81,82).
Didanosine
The AUC of ddI doubles during simultaneous use of ganciclovir. Didanosine has no significant effect on the pharmacokinetics of zidovudine (83).
No clinically relevant interaction occurs between ddI with ritonavir, nevirapine, emtricitabine and nelfinavir (84).
Ribavirine may increase intracellular levels of ddI. The relevance of this is unknown.
Didanosine decreases the bioavailability of ciprofloxacin during simultaneous intake. It is recommended to take ciprofloxacin an hour before or at least 4 hours after ddI (84). Didanosine showed no interaction with indinavir and fluconazole. Ketoconazole and itraconazole increase the AUC of ddI, maar these interactions do not appear te be very relevant.
The AUC of ddI increases by 50% in combination with tenofovir often leading to ddI toxicity (3).
Xanthine oxidase plays a role in the metabolism of didanosine, interactions with inhibitors of xanthine oxidase, like allopurinol, may theoretically decrease the clearance of didanosine.
Emtricitabine
Tenofovir and FTC do not affect each other's pharmacokinetics (85, 86). Emtricitabine is metabolised to a limited extent and is excreted unchanged in the urine through glomerular filtration and active tubular secretion(85). Interactions regarding to inhibition of active tubular secretion cannot be excluded, maar have not been studied (85).
Emcitabrine shows no pharmacokinetic interactions with protease inhibitors or with ddI (85).
Lamivudine
Lamivudine shows few metabolic interactions. The drug is excreted in an unchanged form through glomerular filtration and active tubular secretion (87, 88).
No interaction is seen with ZVD and ddI (87, 88).
Trimethoprim may decrease active tubular secretion, increasing the AUC of lamivudine by 40% (87, 88). Applications of high dose co-trimoxazole in pneumocystis carinii infections should not be combined with lamivudine (87). There is inadequate documentation on a possible interaction with intravenous ganciclovir or foscarnet. This combination should be avoided.
Tenofovir
Tenofovir is mainly excreted uchanged in the urine through glomerular filtration and active tubular secretion (90,91). Interactions regarding to inhibition of active tubular secretion cannot be excluded, but have not been studied (90).
Tenofovir and FTC have no effect on each other's pharmacokinetics (85, 86,91).
The AUC of TDF increases by 30% in combination with lopinavir and ritonavir or atazanavir (92,93). Tenofovir may decrease the AUC of atazanavir by 25%. The AUC of lopinavir increases by 15% by tenofovir. Tenofovir shows no interaction with saquinavir (91).
The AUC of ddI increases by 50% in combination with tenofovir (91). This may increase the risk of pancreatitis and other ddI related toxicity. The AUC of atazanavir decreases by 25% in combination with TDF (86).
Tenofovir showed no interactions with indinavir, methadon, ribavirine or rifampicin (91,93, 94).

Zidovudine

Zidovudine is mainly glucuronidated. The drug may theoretically show interactions with a large number of drugs which are also excreted through glucuronidation, like aspirin, NSAIDs, penicillins and oxazepam. Very limited data on the relevance of these possible interactions is available (95).

The bioavailability of zidovudine may be decreased to a limited extent (22%) by simultaneouse intake with food (96).

The renal clearance of zidovudine decreases by 50% during simultaneous use of co-trimoxazole (96). This interaction is only relevant in disturbed glucuronidation of zidovudine.

Rifampicin lowers the AUC of zidovudine by 50%, an interaction with rifabutin is not very relevant, a 14% decrease of the AUC of zidovudine was seen (96).

The AUC of ZVD increases by 75% in combination with fluconazole (96).

Zidovudine may cause an unpredictable interaction with phenytoin (increase of decrease of the phenytoin levels). Phenytoin levels have to be checked on a regular basis.

Atovaquone increases the AUC of zidovudine by 35%. Valproic acid and methadone may also lead to an increase in the AUC of zidovudine, but little data are available.

Zidovudine is antagonistic in combination with ribavirine or stavudine.

Nephrotoxic or myelosuppressive drugs may increase potential side-effects of ZVD (SPC on zidovudine).

6.3 Approved indications

There are no major differences in the approved indications. The applicability in children is described in 5.5.

Treatment co-infections

Lamivudine, emtricitabine and tenofovir also have anti hepatitis B virus activity. An advantage of these drugs is that "two in one" treatment is possible It is recommended that lamivudine or emtricitabine should be combined with tenofovir (97) in case of hepatitis B co-infection. Only lamivudine is approved for this indication.

6.4 Contra-indications

All drugs are contra-indicated in case of hypersensitivity.

Hypersensitivity to abacavir may be very serious.

6.5 Use in children and elderly

No dose adjustments are necessary in the elderly.

Zidovudine/lamivudine (Combivir) and abacavir/lamivudine (Kivexa) can be used in children from 12 years. The individual components can be used from 3 months.

Lamivudine can be used from 3 months

Didanosine tablets can be used from 6 years.

Tenofovir and emcitabine are only applicable in adults.

6.6 Use in renal and hepatic disease

A dose reduction is necessary in case of renal function impaiment. Abacavir/Lamivudine should not be used when the creatinine clearance is lower than 50 ml/min. Tenofovir/Emtricitabine should bot be used when the creatinine clearance is lower than 30 ml/min.

No dose adjustments are usually necessary in patients with liver disease.

6.7 Use in pregancy and lactation
A variable extent of mitochondrial damage may occur during in utero exposition to nucleoside-analogues. This may lead to hematologic toxicity or metabolic disturbances.
All drugs should be avoided during lactation. None of the combinations is recommended in case of pregnancy, but they are usually not absolutely contra-indicated.

6.8 Special precautions

Zidovudine/Lamivudine (Combivir)	Monitoring of hematologic parameters (ZVD) Lowering of the dosage of ZVD in abnormal hematologic parameters Therapy cessation during signs of pancreatitis (ZVD and 3TC) Lactic acidosis has been described. Therapy should be stopped in case of hyperlactatemia or metabolic acidosis Use with great caution in case of hepatomegaly, hepatitis or risk factors for liverdiseases (3TC) Cessation of L may lead to increased symptoms in patients who also have hepatitis B.
Didanosine/Lamivudine	Great caution with pancreatitis in the anamnesis (ddI and 3TC) Peripheral neuropathy may occur (ddI) Changes in the retina and N.opticus are to be checked in children (ddI) Use with great caution in case of hepatomegaly, hepatitis or riskfactors for liverdiseases (3TC) Lactic acidosis has been described. Therapy should be stopped in case of hyperlactatemia or metabolic acidosis (ddI and 3TC) Patients with hepatitis B or C have an increased risk on serious hepatic side-effects (ddI) Lipodystrophy may occur (ddI) Cessation of L may lead to increased symptoms in patients who also have hepatitis B.
Abacavir/Lamivudine (Kivexa)	Cessation of therapy during signs of pancreatitis (ABC and 3TC) Lactic acidosis has been described. Therapy should be stopped in case of hyperlactatemia or metabolic acidosis Use with great caution in case of hepatomegaly, hepatitis or risk factors for liverdiseases (3TC) Lipodystrophy may occur (3TC) Patients with hepatitis B or C have an increased risk on serious hepatic side-effects Cessation of 3TC may lead to increased symptoms in patients who also have hepatitis B.
Tenofovir/Lamivudine	Tenofovir may lower the BMD (TDF) No not use in case of the HIV-1 K65R mutation (TDF) Lactic acidosis has been described. Therapy should be stopped in case of hyperlactatemia or metabolic acidosis (TDF) Cessation of L may lead to increased symptoms in patients who

	also have hepatitis B. Use with great caution in case of hepatomegaly, hepatitis or risk factors for liverdiseases (3TC) Renal function should be checked. Combination with nephrotoxic drugs is not recommended (3TC)
Tenofovir/Emtricitabine (Truvada)	Do not combine with lamivudine Combination with a third nucleoside analogue is not recommended beause of possible virologic failure. The tablet contains lactose. Renal function should be checked. Combination with nephrotoxisc drugs is not recommended (TDF) No not use in case of the HIV-1 K65R mutation (TDF) Tenofovir may lower the bone mineral density (TDF) Patients with hepatitis B or C have an increased risk on serious hepatic side-effects (TDF) Cessation of TDF/FTC may lead to increased symptoms in patients who also have hepatitis B.
Didanosine/Emtricitabine	Great caution with pancreatitis in the anamnesis (ddI) Peripheral neuropathy may occur (ddI) Changes in the retina and N.opticus are to be checked in children (ddI) Lactic acidosis has been described. Therapy should be stopped in case of hyperlactatemia or metabolic acidosis (ddI) Lipodystrophy may occur (ddI) Patients with hepatitis B of C have an increased risk on serious hepatic side-effects (ddI) Lipodystrophy may occur (ddI)

7. Acquisition cost

Acquisition cost excluded for VAT in Euro ("vergoedingsprijs", Z-Index July 2011)

		Cost per month in Euro
Zidovudine/Lamivudine (Combivir)	2 dd 300/150 mg	379
Didanosine ER (Videx) Lamivudine (Epivir)	1 dd 400 or 250 mg (weight based) 300 mg in 1-2 doses	306/336
Abacavir/Lamivudine (Kivexa, Epzicom)	1 dd 600/300 mg	422
Tenofovir (Viread) Lamivudine (Epivir)	1 dd 245 mg 300 mg in 1-2 doses	510
Tenofovir/Emtricitabine (Truvada)	1 dd 200/245 mg	510
Didanosine ER (Videx) Emtricitabine (Emtriva)	1 dd 400 or 250 mg (weight based) 200 mg 1 dose	313/343

8. Conclusion

Optimal care requires individualized management and ongoing attention to relevant scientific and clinical information. The availability of new antiretroviral drugs since the introduction of the fist cART has expanded treatment choices. Guidelines are presented as recommendations if the supporting evidence warrants routine use in a particular situation and as considerations if data are preliminary or incomplete but suggestive. But the importance of adherence, emerging long-term complications of therapy, recognition and management of antiretroviral failure is often underestimated and there is but to often little data to guide our choices.

The judgement of the relative efficacy and safety of the various NRTI backbones in the treament of HIV infection is hindered by the fact that there are only few direct comparative studies. This makes it difficult to make firm statements concerning the pros and cons of the individual drugs concerning efficacy and safety.

In this InforMatrix manuscript, no firm conclusions are drawn by the authors. The purpose of this manuscript is to facilitate discussion on the properties of each treatment option for HIV by using only clinically relevant selection criteria by providing an up-to-date overview. The InforMatrix program will be made available in an interactive format on www.informatrix.nl. By means of the program, the user can assign a relative weight to each main selection criterion (with a total of 30 points to be distributed) and can judge the properties of each therapeutic option per criterion on the basis of his own personal expertise and/or the present document. Zero to ten points can be assigned to each treatment option on each criterion. The program is freely accessible.

The present InforMatrix manuscript is specific for the Netherlands, because the Dutch available formulations and Dutch prices were used. The most important part of the paper (efficacy, safety and tolerability) is internationally valid. Local adjustments are necessary for an optimal use of the method in other countries. This could also include price-adjustments for the individual hospitals in other countries.

9. References

[1] Bartlett J FM, DeMasi R, Quinn J, et al. An Updated Meta-analysis of Triple Combination Therapy in Antiretroviral-naive HIV-infected Adults. Abstract 586 12th Conference on Retrovirusses and Oportunistic Infections 2006.
[2] Hammond E, McKinnon E, Nolan D. Human immunodeficiency virus treatment-induced adipose tissue pathology and lipoatrophy: prevalence and metabolic consequences. Clin Infect Dis. 2010;51:591-9.
[3] Torti C, Quiros-Roldan E, Regazzi M, et al. Early virological failure after tenofovir + didanosine + efavirenz combination in HIV-positive patients upon starting antiretroviral therapy. Antivir Ther 2005;10:505-13
[4] Mallewa JE, Wilkins E, Vilar J, et al HIV-associated lipodystrophy: a review of underlying mechanisms and therapeutic options. J Antimicrob Chemother. 2008;62:648-60.
[5] Guidelines for the Use of Antiretroviral agents in HIV-1 infected Adults and Adolescents. DHHS Panel December 1, 2009. wwwaidsinfonihgov.
[6] Guidelines of the European AIDS Clinical Society version 5 November 2009, www.europeanaidsclinicalsociety.org

[7] Thompson MA, Aberg JA, Cahn P, et al. Antiretroviral treatment of adult HIV infection: 2010 recommendations of the International AIDS Society-USA panel. JAMA. 2010;304:321-33.

[8] Gulick RM, Ribaudo HJ, Shikuma CM, et al. Triple-nucleoside regimens versus efavirenz-containing regimens for the initial treatment of HIV-1 infection. N Engl J Med. 2004;350:1850-61.

[9] Gras L, Kesselring AM, Griffin JT, et al. CD4 cell counts of 800 cells/mm3 or greater after 7 years of highly active antiretroviral therapy are feasible in most patients starting with 350 cells/mm3 or greater. J Acquir Immune Defic Syndr. 2007;45:183-92.

[10] Smith K, Patel P, Fine DM, et al Randomized, double-blind, placebo-matched, multicenter trial of abacavir/lamivudine or tenofovir/emtricitabine with lopinavir/ritonavir for initial HIV treatment. AIDS 2009;23:1547-56

[11] Sax P, Tierney C, Collier A, and ACTG A5202 Study Team Abacavir-lamivudine versus tenofovir-emtricitabine for initial HIV-1 therapy New Engl J Med 2009;361:2230-40

[12] Daar E, Tierney C, Fischl M, and ACTG A5202 Study Team, ACTG 5202: Final Results of ABC/3TC or TDF/FTC with either EFV or ATV/r in Treatment-naive HIV-infected Patients, Abstract 59LB 17th Conference on Retroviruses and Opportunistic Infections San Francisco, CA, USA, 2010

[13] Gallant J, DeJesus E, Arribas JR, et al. Tenofovir DF, emtricitabine and efavirenz vs zidovudine, lamivudine and EFV for HIV. N Engl J Med 2006;354:251-60

[14] DeJesus E, Herrera G, Teofilo E, et al Abacavir versus Zidovudine combined with lamivudine and efavirenz, for the treatment of antiretroviral-naive HIV-infected adults Clin Infect Dis 2004;48:1038-46

[15] Berenguer J, Gonzales J, Ribera E, et al. Didanosine, lamivudine, and efavirenz vs zidovudine, lamivudine, and efavirenz, for initial treatment of HIV infection: Final analysis of a prospective randomized noninferiority clinical trial, GESIDA 3903 Clin Infect Dis 2008;47:1083-32

[16] Saag M, Cahn P, Raffi F, et al. Efficacy and safety of emtricitabine vs stavudine in combination therapy in antiretroviral-naive patients: a randomized trial JAMA 2004;292:180-90

[17] Cassetti I, Madruga JV, Suleiman JM, et al The safety and efficacy of tenofovir DF in combination with lamivudine and efavirenz through 6 years in antiretroviral-naïve HIV-1-infected patients. HIV Clin Trials 2007;8:164-72

[18] Mallal S, Phillips E, Caras G, et al HLA-B5701 screening for hypersensitivity to abacavir. New Engl J Med 2008;358:568-79

[19] National Institute of Allrgy and Infectious Diseases, Division of AIDS (DAIDS) table for grading severity of adult adverse experiences http://www.niaid.nih.gov

[20] Pappa K, Hernandez J, Ha1 B, et al Abacavir/lamivudine shows robust virologic responses in ART-naïve patients for baseline viral loads (VL) of >100,000c/mL and <100,000c/mL by endpoint used in ACTG5202, Abstract THABO304, XVII International AIDS Conference 2008

[21] Hill AM, Sawyer WS. Effects of NRTI backbone on efficacy of first-line boosted PI-based HAART--meta-analysis of 12 clinical trials in 4896 patients. Abstract H-1254. 48th Annual International Conference on Antimicrobial Agents and Chemotherapy 2008. Washington DC, USA.

[22] Vervoort SC, Borleffs JC, Hoepelman AI, et al Adherence in antiretroviral therapy: a review of qualitative studies. AIDS 2007;21:271-81

[23] Kantor R, Shafer RW, Follansbee S, et al Evolution of resistance to drugs in HIV-1 infected patients failing antiretroviral therapy. AIDS 2004;18:1503-11

[24] Sethi AK, Cellentano DD, Gange SJ, et al Association between adherence to antiretroviral therapy and human immunodeficiency virus drug resistance. Clin Infect Dis 2003;37:1112-8.

[25] Bartlett JA, DeMasi R, Quinn J,et al. Overview of the effectiveness of triple combination therapy in antiretroviral-naïve HIV-1 infected adults. AIDS (2001) 15: 1369-77.

[26] Ammassari A, Trotta MP, Murri R, et al. Correlates and predictors of adherence to HAART: Overview of published literature. J AIDS (2002) 31:S123-7.

[27] Parienti JJ, Bangsberg DR,Verdon R et al Better adherence with once daily antiretroviral therapy Clin Infect Dis 2009;48: 484-8

[28] Spaulding A, Rutherford GW, Siegfried N. Tenofovir or zidovudine in three-drug combination therapy with one nucleoside reverse transcriptase inhibitor and one non-nucleoside reverse transcriptase inhibitor for initial treatment of HIV infection in antiretroviral-naïve individuals. Cochrane Database Syst Rev. 2010:CD008740. Review.

[29] Gottesman BS, Leibovici L, Schapiro JM,et al. Nucleoside reverse transcriptase inhibitors in combination therapy for HIV patients: systematic review and meta-analysis. Eur J Clin Microbiol Infect Dis. 2010;29:779-86.

[30] Elzi L, Marzolini C, Furrer H, et al Swiss HIV Cohort Study.Treatment modification in human immunodeficiency virus-infected individuals starting combination antiretroviral therapy between 2005 and 2008. Arch Intern Med. 2010;170:57-65.

[31] Gill CJ, Griffith JL, Jacobson D, et alRelationship of HIV viral loads, CD4 counts, and HAART use to health-related quality of life. J Acquir Immune Defic Syndr. 2002;30:485-92.

[32] Harrigan PR, Hogg RS, Dong WW, et al Predictors of HIV drug-resistance mutations in a large antiretroviral-naive cohort initiating triple antiretroviral therapy. J Infect Dis 2005;191:339-47.

[33] Van Sighum Virologic failure and drug resistance. Chapter 5 Annual Report 2010 Monitoring of HIV infection in the Netherlands. Stichting HIV Monitoring (Athena cohort) www.hiv-monitoring.nl

[34] Nolan D, Mallal S. Complications associated with NRTI therapy: update on clinical features and possible pathogenic mechanisms. Antivir Ther 2004;9:849-63.

[35] White AJ. Mitochondrial toxicity and HIV therapy. Sex Transm Infect 2001;77:158-73.

[36] Kirian MA, Higginson RT, Fulco PP. Acute onset of pancreatitis with concomitant use of tenofovir and didanosine. Ann Pharmacother 2004;38:1660-63.

[37] Reisler RB, Murphy RL, Redfield RR, Parker RA Incidence of pancreatitis in HIV-1-infected individuals enrolled in 20 adult AIDS clinical trials group studies: lessons learned.J. Acquir Immune Defic Syndr 2005 ;39:159-66.

[38] Smith CJ, Olsen CH, Mocroft A, et al The role of antiretroviral therapy in the incidence of pancreatitis in HIV-positive individuals in the EuroSIDA study. AIDS. 2008 Jan 2;22:47-56.

[39] Kakuda TN. Pharmacology of nucleoside and nucleotide reverse transcriptase inhibitor-induced mitochondrial toxicity. Clin Ther 2000;22:685-708.

[40] Saves M, Raffi F, Capeau J, et al Factors related to lipodystrophy and metabolic alterations in patients with human immunodeficiency virus infection receiving highly active antiretroviral therapy. Clin Infect Dis 2002 34:1396-1405.

[41] Martin A, Smith DE, Carr A, et al Reversibility of lipoatrophy in HIV-infected patients 2 years after switching from a thymidine analogue to abacavir: the MITOX Extension Study. AIDS 2004;18:1029-36.

[42] Moyle G, Sabin C, Cartledge J, et al. A randomized trial of tenofovir DF abacavir as replacement for thymidine analog in persons with lipoatrophy. AIDS 2006;20:2043-50

[43] Arenas-Pinto A, Bhaskaran K, Dunn D, et al. The risk of developing peripheral neuropathy induced by nucleoside reverse transcriptase inhibitors decreases over time: evidence from the Delta trial. Antivir Ther. 2008;13:289-95.

[44] Moore RD, Wong WM, Keruly JC, et al Incidence of neuropathy in HIV-infected patients on monotherapy versus those on combination therapy with didanosine, stavudine and hydroxyurea. AIDS 2000;14:273-78.

[45] Davis CM, Shearer WT. Diagnosis and management of HIV drug hypersensitivity. J. Allergy Clin Immunol 2008;121:826-32

[46] Schiller DS. Identification, management, and prevention of adverse effects associated with highly active antiretroviral therapy. Am J Health Syst Pharm. 2004;61:2507-22.

[47] Zimmermann, A.E, Pizzoferrato T, Bedford J et al., Tenofovir-associated acute and chronic kidney disease: a case of multiple drug interactions. Clin Infect Dis. 2006;42:283-90.

[48] Fux CA, Simcock M, Wolbers M, et al Swiss HIV Cohort Study. Tenofovir use is associated with a reduction in calculated glomerular filtration rates in the Swiss HIV Cohort Study.Antivir Ther. 2007;12:1165-73.

[49] Mocroft A, Kirk O, Reiss P, De Wit S, Sedlacek D, Beniowski M, Gatell J, Phillips AN, Ledergerber B, Lundgren JD; EuroSIDA Study Group. Estimated glomerular filtration rate, chronic kidney disease and antiretroviral drug use in HIV-positive patients. AIDS 2010;24:1667-78.

[50] Izzedine, H.Hulot JS, Vittecoq D, et al. Long-term renal safety of tenofovir disoproxil fumarate in antiretroviral-naive HIV-1-infected patients. Data from a double-blind randomized active-controlled multicentre study. Nephrol Dial Transplant 2005;20:743-6.

[51] Gallant JE, Moore RD. Renal function with use of tenofovir-containing initial antiretroviral regimen. AIDS 2009;23:1971-75

[52] Wever K, van Agtmael MA, Carr A. Incomplete reversibility of tenofovir-related renal toxicity in HIV-infected men. J Acquir Immune Defic Syndr. 2010;55:78-81

[53] Cooper RD, Wiebe N, Smith N, et al Systematic review and meta-analysis: renal safety of tenofovir disoproxil fumarate in HIV-infected patients.Clinical Infect Dis 2010;51:496-505

[54] Guaraldi G, Zona S, Roverato A, et al. Prevalence of poly-pathology is more common in HIV-infected patients than in HIV-negative controls in any age strata. Program and abstracts of the 17th Conference on Retroviruses and Opportunistic Infections; February 16-19, 2010; San Francisco, California. Abstract 727.

[55] DAD Study Group, Friis-Møller N, Reiss P, et al. Class of antiretroviral drugs and the risk of myocardial infarction. N Engl J Med. 2007;356:1723-1735.

[56] Currier JS, Taylor A, Boyd F, et al. Coronary heart disease in HIV-infected individuals. J Acquir Immune Defic Syndr. 2003;33:506-512.

[57] Klein D, Hurley LB, Quesenberry CP Jr, Sidney S. Do protease inhibitors increase the risk for coronary heart disease in patients with HIV-1 infection? J Acquir Immune Defic Syndr. 2002;30:471-7.

[58] Triant VA, Lee H, Hadigan C, et al Increased acute myocardial infarction rates and cardiovascular risk factors among patients with human immunodeficiency virus disease. J Clin Endocrinol Metab. 2007;92:2506-12.

[59] Mary-Krause M, Cotte L, Simon A, et al. Increased risk of myocardial infarction with duration of protease inhibitor therapy in HIV-infected men. AIDS. 2003;17:2479-86.

[60] Bozzette SA, Ake CF, Tam HK, et al Cardiovascular and cerebrovascular events in patients treated for human immunodeficiency virus infection. N Engl J Med. 2003;348:702-10.

[61] Grunfeld C, Delaney JA, Wanke C, et al Preclinical atherosclerosis due to HIV infection: carotid intima-medial thickness measurements from the FRAM study. AIDS. 2009;23:1841-9.

[62] D:A:D Study Group, Sabin CA, Worm SW, et al. Use of nucleoside reverse transcriptase inhibitors and risk of myocardial infarction in HIV-infected patients enrolled in the D:A:D study: a multi-cohort collaboration. Lancet. 2008;371:1417-26.

[63] Worm SW, Sabin C, Weber R, et al. Risk of myocardial infarction in patients with HIV infection exposed to specific individual antiretroviral drugs from the 3 major drug classes: the Data Collection on Adverse Events of Anti-HIV Drugs (D:A:D) study. J Infect Dis. 2010;201:318-30.

[64] Strategies for Management of Anti-Retroviral Therapy/INSIGHT; DAD Study Groups. Use of nucleoside reverse transcriptase inhibitors and risk of myocardial infarction in HIV-infected patients. AIDS. 2008;22:F17-F24.

[65] Martínez E, Larrousse M, Podzamczer D, et al. Abacavir-based therapy does not affect biological mechanisms associated with cardiovascular dysfunction. AIDS. 2010;24:F1-F9.

[66] Bedimo R, Westfall A, Drechsler H, et al Abacavir use and risk of acute myocardial infarction and cerebrovascular disease in the HAART era. Program and abstracts of the 5th International AIDS Society Conference on HIV Pathogenesis, Treatment and Prevention; July 19-22, 2009; Cape Town, South Africa. Abstract MOAB202.

[67] Bartlett JA, Chen SS, Quinn JB. Comparative efficacy of nucleoside/nucleotide reverse transcriptase inhibitors in combination with efavirenz: results of a systematic overview. HIV Clin Trials. 2007;84:221-6. Review.

[68] Brown TT, Qaqish RB. Antiretroviral therapy and the prevalence of osteopenia and osteoporosis: a meta-analytic review. AIDS 2006;20:2165-74

[69] Womack J, Goulet J, Gibert C, and Veterans Aging Cohort Project Team. HIV infection and fragility fracture risk among male veterans. Program and abstracts of the 17th Conference on Retroviruses and Opportunistic Infections; February 16-19, 2010; San Francisco, California. Abstract 129.

[70] Gallant JE, Staszewski S, Pozniak AL, et al. Efficacy and safety of tenofovir DF vs stavudine in combination therapy in antiretroviral-naive patients: a 3-year randomized trial. JAMA. 2004;292:191-201.

[71] Martin A, Bloch M, Amin J, et al. Simplification of antiretroviral therapy with tenofovir-emtricitabine or abacavir-lamivudine: a randomized, 96-week trial. Clin Infect Dis. 2009;49:1591-1601.

[72] Moyle G, Givens N, Pearce H, Compston J. Effects of ART on bone turnover markers and bone density in HIV-infected patients. Antivir Ther. 2009;14(suppl 2):A14.

[73] Stellbrink HJ, Orkin C, Arribas JR, et al. Comparison of changes in bone density and turnover with abacavir-lamivudine versus tenofovir-emtricitabine in HIV-infected adults: 48-week results from the ASSERT study. Clin Infect Dis. 2010;51:963-972.

[74] McComsey G, Kitch D, Daar E, et al. Bone and limb fat outcomes of ACTG A5224s, a substudy of ACTG A5202: a prospective, randomized, partially blinded phase III trial of ABC/3TC or TDF/FTC with EFV or ATV/r for initial treatment of HIV-1 infection. Program and abstracts of the 17th Conference on Retroviruses and Opportunistic Infections; February 16-19, 2010a; San Francisco, California. Abstract 106LB.

[75] Huang J, Hughes M, Riddler S, et al. Effects of randomized regimen and nucleoside reverse transcriptase inhibitor (NRTI) selection on 96 week bone mineral density (BMD): results from ACTG 5142. Program and abstracts of the 18th International AIDS Conference; Vienna, Austria; July 18-23, 2010. Abstract WEAB0304. www.emea.eu and www.fda.gov (latest assessed December 2010)

[76] Opravil M, Ledergerber B, Furrer H, et al Clinical efficacy of early initiation of HAART in patients with asymptomatic HIV infection and CD4 cell l count > 350 x 106/L. AIDS 2002:16:1371-81

[77] d'Arminio Monforte A, Lepri AC, Rezza G, et al Insight into reasons for discontinuation of the first highly active antiretroviral therapy regimen in a cohort of antiretroviral naïve patients. AIDS 2000;14:499-507

[78] Gras L, Smit C. Effects of cART on HIV RNA concentration in plasma, CD4 cell count and toxicity driven therapy changes. Chapter 4 Annual Report 2010 Monitoring of HIV infection in the Netherlands. Stichting HIV Monitoring (Athena cohort) www.hiv-monitoring.nl

[79] Dando TM, Scott LJ. Abacavir plus lamivudine: a review of their combined use in the management of HIV infection. Drugs 2005;65:285-302.

[80] Hervey PS, Perry CM. Abacavir: a review of its clinical potential in patients with HIV infection.Drugs 2000;60:447-79.

[81] Foster RH, Faulds D. Abacavir. Drugs 1998;55:729-736.

[82] Perry CM, Balfour JA. Didanosine. An update on its antiviral activity, pharmacokinetic properties and therapeutic efficacy in the management of HIV disease. Drugs 1996;52:928-62.

[83] Perry CM, Noble S. Didanosine: an updated review of its use in HIV infection. Drugs 1999;58:1099-1135.

[84] Bang LM, Scott LJ. Emtricitabine: an antiretroviral agent for HIV infection. Drugs 2003;63:2413-24.

[85] Dando TM, Wagstaff AJ. Emtricitabine/tenofovir disoproxil fumarate. Drugs 2004;64:2075-82.

[86] Johnson MA, Moore KH, Yuen GJ et al. Clinical pharmacokinetics of lamivudine. Clin Pharmacokinet 1999;36:41-66.

[87] Perry CM, Faulds D. Lamivudine. A review of its antiviral activity, pharmacokinetic properties and therapeutic efficacy in the management of HIV infection. Drugs 1997;53:657-80.

[88] Lea AP, Faulds D. Stavudine: a review of its pharmacodynamic and pharmacokinetic properties and clinical potential in HIV infection. Drugs 1996;51:846-64.

[89] Rana KZ, Dudley MN.   Clinical pharmacokinetics of stavudine. Clin Pharmacokinet 1997;33:276-284.

[90] Kearney BP, Flaherty JF, Shah J.   Tenofovir disoproxil fumarate: clinical pharmacology and pharmacokinetics. Clin Pharmacokinet 2004;43:595-612.

[91] Chapman T, McGavin J, Noble S. Tenofovir disoproxil fumarate. Drugs 2003;63:1597-1608.

[92] Lyseng-Williamson KA, Reynolds after et al.   Tenofovir disoproxil fumarate: a review of its use in the management of HIV infection. Drugs 2005;65:413-32.

[93] Fung HB, Stone EA, Piacenti FJ.   Tenofovir disoproxil fumarate: a nucleotide reverse transcriptase inhibitor for the treatment of HIV infection. Clin Ther 2002;24:1515-48.

[94] Wilde MI, Langtry HD.   Zidovudine. An update of its pharmacodynamic and pharmacokinetic properties, and therapeutic efficacy. Drugs 1993;46:515-78.

[95] Acosta EP, Page LM, Fletcher CV.   Clinical pharmacokinetics of zidovudine. An update. Clin Pharmacokinet 1996;30:251-62.

[96] EASL Clinical Practice Guidelines : Management of chronic hepatitis B. J of Hepatology 2009;50:227-42

Part 2

New Therapy Strategies

4

Cell-Delivered Gene Therapy for HIV

Scott Ledger[1], Borislav Savkovic[2], Michelle Millington[3], Helen Impey[3],
Maureen Boyd[3], John M. Murray[2,4,5] and Geoff Symonds[3,5]
[1]*The Faculty of Medicine, The University of New South Wales, Sydney*
[2]*The School of Mathematics and Statistics, The University of New South Wales, Sydney*
[3]*Calimmune Australia, 405 Liverpool St Darlinghurst, NSW*
[4]*The Kirby Institute, The University of New South Wales, Sydney NSW*
[5]*St Vincent's Institute for Applied Medical Research*
405 Liverpool St Darlinghurst, NSW
Australia

1. Introduction

Gene therapy involves the transfer of genetic material into cells of an individual to treat an underlying illness either through the expression of advantageous genes or the silencing of disadvantageous ones (Flotte 2007; Kohn and Candotti 2009). Gene therapy has been used successfully to treat several diseases, for example SCID-X1 (Cavazzana-Calvo, Hacein-Bey et al. 2000) and SCID-ADA (Aiuti 2004) and holds out promise as a more general treatment regimen (Flotte 2007). One of the driving forces behind the area of research into the treatment of HIV is the resistance to, and side effects of, the current drugs being used. This development of resistance and the need for continuous and ongoing daily medication have been major shortcomings of conventional highly active antiretroviral therapy (HAART) when employed as a treatment against HIV (Perno, Moyle et al. 2008). An additional driving force behind interest in gene therapy is the potential for a one-off treatment that would continue to work for the life of the individual (Symonds, Johnstone et al. 2010). One can envisage gene therapy as a full or partial replacement for HAART, that may help to overcome issues of viral resistance, co-morbidity and attendant compliance (i.e. daily administration of HAART for life).

While HAART is a systemic form of treatment which provides a substantial level of protection to HIV susceptible cells in the body for many years, it is highly susceptible to the development of a resistant HIV quasispecies, that may selectively expand due to the strong evolutionary pressure exerted by HAART (Perno, Moyle et al. 2008). Whereas HAART-based treatments bathe each cell in some level of drug, gene-therapy results in a polar population dynamic consisting of gene protected and unprotected cells. This is due to the fact that it is neither practical nor possible to have a protective gene against HIV introduced into all cells of the body, but rather only a subset of the total cell population is afforded protection (Symonds, Johnstone et al. 2010). This polar dynamic is predicted to provide additional pressures to the suriviving HIV population (Applegate, Birkett et al. 2010). Cells that might be afforded protection include CD4+ T cells and macrophages, which are known to be targets of HIV infection, as well as other cell populations susceptible to HIV infection.

In this chapter we describe the biological and clinical underpinnings of gene-therapy including the therapeutic genes employed for protection against HIV, delivery methods of the vectors carrying these protective genes into the cells, expression cassettes and finally the target cells into which the protective genes are introduced. We then estimate the potential in-vivo protective effects of gene-therapy against HIV.

2. Biological and clinical aspects of gene-therapy

In this section we look at the biological and clinical aspects of gene-therapy. Observations associated with natural immunity that may be utilized in gene-therapy against HIV are discussed in section 2.1. Stages of the HIV infection cycle that may be inhibited by gene-therapy, and the various gene therapeutic that may be employed to this aim, are the subject of section 2.2. Various delivery vectors and promoters that can achieve effective delivery and transcription of the protective gene into the cell to be transduced are the subject of section 2.3. The biological underpinnings of the target cell to be transduced with a protective gene, either CD4+ T cells or Hematopoietic Stem Cells (HSC) are discussed in section 2.4. The clinical aspects of collection of cells for transduction via apheresis and associated preparation regimens are discussed in section 2.5. Finally, Section 2.6 is concerned with clinical trials to-date of anti-HIV gene-therapy and results reported therein.

2.1 CCR5 and the 32-nucleotide deletion mutation: A strong case for gene therapy

Recent additional impetus for gene-therapy for HIV is based upon the earlier observation that some individuals do not become infected upon repeated exposure to HIV (Zimmerman, Buckler-White et al. 1997). Studies of these individuals led to the discovery of a mutation in CCR5, an important co-receptor for HIV attachment to target cells prior to infection. Such a mutation was found to confer natural immunity against HIV (Zimmerman, Buckler-White et al. 1997).

The mutation discovered was found to be a 32 nucleotide deletion (CCR5d32) within the CCR5 gene (Zimmerman, Buckler-White et al. 1997). This mutation was observed to be very common among individuals of European background and it has subsequently been determined that of Caucasian individuals, approximately 10% are heterozygous and 1-3% homozygous for this mutation (Dean, Carrington et al. 1996; Liu, Paxton et al. 1996; Samson, Libert et al. 1996; Agrawal, Lu et al. 2004), with the mutation being almost non-existent in all other populations. There has been considerable speculation regarding the origin and purpose of the mutation. It has been shown that the percentage of CCR5d32 mutation occurring in today's population is roughly comparable to that found in samples from individuals of the Bronze Age (approximately 3000 years ago) (Hummel, Schmidt et al. 2005; Hedrick and Verrelli 2006). There is evidence suggesting that smallpox provided a selective advantage for CCR5d32 (Galvani and Slatkin 2003), indicating that there may be other selective advantages associated with the mutation. The mutation does not seem to present any significant disadvantages to the individuals other than an increased risk of West-Nile disease (Glass, McDermott et al. 2006). Such observations led to an interest in mimicking this natural mutation for HIV-infected individuals via genetic manipulation (i.e. transduction) of cells vulnerable to HIV infection. (see below)

It has been noted that the 32 nucleotide deletion results in 31 new amino acids being coded for, resulting in an active CCR5d32 protein. This protein instead of presenting as CCR5 receptors on the cell surface like the wild-type counterpart, CCR5d32 actually binds to and interacts with CXCR4 receptors (Agrawal, Lu et al. 2004), the other major coreceptor for HIV attachment. This provides an additional protection against HIV infection beyond the mere absence of a functional CCR5 co-receptor, especially when concerning strains capable of utilizing the CXCR4 coreceptor (Agrawal, Lu et al. 2004; Jin, Agrawal et al. 2008). Further evidence towards the beneficial effect of the CCR5d32 protein comes from evidence that a polymorphism in the promoter region in CCR5-/- individuals can affect the protective capabilities of the d32 mutation. It has been demonstrated that an increase in CCR5d32 protein expression will improve resistance to HIV, while decreased CCR5d32 expression reduces the protective effect (Jin, Agrawal et al. 2008).

This CCR5d32 mutation has been successfully utilized in a patient, who suffered from both HIV/AIDS and leukaemia (Hutter, Nowak et al. 2009; Allers, Hutter et al. 2010). This individual, termed the "Berlin patient", had complete ablation of their immune system (to treat the leukemia) before matched allogeneic donor hematopoietic stem cells (HSC) homozygous for the CCR5d32 mutation were transfused into the patient. After one recurrence of leukaemia and a repeat of the treatment (ablation and reconstitution), the patient has had undetectable levels of HIV (and no recurring leukaemia) for more than 3 years without the use of any antiretroviral drugs (Hutter, Nowak et al. 2009; Allers, Hutter et al. 2010). This unique result of "functional" cure of HIV indicates significant potential for the use of gene-therapy to mimic this result by down-regulation of CCR5.

2.2 Choosing a stage of HIV infection cycle to inhibit: Which therapeutic genes hold out promise?

2.2.1 Classes and methods of HIV inhibition

Gene-therapy may be aimed to target various stages of the HIV infection cycle as shown in Figure 1. Class 1 therapy inhibits all steps prior to viral integration into the cellular genome, Class 2 inhibits expression of viral genes and Class 3 inhibits production of new virions once integration and expression has taken place (von Laer, Hasselmann et al. 2006). According to predictions from mathematical modelling, as discussed in section 3.1, Class 1 gene therapies are likely to be the most effective as they inhibit HIV at the first steps, and provide a selective advantage to these cells by avoiding any viral or immunological induced death from infection. Hence many gene therapeutics currently under investigation include components that impair attachment or fusion stages of the viral life-cycle (Symonds, Johnstone et al. 2010).

While all these classes are potential HIV gene therapeutics, practically, the use of multiple therapeutics in combination is likely to be the most effective method. This is analogous to the antiretroviral situation where it does not take long for HIV resistance to emerge against single antiretroviral drugs. These antiretroviral drugs have been shown to be far more effective when used in combination. It is for this reason that gene therapy research has often been focused on the use of multiple gene therapuetics used in conjunction with one-another. As well as the variety of targets being investigated, there is additionally a wide range of methods to achieve inhibition of these targets. The most commonly employed methods to-date include the following:

Antisense (Class 2): Antisense RNA is a synthetic nucleotide sequence that binds to mRNA in order to inhibit its function. This method can be used against a wide range of targets, including the HIV envelope (Levine, Humeau et al. 2006).

Aptamers (Class 2 or 3): Aptamers are single-stranded RNAs or DNAs. They disrupt at the protein level by tightly binding to their target ligand (Que-Gewirth and Sullenger 2007). Aptamers can be used to target a wide array of proteins and as such have potential to be used in multiple settings.

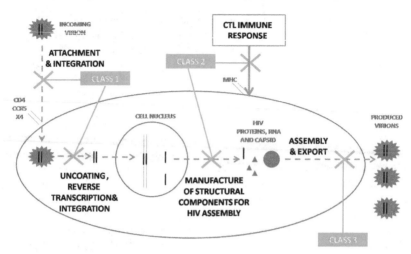

Fig. 1. The three Classes of gene-therapy according to cycle of HIV infection inhibited as defined by von Laer et al(von Laer, Hasselmann et al. 2006; von Laer, Hasselmann et al. 2006). Class 1 inhibits all steps in the infection cycle prior to integration of the HIV RNA into the cellular genome. In particular, Class 1 inhibits either the entry of the HIV virion into the cell (i.e. inhibition of attachment/integration of the HIV virion through the CD4, CCR5 and X4 receptors/coreceptors) or inhibits integration into the cellular genome once a virion has entered the cell (i.e. blocks uncoating, reverse transcription or integration). Class 2 inhibits gene expression and the production of structural components required for the assembly of new HIV virions. Class 2 also results in lower susceptitibliy to cell death through the cytotoxic T lymphocyte (CTL) immune response, as a result of reduced recongnition via the Major Histocompatiblity Complex (MHC). Finally, Class 3 inhibits the assembly and export of virions from the infected cell.

Intracellular Antibodies (Class 1 or 3): Intracellular antibodies, or "intrabodies", are designed to bind to and inactivate target molecules inside host cells (Chen, Bagley et al. 1994). One target which has been used by intrabodies is CCR5, whereby the intrabodies bind to CCR5 and block surface expression (Rossi, June et al. 2007).

Ribozymes (Class 2): Ribozymes are catalytic RNA molecules that have the ability to degrade RNA in a sequence-specific manner (Sun, Wang et al. 1995). When used as anti-HIV agents, they have the potential to target multiple steps, affecting incoming RNA (during infection, in this sense they can act in part as Class1), primary RNA transcripts (from integrated provirus), spliced mRNAs and mature RNA being packaged into virions. These are primarily Class 2 inhibitors and examples are those designed to target the conserved regions of HIV such as the overlapping regions of *vpr* and *tat* reading frames (Mitsuyasu, Merigan et al. 2009). Highly conserved regions are desirable as targets so that sequence specificity is more likely to be maintained.

Short hairpin RNA (Class 1 or 2): Short hairpin RNA is a sequence of RNA that folds back upon itself in a hairpin turn; it can be used to initiate RNA interference and consequently silence gene expression (McIntyre and Fanning 2006). shRNA expression vectors utilise a promoter to drive expression of the shRNA. As an integrated vector, this expression cassette will be passed on to daughter cells, allowing the gene silencing to be maintained *in vivo*. The shRNA hairpin structure is cleaved by the cellular machinery into siRNA which is then bound to the RNA-induced silencing complex. This complex binds to and cleaves mRNAs which match the siRNA that is bound to it (Hannon and Rossi 2004). The use of siRNA for gene silencing has become a method of choice and can be potentially applied to many targets, including down-regulation of CCR5 that will decrease target cell infectivity by HIV and other host receptors as the removal or impairment of these receptors will render HIV non-infectious (Class 1).

Class	Target Site	Why	Goal	How
1	CCR5	Important co-receptor	Remove/prevent expression of CCR5	Zinc-finger, siRNA
1	CD4	Essential receptor for HIV attachment	Remove/prevent expression of CD4	Zinc-finger, siRNA
1	CXCR4	Important co-receptor	Remove/prevent expression of CXCR4	Zinc-finger, siRNA, ribozyme
1	Membrane Fusion (HIV heptad repeat)	Essential for viral entry	Prevent entry of HIV through host-cell membrane	siRNA
2	Tat	Important for Transcription	Disrupt *tat* gene	Tar decoy, siRNA, ribozyme
2	Rev	Important for virion Translation	Disrupt *rev* gene	siRNA, REV mutants
3	Env, Protease, Helicase	Important for virion maturation	Prevent virion maturation	siRNA, Antisense RNA,
3	Gag	Important for virion assembly	Disrupt gag gene	Ribozyme, siRNA

Table 1. A list of some HIV gene therapy targets, the goals and the mechanics of how they are being explored. This table shows a variety of Class 1, 2 and 3 therapies and the range of approaches against targets.

Fusion Inhibitors (Class 1): One fusion inhibitor which has been researched in detail is the maC46 peptide (C46) (Zahn, Hermann et al. 2008). It inhibits viral fusion by interacting with the N-terminal hydrophobic alpha-helix. This prevents changes essential for membrane fusion of the virus and host cell. This fusion inhibitor has been found to be highly effective at blocking HIV replication (Zahn, Hermann et al. 2008).

Zinc Finger Nucleases (ZFNs) (Class 1 or 2): ZFNs bind to targeted open reading frames. Two juxtaposed ZFN's on DNA results in dimerisation of the endonuclease domains, generating a double-stranded break at the targeted DNA (Porteus and Carroll 2005). The mutagenic pathways relied on to repair the DNA breaks result in nucleotide mutations at the break-sites, thus permanently disrupting the gene (Porteus and Carroll 2005). While experiments in mice have shown this method to be effective, there is still a risk of non-target directed mutagenesis. Another limitation of this technique is the inability to add protective genes, as only the effective deletion/inactivation of genes can be performed, thus limiting the applications for the use of ZFNs to applications such as inactivation of CCR5 (Class 1).

2.2.2 Strong arguments for gene-therapy based entry inhibition

Class 1 inhibitors generally act at the level of HIV binding to the target cell (von Laer, Hasselmann et al. 2006). It is expected that this would be the most effective as HIV is blocked from entry to the target cell and any subsequent replication steps cannot take place. An important recent contribution to the argument for Class 1 inhibitors is the discovery of the cause of the so-called 'bystander effect' where apparently non HIV infected cells also succumb to HIV pathogenesis (Doitsh, Cavrois et al. 2010). The observation that productively infected cells are not the only contributors to host-cell death has been noted previously, however the cause of this cell death had remained unknown until Doitsh et al discovered abortive/nonproductive HIV infection in host-cells (approximately 95% of infected cells) and the induction of apoptosis in these cells (Doitsh, Cavrois et al. 2010). This "bystander effect" is likely to have contributed to the lack of success of some antiretroviral therapy methods, including a variety of clinical trials whereby HIV infection was only inhibited after HIV entry, as host-induced apoptosis would greatly reduce the effectiveness of treatment. This effect indicates a crucial additional benefit of entry-inhibitors over other classes of antiviral treatment.

One of the resistance mechanisms developed by HIV against the antiretroviral CCR5 antagonists, such as maraviroc, is not just the use of other co-receptors such as CXCR4, it is the use of maraviroc-bound CCR5 receptors (Westby, Smith-Burchnell et al. 2007). This mechanism of resistance would not be available against cells containing a down-regulation, or mutation-mediated deletion of the CCR5 receptor produced by gene therapy. An added bonus of the use of attachment and/or fusion inhibitors is that they do not provide cross-resistance with other treatment methods such as protease and integration inhibitors.

2.3 Vectors, delivery methods and promoters: Delivering the protective gene into the cell

The therapeutic used in gene therapy must be carried within a suitable vector or delivery system; for HIV gene therapy these vectors should generally be capable of integrating into the host cells with minimal risk of generation of replication competent lentivirus or insertional mutagenesis (Wu, Wakefield et al. 2000; Symonds, Johnstone et al. 2010). The vector must also be non-toxic to the host while allowing the expression of the relevant gene(s). There are many techniques and delivery vectors which can be utilized for this purpose. Examples of the most commonly used delivery vectors are shown in Table 2.

Transposon-based delivery systems consist of a synthetic transposon and an associated transposase and work via a cut-and-paste mechanism whereby the transposase recognises the inverted direct sequences in the transposon, and then the transposon is excised and later integrated into a target DNA region (Tamhane and Akkina 2008). They can, for example, be used to carry shRNAs.

Delivery Vector	Advantage	Disadvantage
Transposons	Can provide permanent expression of multiple genes	Potential for insertional mutagenesis
Plasmid DNA Nucleofection	Treatment has been highly effective (Holt, Wang et al. 2010)	Slight increase in apoptosis of HSCs (Holt, Wang et al. 2010)
Murine Leukaemia Virus	Little/no adverse effects (Amado, Mitsuyasu et al. 2004; Macpherson, Boyd et al. 2005)	Can only infect actively replicating cells (Roe, Reynolds et al. 1993) May induce insertional mutagenesis (Symonds, Johnstone et al. 2010)
Adenovirus	Can infect non-replicating cells (Zhang, Sankar et al. 1998)	Innate immune response (Liu and Muruve 2003)
Lentivirus	Can infect non-replicating cells (Zufferey, Dull et al. 1998), Does not effect proliferation or differentiation of HSCs (Gervaix, Schwarz et al. 1997)	Slight risk of insertional mutagenesis (Philippe, Sarkis et al. 2006)
Conditionally replicating virus	Higher transduction efficiency	Risk of mutation/recombination

Table 2. A variety of commonly used delivery vectors and their associated advantages and disadvantages.

Nucleofection of DNA involves directly adding the DNA into the targeted cells by disrupting the cell membrane through electroporation. While this is not an ever-present biological vector as those mentioned above, it is more of an event-based vector which can provide a method of entry either for less entry-capable vectors, or plasmid DNA (Aluigi, Fogli et al. 2006).

Viral delivery vectors are typically made from the backbone of suitable viruses, whereby pathogenic, and (often) replication-mediating genes are removed, and only the essential genes remain (Kootstra and Verma 2003). The therapeutic gene(s) being used is/are then added to the viral backbone. The virus is then able to infect host cells as would its natural counterpart. However without the ability to replicate or express harmful genes. It is used only to integrate into the host genome and allow the therapeutic gene to be active.

One of the main concerns regarding gene therapies is the potential for insertional mutagenesis. This has been shown to occur in SCID-X1 trials (Howe, Mansour et al. 2008) where the insertional mutagenesis led to myeloproliferation/leukemia (Howe, Mansour et al. 2008). While insertional mutagenesis events have occurred in this and a few other gene therapy trials eg CGD (Stein, Ott et al. 2010), they have not occurred in HIV gene therapy trials, and a great deal of effort is undertaken to ensure that this event does not occur.

To ensure efficient transcription of the therapeutic gene, a suitable promoter is required. A promoter is a region of DNA that facilitates the transcription of nearby downstream gene(s), and is essential for the efficient expression of the desired gene(s). The choice of the promoter to be used in gene therapies is highly important, and various promoters have been tested in laboratory studies and clinical trials. Promoters currently in use in HIV gene therapy studies are quite diverse and include U6 (human derived), T7 (bacteriophage derived), and Ubc (Human ubiquitin c) (Anderson, Banerjea et al. 2003; Boden, Pusch et al. 2003; Weber and Cannon 2007):

There have been studies using different promoters in HIV gene therapy work-up and many have been shown to be effective. However, due to the many different therapeutic genes, their delivery vectors, and the cells targeted for transduction, it is difficult to determine which promoters are the most effective and as such, each needs to be tested.

It has been noted that a highly expressive promoter may not be the ideal candidate, as many highly efficient promoters can have other side-effects. As noted above, of key concern is the trans-activation (insertional mutagenesis) of nearby cellular genes (Weber and Cannon 2007), potentially leading to oncogenic effects by over-expression of important proteins.

2.4 Transduction targets: Which cells should be protected against HIV?

HIV infection is typically characterized by CD4+ T cell infection and depletion. In addition, other cells are also infected by HIV, including macrophages and monocytes and most recently there have been reports of hematopoietic stem cell (HSC) infection (Stanley, Kessler et al. 1992; Carter, Onafuwa-Nuga et al. 2010; Carter, McNamara et al. 2011). In the case of gene therapy for HIV the two most common cell types that have been transduced to date with the therapeutic relevant gene are CD4+ T lymphocytes and HSC. Transduction of these cells is expected to provide the best outcome due to CD4+ T cells being the main targets of HIV infection and the ability of HSC to differentiate into all susceptible cells. In this subsection we discuss the biological aspects of transducing either CD4+ T cells or HSC with a protective gene.

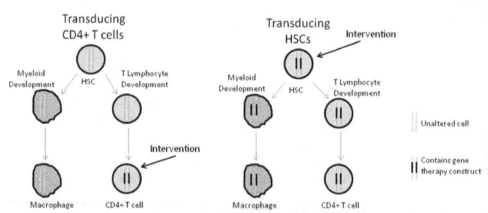

Fig. 2. Two ways of achieving cell populations protected against HIV as a result of either transducing CD4+ T cells or HSC. If the CD4+ T cell population is transduced with a protective gene (left), then protection against HIV is only afforded to CD4+ T cells. If on the other hand HSC are transduced with a protective gene (right), then the protected gene is retained by all cells derived from the HSC via differentiation through the myeloid (e.g macrophage) and lymphoid lineages (e.g CD4+ T cell). The approach of transducing HSC thus provides protection against HIV to a broader class of cells.

2.4.1 Transduction of CD4+ T cells

The use of CD4+ T cells as target cells for HIV gene therapy has been explored in several studies (see section relating to clinical trials). Isolation and transduction of CD4+ T cells is relatively simple. The key advantage of targeting CD4+ T cells is the ease with which they may be accessed. As they largely populate and regularly traffic through peripheral blood, no stimulatory factors are required to mobilize them prior to collection. Conceptually it can be envisaged that the introduction of a protected population of CD4+ T lymphocytes should have impact as these are the cells specifically depleted by HIV infection; the greater the severity of HIV infection the greater the CD4+ T lymphocyte decline.

One such study involving the therapy of CD4+ T cells was performed by Levine in 2006 (Levine, Humeau et al. 2006) whereby peripheral blood CD4+ T cells were harvested from each subject by apheresis. The collected samples were then depleted of CD8+ cells and monocytes, transduced with the gene construct *ex vivo*, activated via CD3 and CD28 costimulation and expanded before being re-infused into the patients. This method of therapy was shown to be both safe in treatment, and effective in delivery of the therapeutic gene (Levine, Humeau et al. 2006; Brunstein, Miller et al. 2011).

Predicted in-vivo dynamics of CD4+ T cell transduction, based on mathematical modelling, are discussed in section 3.2.1.

2.4.2 Transduction of hematopoietic stem cells (HSC)

Due to the range of cells which HIV infects, it is thought to be a significant advantage to transduce HSC, as these cells provide a continuous supply (following differentiation) into a range of immunological cells (monocytes, macrophages, CD4+ T cells, CD8+ cells, dendritic cells, microglial cells) which may thus be protected against HIV infection (Carter and Ehrlich 2008). A delay in the newly 'protected cell' production would be expected, thus delaying the effect of the therapeutic gene(s). However, there can still be a significant production of CD4+ T lymphocytes, the supply of which has been predicted to be a rate of approximately 1.65 cells/μL of blood/day (due to thymic reconstitution) (Murray, Kaufmann et al. 2003). This results in the production of a stable population of protected cells which could impact on CD4+ T cell number and viral load.

While CD4+ T cells (and other cell types common in peripheral blood) can be obtained relatively simply prior to transduction by apheresis from peripheral blood, HSC must first be mobilised from the bone marrow (discussed in detail below). This creates an additional component to the treatment process. Currently the most common method for the mobilisation of HSC is the use of granulocyte colony stimulating factor (G-CSF), a treatment that usually spans 4-5 days before the apheresis of peripheral blood can begin. Predicted in-vivo dynamics of HSC transduced with a protective gene are discussed in section 3.2.2.

2.5 Collection of cells for transduction: Apheresis and treatment methods for optimized and high-volume cell collection

Current gene therapy protocols for HIV require the isolation of the relevant cells to be transduced, generally following apheresis (Symonds, Johnstone et al. 2010). Apheresis is the process of removing mononuclear cells from blood and returning neutrophils, platelets, plasma and red blood cells to the donor, in order to collect more of one particular part of the blood than could be separated from a unit of whole blood. Apheresis allows for the collection of large quantities of cells, and in the case of gene therapies for HIV, total lymphocytes, CD4+ cells, or HSC are the cell types collected.

It is common practice to use a stimulating agent such as G-CSF in order to increase the quantity of HSC in the peripheral blood. The resulting increase in cell numbers in peripheral blood is due to redistribution of cells from other compartments of the body (i.e bone marrow and lymph tissue). The use of G-CSF and other stimulating factors is essential when HSC (largely inhabiting the bone marrow) are to be transduced with the therapeutic gene. Various trials have shown HSC cell counts in peripheral blood increase 20-50-fold over the course of GCSF administration (Lane, Law et al. 1995; Law, Lane et al. 1999; Valgimigli, Rigolin et al. 2005).

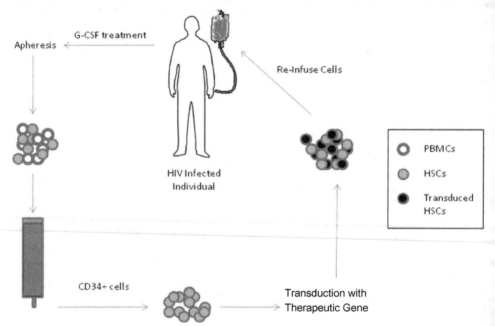

Fig. 3. Illustration of the clinical aspects of therapeutic apheresis (for HSC harvesting), and the subsequent processes of transduction and reinfusion. The HIV infected individual is first administered G-CSF in order to effect mobilization of HSC from bone marrow into peripiheral blood. The mobilized HSC are then collected from peripheral blood and subsequently transduced with a protective gene. The transduced HSC are then reinfused into the patient.

A technique known as myeloablation has been utilized in some clinical trials (before the transduced cell infusion) in order to improve engraftment of the gene-containing cells (Strayer, Akkina et al. 2005). This procedure involves the killing of HSC, thereby reducing the endogenous non-transduced cells, thereby creating more space for the transduced cell population.

2.6 Important studies involving gene-therapy: Promising results and insights
Several mouse studies and clinical trials have been conducted in the area of HIV gene therapy, with several different therapuetic targets.

Target/Mechanism of Action	Construct	Results	Reference
Rev	Inhibitory Rev protein, Rev M10, delivered to CD4+ cells by gold particles	Preferential survival of cells with construct. Limited duration of engraftment.	(Woffendin, Ranga et al. 1996)
Rev	Inhibitory Rev protein, Rev M10, delivered to CD4+ cells by retroviral vector	More persistent engraftment compared with gold particle delivery. No change	(Ranga, Woffendin et al. 1998)
Rev	"Humanized" dominant-negative REV protein (huM10) and nontranslated marker gene (FX) as an internal control in retroviral vector	Gene marking in first months, then low or undetectable except in one patient when viral load increased. No serious adverse events.	(Podsakoff, Engel et al. 2005)
rev/TAR	Trans-dominant rev with or without antisense TAR and control (neo) gene in CD4+ T lymphocytes	Long term survival of cells at low level. Preferential survival of gene-containing cells in a patient with high viral load.	(Morgan, Walker et al. 2005)
RRE decoy	Retroviral-mediated transfer of an RRE decoy gene into bone marrow CD34+ cells	No adverse effects. 2 subjects' cells detected containing both the RRE and LN vectors on the day after cell infusion. All subsequent samples negative for the L-RRE-neo vector. Cells containing the control LN vector detected up to 330 days.	(Kohn, Bauer et al. 1999; Bauer, Selander et al. 2000)
Env antisense	Single infusion of VRX496™, a lentiviral construct encoding an antisense targeting HIV env, in CD4+ T cells	CD4+ counts increased in 4/5 patients, viral loads stable, prolonged engraftment. Well tolerated. Transient vector mobilization. Safe to date.	(Levine, Humeau et al. 2006)
rev/tat ribozyme	tat and tat/rev ribozyme in CD34+cells in autologous CD34+ cells and empty vector backbone in two patient groups with and without ablation	Trial 1 - 3/5 patients showed low-frequency marking of PBMC with ribozyme and vector backbone. Trial 2 – gene marked cells detected after infusion and to one year, and RNA expression detected.	(Michienzi, Castanotto et al. 2003)

Target/Mechanism of Action	Construct	Results	Reference
tat/vpr ribozyme	Phase I study: Moloney murine leukaemia retroviral vector encoding a ribozyme vs control LNL6 vector in CD34+ HPSC	de novo production of myeloid and lymphoid cells. Degree of persistence of gene-containing cells dependent on transduced cell dose	(Amado, Mitsuyasu et al. 1999; Amado, Mitsuyasu et al. 2004)
tat/vpr ribozyme	Retroviral vector encoding a ribozyme vs control LNL6 vector to transduce T lymphocytes, predominantly CD4+ T lymphocytes	Safe and feasible procedure. Long-term survival of genetically modified T-lymphocytes.	(Macpherson, Boyd et al. 2005)
tat/vpr ribozyme	Phase II study: Moloney murine leukaemia virus-based, replication-incompetent gamma retroviral vector with gene encoding a ribozyme vs placebo in CD34+ cells	No significant difference mean plasma viral load at primary end-point but lower TWAUC. No safety concerns.	(Mitsuyasu, Merigan et al. 2009)
Fusion inhibitor	Gene encoding membrane anchored peptide C46 fusion inhibitor delivered by retroviral vector in T cells.	Increased CD4. No significant change in viral load (except after treatment change). Modified cells detected at one year. Low level marking. No major toxicity	(van Lunzen, Glaunsinger et al. 2007)
CCR5	CCR5-specific zinc finger nuclease based product, SB-728-T, in autologous CD4+ T cells. Two phase 1 trials with various dosing regimens in different patient groups.	Preliminary data on 1 patient only ZFN-modified cells persisted in circulation and observed in GALT. Suggested delay in return of viral load after structured treatment interruption.	(2009)
Tat/rev, CCR5, TAR decoy	Tat/rev short hairpin RNA, TAR decoy and CCR5 ribozyme expressed from a self-inactivating lentiviral vector transduced in CD34+ cells, along with standard unmanipulated HPCs in 4 patients with HIV and non-Hodgkin's lymphoma	Engraftment by 11 days. Low levels of gene marking observed up to 24 months as was expression of siRNA and CCR	(DiGiusto, Krishnan et al. 2010)

Target/Mechanism of Action	Construct	Results	Reference
Modified T-cell receptor	Autologous infusion of CD4+ and CD8+ T cells modified by CD4ζ in a murine moloney leukaemia virus backbone given +/- IL-2.	Gene-modified cells followed and detected to 12 months with no difference due to IL-2. No significant change in plasma viral load. CD4ζ signal detected in rectal biopsy.	(Mitsuyasu, Anton et al. 2000)

Table 3. (Apapted from Symonds et al (Symonds, Johnstone et al. 2010)): A list of HIV gene therapy clinical trials and their outcomes. Each of these studies vary in their gene therapy target, and method of targeting the specific region.

To date, as shown in Table 3, several different gene therapies have entered Phase 1 clinical trials, and some into Phase 2) indicating the safety of a range of HIV gene therapeutics including antisense, ribozymes, decoys, intracellular antibodies and zinc fingers targeting CCR5.

3. Protective effects of anti-HIV gene-therapy: Predictions from mathematical modeling

In gene-therapy research, mathematical modelling has been employed to predict the protective effects of anti-HIV gene-therapy (von Laer, Hasselmann et al. 2006; von Laer, Hasselmann et al. 2006). In this section we review current results on mathematical modelling, with respect to predictions of the *in-vivo* anti-HIV protective effects. Mathematical models deal with the complex interactions between gene-therapy, the immune system and HIV infection (Perelson, Essunger et al. 1997). Given the relative sparsity of current clinical trial data of gene-therapy for HIV, and the long time-spans over which predictions are to be made (i.e. over many years) mathematical modelling can provide predictions on the likely *in-vivo* effectiveness of current and future gene-therapies. Modelling work to-date has led to important insights regarding key design factors as well as parameters that should be optimized in order to maximize the effectiveness of therapy (von Laer, Hasselmann et al. 2006; von Laer, Hasselmann et al. 2006). In this section we review current results and key insights.

3.1 Why is Class 1 gene-therapy the most promising approach?

As discussed previously, three different broad stages of the HIV infection cycle may be targeted for inhibition of HIV infection (Figure 1) with the inhibitors referred to as Class 1, 2, and 3 (von Laer, Hasselmann et al. 2006; von Laer, Hasselmann et al. 2006). It is of interest whether inhibiting earlier stages (via Class 1), intermediate stages (via Class 2) or later stages (via Class 3) of the infection cycle might provide maximum effectiveness of the therapy. Is it more desirable to prevent HIV entry and integration into the cellular genome via Class 1, to inhibit the production of structural components for HIV assembly via Class 2, or to inhibit the assembly/export of new HIV virions via Class 3? This question has been addressed by a number of investigators (von Laer, Hasselmann et al. 2006; von Laer, Hasselmann et al. 2006; Applegate, Birkett et al. 2010), subject to a variety of modelling assumptions reflecting differing levels of complexity of the interaction between HIV, gene-therapy and the immune system.

Investigations to-date have demonstrated that Class 1 protection appears to be highly desirable in terms of reducing viral loads and increasing CD4+ T cell counts (von Laer, Hasselmann et al. 2006; Applegate, Birkett et al. 2010; Aviran, Shah et al. 2010). The underlying reason for the superiority of Class 1 therapy (over Class 2 and Class 3) has been attributed to the high selective advantage of the protected cell population conferred by Class 1 inhibition (von Laer, Hasselmann et al. 2006; von Laer, Hasselmann et al. 2006; Applegate, Birkett et al. 2010). Since Class 1 inhibits all steps prior to viral integration into the cellular genome (Figure 1), any cell containing the protective gene is less likely to be infected than a non-protected cell. Consequently, Class 1 promotes the survival and expansion of the protected non-infected cells, whereas the non-protected cells are more prone to infection and selective killing through cytopathic effects associated either with the virus or the CTL immune response (von Laer, Hasselmann et al. 2006; von Laer, Hasselmann et al. 2006).

In contrast to Class 1 agents, Class 2 and Class 3 therapies have been shown to require much higher degrees of inhibition in order to achieve clinically significant effects (von Laer, Hasselmann et al. 2006; von Laer, Hasselmann et al. 2006; Applegate, Birkett et al. 2010). Class 2 inhibits cytopathic effects associated with the viral infection and the CTL immune response (Figure 1). Any infected cell with Class 2 protection is therefore longer-lived and also has a reduced viral production rate compared to an unprotected and infected cell (von Laer, Hasselmann et al. 2006; von Laer, Hasselmann et al. 2006; Applegate, Birkett et al. 2010). Class 2 consequently confers a selective survival advantage to the infected cells containing the protective gene relative to other infected cells, but not to non-infected cells containing the protective gene (as is the case with Class 1). In contrast, Class 3 only inhibits the export of new HIV virions from an infected cell and thus provides minimal selective advantage (von Laer, Hasselmann et al. 2006; von Laer, Hasselmann et al. 2006). Hence Class 1 is the only class that confers a selective survival advantage to non-infected cells containing the protective gene (von Laer, Hasselmann et al. 2006; von Laer, Hasselmann et al. 2006; Applegate, Birkett et al. 2010).

Collectively therefore, modelling work to-date implies that Class 1 is essential due to the selective survival advantage conferred to the protected and non-infected cells. Still, it is important to note that augmenting Class 1 with Class 2 and/or Class 3 protection might further increase the effectiveness of therapy (von Laer, Hasselmann et al. 2006; von Laer, Hasselmann et al. 2006; Applegate, Birkett et al. 2010). Recent findings relating to the "Bystander Effect", as discussed previously in section 2.2.2, have lent further support to arguments relating to Class 1 inhibition (Doitsh, Cavrois et al. 2010), as abortive infections (HIV virion enters the cell, but does not integrate into cellular genome) comprise 95% of all cell death resulting from HIV infection.

3.2 Two different transduction approaches: To transduce CD4+ T cells or HSC with a protective gene?

As discussed previously in section 2.4, it is possible to either transduce CD4+ T cells with a protective gene (for an immediately protected population of CD4+ T cells) or to transduce HSC, that provide protection to CD4+ T cells following differentiation through the lymphoid line and to monocyte/macrophages following differentiation throught the myeloid line. While the relative merits of each approach have attracted substantial interest, the long-term quantitative advantages and disadvantages of each approach in the clinical setting remain to be elucidated. Consequently, investigators have turned to predictions from mathematical modelling in order to shed light on the in-vivo dynamics of the two approaches. In this section, we review the predictions from such modelling work to-date.

3.2.1 Transducing CD4+ T cells with a protective gene: Can we achieve establishment of a sufficiently large and sufficiently "receptor-diverse" CD4+ T cell population that is protected against HIV?

Expansion of numbers of CD4+ T cells containing a protective gene is subject to the rate-limiting step of homeostatic cell division and proliferation (von Laer, Hasselmann et al. 2006). Thus it is important to determine how quickly a substantial CD4+ T cell population could expand from a small initial fraction of protected cells. Such considerations are motivated by the fact that it is currently feasible and practical to transduce only a portion of the total CD4+ T cell population (Dropulic and June 2006; von Laer, Baum et al. 2009), so that expansion of the protected CD4+ T cell population will have to rely on in vivo mechanisms.

While modelling has shown that a small fraction of initially transduced cells could potentially result in significant expansion of the protected CD4+ T cell population, reductions of viral load, and also a delay in the onset of AIDS (Lund, Lund et al. 1997; Leonard and Schaffer 2006; von Laer, Hasselmann et al. 2006; Aviran, Shah et al. 2010), most of these models have assumed a strong feedback mechanism upregulating cellular proliferation when numbers fall below a normal level. Whereas such homeostatic mechanisms are believed to contribute to the maintenance of T cell numbers in healthy individuals (Khaled and Durum 2002), the speed with which they occur is likely to be significantly slower in practice. Current clinical trials have not produced CD4+ T cell expansions at rates as fast as predicted by mathematical modelling (Dropulic and June 2006; von Laer, Baum et al. 2009).

Current estimates of T lymphocyte division put the normal rate at approximately 1 division every 3.5 years for naive T cells and 1 division every 22 weeks for memory T cells (McLean and Michie 1995). If the transduced CD4+ T cells are to expand in vivo, then such time-scales should provide an indication of the slow nature of any in vivo expansion of the transduced CD4+ T cell population unless driven by strong selective pressure by HIV.

More realistic upper bounds on rates of CD4+ T cell expansion in-vivo under gene-therapy may be obtained by consideration of CD4+ T cell reconstitution on HAART (Byakwaga, Murray et al. 2009). Reconstitution of the CD4+ T cell population under HAART appears relatively slow with average increases of approximately 300 cells/µL observed after about 6 years (Byakwaga, Murray et al. 2009). Given that reconstitution on HAART usually only takes place under complete viral suppression (as opposed to gene-therapy where a measurable viral population may be present), it appears likely that the expansion rates of the protected CD4+ T cell population under gene-therapy may be substantially slower. Unlike the situation with HAART high viral levels may be preferable in early stages of gene therapy to act as a driving force for the expansion of a protected CD4+ T cell population via a selective mechanism.

Several additional factors might further inhibit the expansion of the protected CD4+ T cell population in-vivo. First, unless sufficient selective survival advantage is conferred to the protected CD4+ T cell population, the protected cell population might not expand substantially in-vivo. Second, the transduced CD4+ T-cells might have increased death rates or decreased proliferative ability due to interference of the protective gene with normal cell functionality (Dropulic and June 2006; von Laer, Baum et al. 2009; Tayi, Bowen et al. 2010). Third, the unprotected de-novo CD4+ T-cells exported from the thymus might effectively dilute the transduced CD4+ T-cells in the periphery (Aviran, Shah et al. 2010). This latter problem may potentially be addressed by subsequent "booster" treatments involving repeated infusions of transduced CD4+ T cells or by also using HSC.

An additional disadvantage associated with the direct transduction of CD4+ T cells is that peripheral expansion of their number does not necessarily correspond to an equivalent expansion in the T cell repertoire (Nikolich-Zugich, Slifka et al. 2004; Allen, Turner et al. 2011; Wiegers, Kaufmann et al. 2011). This is important as any resulting "gaps" in the T cell repertoire may result in increased probability of immune system evasion by pathogens and consequently in increased risk of infection or morbidity (Nikolich-Zugich, Slifka et al. 2004; Allen, Turner et al. 2011; Wiegers, Kaufmann et al. 2011).

Hence although direct transduction of CD4+ T cells results in a faster appearance in peripheral blood of a protected component of this susceptible population, there may be disadvantages in that these may not provide a diverse immune response and other cell populations will not protected.

3.2.2 Transducing HSC with a protective gene: Increasing T cell receptor repertoire and broadening class of protected cells

An alternative to transducing CD4+ T cells directly is to instead transduce HSC. In this case, the production of de-novo CD4+ T cells containing the protective gene occurs as a result of HSC differentiation through the lymphoid line and subsequent export from the thymus (Symonds, Johnstone et al. 2010).

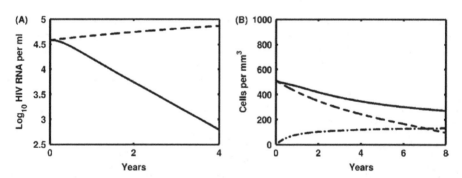

Fig. 4. Modelling predictions by Murray et al.(Murray, Fanning et al. 2009) regarding comparison of the scenario that 20% of all HSC in the bone marrow are transduced with a tat-vpr specific anti-HIV ribozyme (OZ1) versus the scenario that no gene-therapy treatment is received. Reproduced with permission from Murray et al.(Murray, Fanning et al. 2009). The patient was assumed HAART-naive. The time-scale on the horizontal ordinate denotes the time since receiving gene-therapy at year 0. (A) Treatment with OZ1, $\log_{10}$ HIV RNA copies/ml (solid line); No treatment, $\log_{10}$ HIV RNA copies/ml (dashed line). (B) Treatment with OZ1, total CD4+ T lymphocytes/mm³ (solid line), OZ1+CD4+ T lymphocytes/mm³ (dash–dot line); No treatment , total CD4+ T lymphocytes/mm³ (dashed line).

Transducing HSC with a protective gene has two distinct advantages. First, the export of protected de-novo CD4+ T cells from the thymus results in a diversification of the T cell receptor repertoire (Allen, Turner et al. 2011; Wiegers, Kaufmann et al. 2011). Consequently the expanded CD4+ T cell population containing the protective gene exhibits more 'extensive" TCR coverage over time, reducing the risk that pathogens might evade the immune response (Nikolich-Zugich, Slifka et al. 2004; Allen, Turner et al. 2011; Wiegers, Kaufmann et al. 2011). Secondly, HSC differentiate into a broad range of cells (besides CD4+ T cells), including macrophages that are susceptible to HIV infection and that may represent important latent HIV reservoirs (Chun, Carruth et al. 1997; Chun, Stuyver et al. 1997; Crowe and Sonza 2000). Consequently, HSC transduction provides protection against HIV to a broader class of cells than just CD4+ T cells.

The transduction of HSC does not immediately provide a protected population of CD4+ T cells in the periphery, but rather the protected CD4+ T cell population is established relatively slowly as HSC differentiate and are exported from the thymus (Symonds, Johnstone et al. 2010). Thymic production of CD4+ T cells has been estimated at approximately 1.65 cells/μL/day (Murray, Kaufmann et al. 2003) in peripheral blood. Assuming that a percentage P of total HSC in the bone marrow is transduced, then one would correspondingly expect that CD4+ T cells containing the protective gene would be exported at a rate of 1.65 x P cells/μL/day from the thymus (Murray, Fanning et al. 2009). Such numbers provide estimates of rates at which the establishment of a protected CD4+ T cell population might take place in-vivo in peripheral blood.

Achieving high engraftment efficiencies of HSC in the bone marrow is important. While a number of clinical trials in which HSC were transduced reported indications of clinical effect against HIV (Symonds, Johnstone et al. 2010), engraftment percentages in the bone marrow have been relatively low (Dropulic and June 2006; Mitsuyasu, Merigan et al. 2009; von Laer, Baum et al. 2009; Symonds, Johnstone et al. 2010). Such results underscore the need for more effective methods of cell harvesting, transduction and homing, that achieve higher engraftment efficiencies. Increased engraftment percentages should lead to more substantial clinical effects in terms of protection against HIV (Mitsuyasu, Merigan et al. 2009; Murray, Fanning et al. 2009).

Despite relatively low engraftment efficiencies to-date, it is of practical interest for future research directions to determine what engraftment percentages might suffice for clinically meaningful effects of the therapy. This question was addressed in recent modelling work (Murray, Fanning et al. 2009), that considered HSC transduction with a *tat-vpr* specific anti-HIV ribozyme (OZ1) employed in a recent phase 2 clinical trial (Mitsuyasu, Merigan et al. 2009). Under the assumption that 20% of all HSC in the bone marrow are transduced (i.e. engraftment percentage P = 20%), and that correspondingly 20% of CD4+ T cells exported from the thymus contain the protective gene, the modelling predicted reductions of 0.5 log_{10} in viral load for a HAART-naive individual after 1 year (Figure 4 A). Benefits in terms of forestalment of onset of AIDS at 8 years post-infection were also estimated (Figure 4 B). Slighly less prononunced effects were observed for patients that were concurrently enrolled on HAART (Murray, Fanning et al. 2009). Such results are encouraging and indicate that relatively modest engraftment percentages could achieve a clinically relevant effect. Consequently full bone marrow ablation may be unnecessary.

3.3 Resistance development under gene-therapy: How does it differ from HAART?

Systemic antiretroviral therapy bathes each cell in some level of the drugs being used depending on the penetration of the individual drugs to that region of the body, their concentration, pharmacokinetics and timing between dosages (Abdel-Rahman and Kauffman 2004). The clinical management of the combinations of drugs used in a regimen is an important part of successful treatment through suppressing the development of drug resistance. Early in the development of antiretroviral drugs there were few agents available and by necessity these were applied as monotherapy leading to the failure of these and subsequent drugs from the same class. Current HAART regimens involve three drugs from at least 2 drug classes to limit the likelihood that mutations in the HIV quasispecies will be present prior to the commencement of therapy or will develop subsequently.

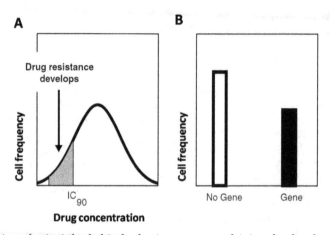

Fig. 5. Illustration of principles behind selection pressures driving the development of resistance with antiretroviral therapy and with gene-therapy. Adapted with permission from Applegate et al.(Applegate, Birkett et al. 2010). (A) The horizontal ordinate denotes the concentration of antiretroviral drug received, and the vertical ordinate denotes the frequency of cells receiving the antiretroviral drug concentration. The selection pressure driving resistance in systemic antiretroviral therapy results from bathing each cell in some drug concentration. This provides a "continuous spectrum" for selection of HIV escape mutants, since many cells will receive suboptimal drug concentrations allowing viral replication and the preferential development of drug-resistant strains (as shown by shaded region indicated by the arrow). (B) The horizontal ordinate splits the cell population into two parts of either having a protective gene or not. The vertical ordinate denotes the frequency of cells containing the gene and not containing the gene. The bipartite distribution of protected and unprotected results provides a different selection environment whereby sufficient wild-type replication takes place in the non-protected population (i.e. no gene), thus mitigating the escape of viral mutants.

Similar concerns exist for the development of resistance to HIV gene therapy (Leonard and Schaffer 2006; Applegate, Birkett et al. 2010). The quasispecies nature of HIV and its high mutation rate imply the existence of every single mutation to any agent prior to the start of therapy. If there is sufficient viral replication under therapy, even for a reasonably short period, there is the chance that these singly resistant clones will evolve into variants with additional mutations and that are highly resistant to therapy. HIV gene therapy seems to fall into the classification of approaches that lend themselves to the development of resistance: not all cells will contain the therapy and so there will be considerable viral replication, and this will be even more evident for gene therapy delivered to HSC since it will take some time for the protected CD4+ T cells to mature from the HSC and appear in the periphery (Applegate, Birkett et al. 2010). However there is a considerable difference between gene therapy and a systemic treatment that is not suitably suppressive.

Unless myeloablation is conducted to eliminate endogenous non-gene containing HSC and T cells, it is expected that there will always be a sizeable proportion of HSC and CD4+ T cells that do not contain the therapy. Achieving 20% gene transduced HSC without ablation may be an upper bound (this remains to be tested). Similar limitations exist for those trials that instead transduce peripheral CD4+ T cells. At any time there is an estimated 2% of total T cells in peripheral blood and not all T cells are likely to traffic to this compartment. So large-scale apheresis of CD4+ T cells from peripheral blood will remove, and be able to infuse, only a fraction of their total.

Hence gene therapy will partition HIV-susceptible cells into a bipartite population: those containing the therapy and those that do not. This 0-1 distribution is very different from the continuous distribution of drug concentration within cells for an individual receiving antiretroviral therapy (Figure 5). In this situation gene therapy is less likely to lead to the development of resistance (Applegate, Birkett et al. 2010). However there is a trade-off in that it is also less suppressive for the same reason. As cells containing gene therapy become more widespread in the body of an infected individual they will exert more pressure on the virus and select for resistance (Leonard and Schaffer 2006). For this reason the same general principles that apply to antiretroviral therapy are also valid in this context. Gene therapy should target multiple viral and cellular mechanisms.

Mathematical modelling of gene therapy delivered to HSC that targets multiple mechanisms with reasonable efficacy and where the resistant virus is also less fit than wild-type determined that this therapy will reduce virus and maintain a viable T cell population for extended periods without the expansion of resistant virus (Applegate, Birkett et al. 2010). However there were important qualifications to the extent of this success. Primarily the gene therapy needs to be Class 1 and inhibit infection of cells. Additionally the likelihood of resistance to a particular component of the therapy and the fitness cost that incurs will also contribute to the speed at which virus overcomes the therapy.

3.4 Future perspectives: What can we expect from gene-therapy against HIV?

Gene therapy holds out high promise as an effective therapy against HIV. The definition of success of gene-therapy treatment may vary, depending on a variety of circumstances. As discussed in Section 2.1, an obvious success would be one similar to that of the Berlin Patient whereby an individual would be completely and sustainably cured of HIV and have their immune system restored to "normal" levels. It is however important to provide more practical goals, as it is not likely that a "cure" will be achieved with all patients, and as such, more "modest" goals might be more practical and more realistic. Removing the need for an individual to be on HAART would be defined as success, as this can save the individual from life-long drug regimens often with considerable side-effects (Yeni 2006). Another "successful" outcome might consists in preservation of immune system functionality depite the presence of measurable viral loads, as observed during SIV infection in its natural hosts (Liovat, Jacquelin et al. 2009; Pandrea, Silvestri et al. 2009).

As discussed in section 3.2.2 above, predictions from mathematical modelling indicate that full ablation of the immune system need not be necessary in order for clinically significant effects to be observed (Murray, Fanning et al. 2009). Assuming HSC engraftment percentages of about 20%, it has been predicted that substantial viral control may be achieved and CD4+ T cell counts maintained above the critical limit of 200 cells/μL (Murray, Fanning et al. 2009). The major challenge to achieving substantial clinical effect thus relates to achieving sufficient engraftment percentages.

Gene therapy will have varying degrees of effectiveness depending on the circumstances of the individual. The length of time for which an individual has been infected with HIV is an important factor to consider when providing gene therapy treatment. Due to the tropism of HIV in an infected individual changing over the duration of infection from CCR5-tropic to CXCR4-tropic, any treatment targeting CCR5 would be best used on patients in fairly early-phase infection (Mosier 2009). For gene-therapy aiming to transduce HSC, it also appears reasonable to expect that the therapeutic effects in younger patients will be more pronounced due to their greater rates of thymic activity (Pido-Lopez, Imami et al. 2001). Futhermore, patients on HAART, patients for whom available antiretroviral therapies have been exhausted and patients suffering severe HAART-associated side-effects should also benefit, given that gene-therapy provides an alternative layer of protection via cell-mediated immunity in addition to antiretroviral therapies (Symonds, Johnstone et al. 2010).

Finally, as discussed in section 3.2, both HSC and CD4+ T cells represent feasible targets for transduction. While CD4+ T cell transduction may suffer from limitations due to a restricted T cell receptor repertoire and not protecting other susceptible cell population, it will however provide an immediate protected population. Conversely HSC are limited by the degree of thymic production and bone marrow engraftment, yet have the potential to generate a long-lasting array of HIV protected immune cells. Thus it appears that most effective therapies might employ a combination of these two approaches in order to provide optimum protection, possibly employing infusions of transduced cells.

4. Conclusion

In this chapter we discussed the current biological underpinnings of gene-therapy against HIV, as well as predictions from mathematical modelling of the clinical effects achievable through gene-therapy.

We discussed the various biological and clinical aspects relating to HIV gene therapy. An indication of the possible effectiveness of gene therapy was provided in terms of the naturally occurring mutation, CCR5d32, which provides extremely high levels of resistance against HIV infection. Most importantly however, the utilisation of this mutation in a bone marrow transplant, ridding an individual of any measurable HIV levels, indicates the capability of using gene therapy to functionally "cure" people of HIV. An assessment of the target areas of HIV gene therapy was conducted, indicating not only the possibility, but also a clear need to target multiple aspects of HIV infection (favourably entry stage), in order to prevent the emergence of resistance. The various options for delivery methods were discussed, indicating a range of techniques by which to introduce the therapeutic gene. Each of these methods exhibit their own advantages and disadvantages, however all are valid options in a variety of situations, with lentiviral vectors showing some of the most promise. The options for the ideal cell-type to target were discussed, indicating validity of using either CD4+ T cells for their immediate effect or HSC for the more sustained and broad spectrum protection. However it is also critical to consider the combination of these as an option in gene therapy. The aspects and priniciples of apheresis, ablation, and G-CSF-induced mobilisation were discussed, indicating their role in treatments. With mobilisation being crucial for the efficient transduction of HSC, and ablation of non-tranduced cells having the potential to provide a significant proportional increase in the amount of protected cells, both are critical when designing treatment regimens. Finally, clinical trials whereby HIV gene therapy has been conducted, and the outcomes of these trials were summarised, highlighting the high safety levels associated with gene therapuetics. Due to the observed high safety in these studies, with the promise of reasonable levels of efficacy and a proof of concept (in the Berlin Patient), HIV gene therapies are a very promising area of HIV research.

In the final sections we discussed predictions obtained from mathematical modelling regarding the in-vivo effectiveness of gene-therapy. We outlined why HIV virion entry inhibition via Class 1 gene-therapy has been shown to be essential in terms of achieving clinically meaningful effects. We explained how the selective survival advantage conferred to non-infected cells containing the Class 1 protective gene is the key factor contributing to the success of Class 1 therapy. We saw that transduction of CD4+ T cells provides an immediately protected CD4+ T cell population, but that in-vivo expansion of the protected cells may be a slow process and does not result in increased T cell receptor diversity in the expanded population. In contrast, transduction of HSC results in higher T cell receptor diversity, and in protection of a broader range of cells than solely CD4+ T cells. We also discussed the differences in viral resistance development under HAART and under gene-therapy. While HAART bathes each cell in some drug concentration, resulting in suboptimal dosages for many cells and consequent promotion in escape of viral mutants, gene-therapy partitions the cell population into protected (contains gene) and unprotected (does not contain gene) cell populations. We outlined how this bi-partite distribution promotes the expansion of a cell population protected against HIV, while at the same time mitigating risks of viral mutation escape as a result of sufficient wild-type viral replication in the non-protected cell population. Finally, we discussed future perspectives outlining how gene-therapy promises to achieve sufficient preservation of immune system functionality (without HAART-associated toxicity and non-adherence issues) resulting in forestallement of AIDS and thereby achieving similar effects as observed during SIV infection in its natural hosts. We also outlined how gene-based therapies may be employed in conjunction or disjunction with HAART depending on individual patient circumstances and viral tropism in the infected individual.

In conclusion, based on the clinical results and mathematical modeling work to-date, further clinical investigation of gene-therapy is more than justified, as gene-therapy holds high promise in terms of controlling HIV infection, preserving immune system functionality, and prevention of the onset of AIDS.

5. References

(2009). "Trial watch: novel HIV gene therapy enters Phase I trial." Nat Rev Drug Discov 8(4): 267.

Abdel-Rahman, S. M. and R. E. Kauffman (2004). "The integration of pharmacokinetics and pharmacodynamics: understanding dose-response." Annu Rev Pharmacol Toxicol 44: 111-136.

Agrawal, L., X. Lu, et al. (2004). "Role for CCR5Delta32 protein in resistance to R5, R5X4, and X4 human immunodeficiency virus type 1 in primary CD4+ cells." J Virol 78(5): 2277-2287.

Aiuti, A. (2004). "Gene therapy for adenosine-deaminase-deficient severe combined immunodeficiency." Best Pract Res Clin Haematol 17(3): 505-516.

Allen, S., S. J. Turner, et al. (2011). "Shaping the T-cell repertoire in the periphery." Immunol Cell Biol 89(1): 60-69.

Allers, K., G. Hutter, et al. (2010). "Evidence for the cure of HIV infection by CCR5{Delta}32/{Delta}32 stem cell transplantation." Blood.

Aluigi, M., M. Fogli, et al. (2006). "Nucleofection is an efficient nonviral transfection technique for human bone marrow-derived mesenchymal stem cells." Stem Cells 24(2): 454-461.

Amado, R. G., R. T. Mitsuyasu, et al. (2004). "Anti-human immunodeficiency virus hematopoietic progenitor cell-delivered ribozyme in a phase I study: myeloid and lymphoid reconstitution in human immunodeficiency virus type-1-infected patients." Hum Gene Ther 15(3): 251-262.

Amado, R. G., R. T. Mitsuyasu, et al. (1999). "A phase I trial of autologous CD34+ hematopoietic progenitor cells transduced with an anti-HIV ribozyme." Hum Gene Ther 10(13): 2255-2270.

Anderson, J., A. Banerjea, et al. (2003). "Potent suppression of HIV type 1 infection by a short hairpin anti-CXCR4 siRNA." AIDS Res Hum Retroviruses 19(8): 699-706.

Applegate, T. L., D. J. Birkett, et al. (2010). "In silico modeling indicates the development of HIV-1 resistance to multiple shRNA gene therapy differs to standard antiretroviral therapy." Retrovirology 7: 83.

Aviran, S., P. S. Shah, et al. (2010). "Computational models of HIV-1 resistance to gene therapy elucidate therapy design principles." PLoS Comput Biol 6(8).

Bauer, G., D. Selander, et al. (2000). "Gene therapy for pediatric AIDS." Ann N Y Acad Sci 918: 318-329.

Boden, D., O. Pusch, et al. (2003). "Promoter choice affects the potency of HIV-1 specific RNA interference." Nucleic Acids Res 31(17): 5033-5038.

Brunstein, C. G., J. S. Miller, et al. (2011). "Infusion of ex vivo expanded T regulatory cells in adults transplanted with umbilical cord blood: safety profile and detection kinetics." Blood 117(3): 1061-1070.

Byakwaga, H., J. M. Murray, et al. (2009). "Evolution of CD4+ T cell count in HIV-1-infected adults receiving antiretroviral therapy with sustained long-term virological suppression." AIDS Res Hum Retroviruses 25(6): 756-776.

Carter, C. A. and L. S. Ehrlich (2008). "Cell biology of HIV-1 infection of macrophages." Annu Rev Microbiol 62: 425-443.

Carter, C. C., L. A. McNamara, et al. (2011). "HIV-1 utilizes the CXCR4 chemokine receptor to infect multipotent hematopoietic stem and progenitor cells." Cell Host Microbe 9(3): 223-234.

Carter, C. C., A. Onafuwa-Nuga, et al. (2010). "HIV-1 infects multipotent progenitor cells causing cell death and establishing latent cellular reservoirs." Nat Med 16(4): 446-451.

Cavazzana-Calvo, M., S. Hacein-Bey, et al. (2000). "Gene therapy of human severe combined immunodeficiency (SCID)-X1 disease." Science 288(5466): 669-672.

Chen, S. Y., J. Bagley, et al. (1994). "Intracellular antibodies as a new class of therapeutic molecules for gene therapy." Hum Gene Ther 5(5): 595-601.

Chun, T. W., L. Carruth, et al. (1997). "Quantification of latent tissue reservoirs and total body viral load in HIV-1 infection." Nature 387(6629): 183-188.

Chun, T. W., L. Stuyver, et al. (1997). "Presence of an inducible HIV-1 latent reservoir during highly active antiretroviral therapy." Proc Natl Acad Sci U S A 94(24): 13193-13197.

Crowe, S. M. and S. Sonza (2000). "HIV-1 can be recovered from a variety of cells including peripheral blood monocytes of patients receiving highly active antiretroviral therapy: a further obstacle to eradication." J Leukoc Biol 68(3): 345-350.

Dean, M., M. Carrington, et al. (1996). "Genetic restriction of HIV-1 infection and progression to AIDS by a deletion allele of the CKR5 structural gene. Hemophilia Growth and Development Study, Multicenter AIDS Cohort Study, Multicenter Hemophilia Cohort Study, San Francisco City Cohort, ALIVE Study." Science 273(5283): 1856-1862.

DiGiusto, D. L., A. Krishnan, et al. (2010). "RNA-based gene therapy for HIV with lentiviral vector-modified CD34(+) cells in patients undergoing transplantation for AIDS-related lymphoma." Sci Transl Med 2(36): 36ra43.

Doitsh, G., M. Cavrois, et al. (2010). "Abortive HIV infection mediates CD4 T cell depletion and inflammation in human lymphoid tissue." Cell 143(5): 789-801.

Dropulic, B. and C. H. June (2006). "Gene-based immunotherapy for human immunodeficiency virus infection and acquired immunodeficiency syndrome." Hum Gene Ther 17(6): 577-588.

Flotte, T. R. (2007). "Gene therapy: the first two decades and the current state-of-the-art." J Cell Physiol 213(2): 301-305.

Galvani, A. P. and M. Slatkin (2003). "Evaluating plague and smallpox as historical selective pressures for the CCR5-Delta 32 HIV-resistance allele." Proc Natl Acad Sci U S A 100(25): 15276-15279.

Gervaix, A., L. Schwarz, et al. (1997). "Gene therapy targeting peripheral blood CD34+ hematopoietic stem cells of HIV-infected individuals." Hum Gene Ther 8(18): 2229-2238.

Glass, W. G., D. H. McDermott, et al. (2006). "CCR5 deficiency increases risk of symptomatic West Nile virus infection." J Exp Med 203(1): 35-40.

Hannon, G. J. and J. J. Rossi (2004). "Unlocking the potential of the human genome with RNA interference." Nature 431(7006): 371-378.

Hedrick, P. W. and B. C. Verrelli (2006). ""Ground truth" for selection on CCR5-Delta32." Trends Genet 22(6): 293-296.

Holt, N., J. Wang, et al. (2010). "Human hematopoietic stem/progenitor cells modified by zinc-finger nucleases targeted to CCR5 control HIV-1 in vivo." Nat Biotechnol.

Howe, S. J., M. R. Mansour, et al. (2008). "Insertional mutagenesis combined with acquired somatic mutations causes leukemogenesis following gene therapy of SCID-X1 patients." J Clin Invest 118(9): 3143-3150.

Hummel, S., D. Schmidt, et al. (2005). "Detection of the CCR5-Delta32 HIV resistance gene in Bronze Age skeletons." Genes Immun 6(4): 371-374.

Hutter, G., D. Nowak, et al. (2009). "Long-term control of HIV by CCR5 Delta32/Delta32 stem-cell transplantation." N Engl J Med 360(7): 692-698.

Jin, Q., L. Agrawal, et al. (2008). "CCR5Delta32 59537-G/A promoter polymorphism is associated with low translational efficiency and the loss of CCR5Delta32 protective effects." J Virol 82(5): 2418-2426.

Khaled, A. R. and S. K. Durum (2002). "Lymphocide: cytokines and the control of lymphoid homeostasis." Nat Rev Immunol 2(11): 817-830.

Kohn, D. B., G. Bauer, et al. (1999). "A clinical trial of retroviral-mediated transfer of a rev-responsive element decoy gene into CD34(+) cells from the bone marrow of human immunodeficiency virus-1-infected children." Blood 94(1): 368-371.

Kohn, D. B. and F. Candotti (2009). "Gene therapy fulfilling its promise." N Engl J Med 360(5): 518-521.

Kootstra, N. A. and I. M. Verma (2003). "Gene therapy with viral vectors." Annu Rev Pharmacol Toxicol 43: 413-439.

Lane, T. A., P. Law, et al. (1995). "Harvesting and enrichment of hematopoietic progenitor cells mobilized into the peripheral blood of normal donors by granulocyte-macrophage colony-stimulating factor (GM-CSF) or G-CSF: potential role in allogeneic marrow transplantation." Blood 85(1): 275-282.

Law, P., T. A. Lane, et al. (1999). "Mobilization of peripheral blood progenitor cells for human immunodeficiency virus-infected individuals." Exp Hematol 27(1): 147-154.

Leonard, J. N. and D. V. Schaffer (2006). "Antiviral RNAi therapy: emerging approaches for hitting a moving target." Gene Ther 13(6): 532-540.

Levine, B. L., L. M. Humeau, et al. (2006). "Gene transfer in humans using a conditionally replicating lentiviral vector." Proc Natl Acad Sci U S A 103(46): 17372-17377.

Liovat, A. S., B. Jacquelin, et al. (2009). "African non human primates infected by SIV - why don't they get sick? Lessons from studies on the early phase of non-pathogenic SIV infection." Curr HIV Res 7(1): 39-50.

Liu, Q. and D. A. Muruve (2003). "Molecular basis of the inflammatory response to adenovirus vectors." Gene Ther 10(11): 935-940.

Liu, R., W. A. Paxton, et al. (1996). "Homozygous defect in HIV-1 coreceptor accounts for resistance of some multiply-exposed individuals to HIV-1 infection." Cell 86(3): 367-377.

Lund, O., O. S. Lund, et al. (1997). "Gene therapy of T helper cells in HIV infection: mathematical model of the criteria for clinical effect." Bull Math Biol 59(4): 725-745.

Macpherson, J. L., M. P. Boyd, et al. (2005). "Long-term survival and concomitant gene expression of ribozyme-transduced CD4+ T-lymphocytes in HIV-infected patients." J Gene Med 7(5): 552-564.

McIntyre, G. J. and G. C. Fanning (2006). "Design and cloning strategies for constructing shRNA expression vectors." BMC Biotechnol 6: 1.

McLean, A. R. and C. A. Michie (1995). "In vivo estimates of division and death rates of human T lymphocytes." Proc Natl Acad Sci U S A 92(9): 3707-3711.

Michienzi, A., D. Castanotto, et al. (2003). "RNA-mediated inhibition of HIV in a gene therapy setting." Ann N Y Acad Sci 1002: 63-71.

Mitsuyasu, R. T., P. A. Anton, et al. (2000). "Prolonged survival and tissue trafficking following adoptive transfer of CD4zeta gene-modified autologous CD4(+) and CD8(+) T cells in human immunodeficiency virus-infected subjects." Blood 96(3): 785-793.

Mitsuyasu, R. T., T. C. Merigan, et al. (2009). "Phase 2 gene therapy trial of an anti-HIV ribozyme in autologous CD34+ cells." Nat Med 15(3): 285-292.

Morgan, R. A., R. Walker, et al. (2005). "Preferential survival of CD4+ T lymphocytes engineered with anti-human immunodeficiency virus (HIV) genes in HIV-infected individuals." Hum Gene Ther 16(9): 1065-1074.

Mosier, D. E. (2009). "How HIV changes its tropism: evolution and adaptation?" Curr Opin HIV AIDS 4(2): 125-130.

Murray, J. M., G. C. Fanning, et al. (2009). "Mathematical modelling of the impact of haematopoietic stem cell-delivered gene therapy for HIV." J Gene Med 11(12): 1077-1086.

Murray, J. M., G. R. Kaufmann, et al. (2003). "Naive T cells are maintained by thymic output in early ages but by proliferation without phenotypic change after age twenty." Immunol Cell Biol 81(6): 487-495.

Nikolich-Zugich, J., M. K. Slifka, et al. (2004). "The many important facets of T-cell repertoire diversity." Nat Rev Immunol 4(2): 123-132.

Pandrea, I., G. Silvestri, et al. (2009). "AIDS in african nonhuman primate hosts of SIVs: a new paradigm of SIV infection." Curr HIV Res 7(1): 57-72.

Perelson, A. S., P. Essunger, et al. (1997). "Dynamics of HIV-1 and CD4+ lymphocytes in vivo." AIDS 11 Suppl A: S17-24.

Perno, C. F., G. Moyle, et al. (2008). "Overcoming resistance to existing therapies in HIV-infected patients: the role of new antiretroviral drugs." J Med Virol 80(4): 565-576.

Philippe, S., C. Sarkis, et al. (2006). "Lentiviral vectors with a defective integrase allow efficient and sustained transgene expression in vitro and in vivo." Proc Natl Acad Sci U S A 103(47): 17684-17689.

Pido-Lopez, J., N. Imami, et al. (2001). "Both age and gender affect thymic output: more recent thymic migrants in females than males as they age." Clin Exp Immunol 125(3): 409-413.

Podsakoff, G. M., B. C. Engel, et al. (2005). "Selective survival of peripheral blood lymphocytes in children with HIV-1 following delivery of an anti-HIV gene to bone marrow CD34(+) cells." Mol Ther 12(1): 77-86.

Porteus, M. H. and D. Carroll (2005). "Gene targeting using zinc finger nucleases." Nat Biotechnol 23(8): 967-973.

Que-Gewirth, N. S. and B. A. Sullenger (2007). "Gene therapy progress and prospects: RNA aptamers." Gene Ther 14(4): 283-291.

Ranga, U., C. Woffendin, et al. (1998). "Enhanced T cell engraftment after retroviral delivery of an antiviral gene in HIV-infected individuals." Proc Natl Acad Sci U S A 95(3): 1201-1206.

Roe, T., T. C. Reynolds, et al. (1993). "Integration of murine leukemia virus DNA depends on mitosis." EMBO J 12(5): 2099-2108.

Rossi, J. J., C. H. June, et al. (2007). "Genetic therapies against HIV." Nat Biotechnol 25(12): 1444-1454.

Samson, M., F. Libert, et al. (1996). "Resistance to HIV-1 infection in caucasian individuals bearing mutant alleles of the CCR-5 chemokine receptor gene." Nature 382(6593): 722-725.

Stanley, S. K., S. W. Kessler, et al. (1992). "CD34+ bone marrow cells are infected with HIV in a subset of seropositive individuals." J Immunol 149(2): 689-697.

Stein, S., M. G. Ott, et al. (2010). "Genomic instability and myelodysplasia with monosomy 7 consequent to EVI1 activation after gene therapy for chronic granulomatous disease." Nat Med 16(2): 198-204.

Strayer, D. S., R. Akkina, et al. (2005). "Current status of gene therapy strategies to treat HIV/AIDS." Mol Ther 11(6): 823-842.

Sun, L. Q., L. Wang, et al. (1995). "Target sequence-specific inhibition of HIV-1 replication by ribozymes directed to tat RNA." Nucleic Acids Res 23(15): 2909-2913.

Symonds, G. P., H. A. Johnstone, et al. (2010). "The use of cell-delivered gene therapy for the treatment of HIV/AIDS." Immunol Res 48(1-3): 84-98.

Tamhane, M. and R. Akkina (2008). "Stable gene transfer of CCR5 and CXCR4 siRNAs by sleeping beauty transposon system to confer HIV-1 resistance." AIDS Res Ther 5: 16.

Tayi, V. S., B. D. Bowen, et al. (2010). "Mathematical model of the rate-limiting steps for retrovirus-mediated gene transfer into mammalian cells." Biotechnology and Bioengineering 105(1): 195-209.

Valgimigli, M., G. M. Rigolin, et al. (2005). "Use of granulocyte-colony stimulating factor during acute myocardial infarction to enhance bone marrow stem cell mobilization in humans: clinical and angiographic safety profile." Eur Heart J 26(18): 1838-1845.

van Lunzen, J., T. Glaunsinger, et al. (2007). "Transfer of autologous gene-modified T cells in HIV-infected patients with advanced immunodeficiency and drug-resistant virus." Mol Ther 15(5): 1024-1033.

von Laer, D., C. Baum, et al. (2009). "Antiviral gene therapy." Handb Exp Pharmacol(189): 265-297.

von Laer, D., S. Hasselmann, et al. (2006). "Gene therapy for HIV infection: what does it need to make it work?" The Journal of Gene Medicine 8(6): 658-667.

von Laer, D., S. Hasselmann, et al. (2006). "Impact of gene-modified T cells on HIV infection dynamics." J Theor Biol 238(1): 60-77.

Weber, E. L. and P. M. Cannon (2007). "Promoter choice for retroviral vectors: transcriptional strength versus trans-activation potential." Hum Gene Ther 18(9): 849-860.

Westby, M., C. Smith-Burchnell, et al. (2007). "Reduced maximal inhibition in phenotypic susceptibility assays indicates that viral strains resistant to the CCR5 antagonist maraviroc utilize inhibitor-bound receptor for entry." J Virol 81(5): 2359-2371.

Wiegers, G. J., M. Kaufmann, et al. (2011). "Shaping the T-cell repertoire: a matter of life and death." Immunol Cell Biol 89(1): 33-39.

Woffendin, C., U. Ranga, et al. (1996). "Expression of a protective gene-prolongs survival of T cells in human immunodeficiency virus-infected patients." Proc Natl Acad Sci U S A 93(7): 2889-2894.

Wu, X., J. K. Wakefield, et al. (2000). "Development of a novel trans-lentiviral vector that affords predictable safety." Mol Ther 2(1): 47-55.

Yeni, P. (2006). "Update on HAART in HIV." J Hepatol 44(1 Suppl): S100-103.

Zahn, R. C., F. G. Hermann, et al. (2008). "Efficient entry inhibition of human and nonhuman primate immunodeficiency virus by cell surface-expressed gp41-derived peptides." Gene Ther 15(17): 1210-1222.

Zhang, L., U. Sankar, et al. (1998). "The Himar1 mariner transposase cloned in a recombinant adenovirus vector is functional in mammalian cells." Nucleic Acids Res 26(16): 3687-3693.

Zimmerman, P. A., A. Buckler-White, et al. (1997). "Inherited resistance to HIV-1 conferred by an inactivating mutation in CC chemokine receptor 5: studies in populations with contrasting clinical phenotypes, defined racial background, and quantified risk." Mol Med 3(1): 23-36.

Zufferey, R., T. Dull, et al. (1998). "Self-inactivating lentivirus vector for safe and efficient in vivo gene delivery." J Virol 72(12): 9873-9880.

5

Gene Therapy for HIV-1 Infection

Lisa Egerer, Dorothee von Laer and Janine Kimpel
Innsbruck Medical University, Department of Hygiene,
Microbiology and Social Medicine, Division of Virology, Innsbruck
Austria

1. Introduction

The introduction of the highly active antiretroviral therapy (HAART) for the treatment of HIV-1-infection has dramatically improved the quality of life and the survival of HIV-infected patients. HAART can effectively suppress virus replication and thereby helps to preserve immune functions. However, as HIV-1 persists in latently infected reservoirs (Finzi et al., 1997), complete eradication of the virus by antiretroviral drugs has never been achieved and life-long treatment is required. Moreover, emerging viral resistance and drug toxicity restrict long-term therapeutic efficacy (Brinkman et al., 1999; Vigouroux et al., 1999). As a consequence, HAART has not had a major impact on the global prevalence of HIV-infection and there is no vaccine in sight that could prevent further virus spread.

In addition to HAART and vaccines, gene therapy approaches for HIV-1 infection have been under investigation for more than two decades. Gene therapy could theoretically overcome the limitations of standard antiretroviral drug therapy and facilitate sustained suppression of virus replication after only few treatment cycles. Moreover, the choice of adequate genes or combinations of genes and expression systems could greatly reduce toxicity and prevent the generation of resistant virus strains. Although gene therapy is an expensive and technically challenging therapy today, future developments could simplify the procedures involved and bring down costs. Two basic gene therapeutic strategies for immune reconstitution of AIDS patients have been developed and the safety and efficacy of different approaches have been examined in preclinical and clinical studies. The first strategy aims to specifically kill HIV-infected cells by enhancing the antiviral host immune responses. The second approach, termed 'intracellular immunization', is based on the expression of antiviral genes that prevent HIV-1 replication in its target cells. Furthermore, therapeutic or prophylactic vaccination strategies that aim to enhance anti-HIV immunity and use DNA or viral vectors to express the viral antigens can formally be classified as gene therapy approaches. However, such vaccination strategies are not in the scope of this review.

2. Enhancing HIV-specific immunity: Adoptive transfer of CD8$^+$ T cells

The striking ability of HIV-1 to evade control by the host immune system is a fundamental problem in AIDS pathogenesis. Although most patients develop natural anti-HIV immune responses, the virus does not possess the immunogenicity to mount long-lasting responses strong enough to entirely suppress replication and to allow complete virus eradication from the body. In fact, most affected individuals initially develop immunodominant CD8$^+$ T cell (cytotoxic T lymphocyte, CTL) responses during the acute phase of HIV-1 infection, resulting in transient virus control and a decrease in plasma viremia (Borrow et al., 1994). The importance of CTLs was further confirmed in experiments with SIV-infected non-human primates, where acute infection could not be controlled in animals depleted of CD8[+] T lymphocytes (Schmitz et al., 1999). There is a strong negative correlation between emergence of virus-specific CTLs and the viral set point, as patients with strong early CTL responses show significantly lower viral set points and a slower disease progression (Streeck et al., 2009). However, later, during the chronic phase of HIV-1 infection generation of CD8[+] T cell responses seems to be impaired and dysfunctional CTLs fail to control virus replication in most patients. In contrast, long-term non-progressors – individuals which are HIV-1 seropositive, but do not progress to AIDS – retain high levels of virus-specific T cells, indicating that functional CTL responses are crucial for efficient virus control also in chronic infection (Rinaldo et al., 1995).

One reason for the failure of HIV-specific immunity during the chronic stage of infection may be the high variability of the virus resulting from a high replication rate and error-prone reverse transcription (Phillips et al., 1991). Moreover, HIV-1 attacks the immune system itself, the CD4[+] helper T cell being its major target cell. This results in the preferential infection and a massive loss of HIV-specific CD4[+] T cells already early upon infection, as the virus-specific helper cells migrate to the site of infection where they become activated thereby becoming more susceptible to HIV-1 infection (Demoustier et al., 2002; Douek et al., 2002). Yet, virus-specific CD4[+] T cells are urgently needed to help generating strong, durable immune responses and their absence impairs CTL activation and maturation (Kemball et al., 2007; Matloubian et al., 1994). In addition, progressive exhaustion of virus-specific CD8[+] T cells is a hallmark of the chronic immune activation during ongoing HIV-1 infection. Here, the constant antigen persistence prevents contraction of the effector T cell pool and development of long-lived memory cells. Instead, a stepwise exhaustion characterized by metabolic and transcriptional changes, reduced cytokine and chemokine secretion, loss of proliferation capacity and cytolytic activity is observed, resulting in impaired CTL effector functions and finally apoptosis (Shankar et al., 2000; Trimble & Lieberman, 1998).

Boosting of the natural CTL responses against HIV-1 by cell and gene therapeutic strategies may help to overcome these problems. For this purpose two different strategies have been developed; the adoptive transfer of autologous antigen-specific T cells after *ex vivo* selection and expansion, and the infusion of genetically armed CD8[+] T cells expressing HIV-specific T cell receptors (TCRs). A therapy combining these approaches with the protection of CD4[+] T cells to preserve important T-helper cell functions could potentially impact infection dynamics and ultimately facilitate clearance of the virus.

The adoptive transfer of autologous, antigen-specific CD8[+] T cell clones has been used successfully to treat persistent viral infections and cancer. The allogeneic organ transplantation from cytomegalovirus or Epstein-Barr virus seropositive donors, for instance, is associated with risks for the recipient, if untreated. Co-transplantation of virus-antigen-specific T cells isolated from the donor and expanded *in vitro*, enhanced T cell immunity to the viruses and prevented adverse effects in the immunosuppressed recipients (Heslop et al., 1996; Walter et al., 1995). For HIV-1, however, the transfer of *ex vivo* expanded virus-specific CTLs had only limited success in patients so far. In a study reported by Brodie et al. autologous Gag-specific CTLs were isolated and reinfused into HIV-positive individuals (Brodie et al., 1999). The CTLs engrafted in the patients and were found to migrate to the lymph nodes, which are the major sites of HIV-1 replication (Brodie et al.,

000; Hufert et al., 1997). However, although the CTLs were capable of lysing HIV-1 infected ells *in vivo*, only a transient effect on virus replication was observed (Brodie et al., 1999; Brodie et al., 2000). A major problem of this therapeutic concept is that the CTLs isolated rom patients with advanced disease are often exhausted and terminally differentiated and ack full effector functions. As *in vitro* expansion of these cells is accompanied with a further oss of function, the transferred cell numbers may be insufficient to induce long-term effects. Methods that allow generation of large numbers of fully functional CTLs therefore would be equired to facilitate success of this promising therapy approach.

An alternative to the isolation and expansion of existing antigen-specific T cells from a patient, is the genetic modification of cells resulting in the expression of recombinant HIV-specific receptors. The cell types used for this genetic 'redirection' can be peripheral blood T ells, but also hematopoietic stem cells (HSC), which can afterwards differentiate into immune cells targeting HIV-1. As the isolation and manipulation of T cells is currently easier to perform compared to stem-cell modification, all studies that have been conducted o far used peripheral blood T cells. The receptors used to redirect the immune cells to target HIV-1 can either be natural T cell receptors or artificial chimeric antigen receptors (CARs). For the natural TCRs, CTL clones with high avidity TCRs specific for the target antigens are selected *in vitro*. The alpha and beta chains of these TCRs are then cloned and used to ransduce patient T cells. This approach has been used successfully in the clinic to treat patients with melanoma, where in some cases tumor regression has been observed (Morgan et al., 2006). The isolation and cloning of high-avidity HIV-specific TCRs is also feasible. oseph and colleagues constructed a lentiviral vector expressing a TCR specific for the HIV-1 Gag epitope SL9. Transduction of human primary T cells led to the conversion of peripheral blood CD8+ T cells into HIV-specific CTLs (Joseph et al., 2008). These CTLs exerted anti-HIV activity *in vitro* and *in vivo* in a humanized mouse model. In a similar study, an SL9-specific TCR with enhanced affinity was shown to efficiently mediate control of HIV-1 *in vitro* (Varela-Rohena et al., 2008). Currently this approach is evaluated in a phase I clinical trial (www.ClinicalTrials.gov; identifier: NCT00991224). The use of natural TCRs to generate virus-specific CTLs is limited by the major histocompatibility complex (MHC)-restriction of the TCR. TCRs recognize peptides only if they are presented on a specific type of MHC. Therefore, T cells expressing a given TCR can only be used for treatment of MHC-matched patients. The clinical trial described above, for instance, can only include patients with the HLA-type A*02. For a broader application of this therapy concept a set of TCRs would be required that allows treatment of patients with various haplotypes. Besides, in gene modified CTLs, the genetically transferred TCR can mispair with the endogenous TCR, which may affect its function and lead to autoimmunity. Another drawback of the approach is the downregulation of MHC molecules in HIV-infected cells, which impedes the presentation of viral peptides and recognition by the CTLs (Sommermeyer et al., 2006).

CARs are chimeric antigen receptors composed of an extracellular antigen binding motive connected to an intracellular signal transduction domain via a flexible linker and a transmembrane domain. The antigen binding motive usually is an antigen-specific single-chain variable fragment derived from a monoclonal antibody, while the signal transduction part comes from the CD3 ζ-chain. CARs trigger an MHC-independent antigen recognition (Eshhar et al., 2001). Two CARs with HIV-1 specificity have been developed by Roberts and colleagues (Roberts et al., 1994). The antigen-binding part consists either of the gp120 binding domain from human CD4 or an antibody against gp41. T cells transduced with either of the receptors specifically recognized and killed HIV-infected cells *in vitro*. The receptor containing CD4 has been tested in three clinical trials. In these studies local effects on virus replication were observed, but unfortunately there was no overall change in viral load (Deeks et al., 2002; Mitsuyasu et al., 2000; Walker et al., 2000).

3. Intracellular immunization: Protection of CD4$^+$ T cells

The second gene therapeutic strategy for HIV-1 infection was termed 'intracellular immunization' (Baltimore, 1988) and involves the expression of an antiviral gene in cells susceptible to HIV-1 infection. The target cells for intracellular immunization strategies therefore are mainly peripheral T cells or hematopoietic stem cells. The gene product can either be a protein or an RNA that inhibits HIV-1 replication by interfering with crucial steps of the viral life cycle or by targeting a cellular factor required for virus replication. Efficient genetic protection of the HIV-1 target cell population, i.e. mainly CD4$^+$ T-helper cells, will deprive the virus of the possibility to produce progeny and is therefore expected to result in a drop of viral load and a regeneration of T cell counts. An additional antiviral effect can be achieved, if sufficient T-helper cell clones specific for HIV-1 antigens are protected against viral infection. These gene-protected CD4$^+$ T cells could support the immunologic control of viral replication, without risking infection facilitated by HIV-1 antigen activation. As mentioned above, previous studies have shown that HIV-specific T-helper cell clones, which are crucial for an effective immune control of HIV-1 replication, are preferentially infected by HIV and lost during the course of the disease (Douek et al., 2002).

3.1 Antiviral proteins

Various types of anti-HIV proteins have been developed over the past years. Dominant-negative forms of both, viral proteins and cellular proteins required for virus replication have been described. These dominant-negative mutant proteins antagonize the activity of their corresponding wild-type proteins and thus prevent viral replication. A transdominant form of the HIV-1 Rev protein, RevM10, has been extensively studied *in vitro* and *in vivo*. RevM10 prevents the export of genomic viral RNA from the nucleus and as a result inhibits production of progeny virus (Malim et al., 1989). In clinical trials genetic modification of CD4$^+$ T cells and CD34$^+$ hematopoietic stem cells with RevM10 has been shown to be safe and provide some selective survival advantage. However, no sustained absolute accumulation of gene-modified cells and accordingly no antiviral effect was observed (Morgan et al., 2005; Podsakoff et al., 2005; Ranga et al., 1998; Woffendin et al., 1996). Furthermore, transdominant mutants of HIV-1 Tat that prevent Tat transactiviation have been developed (Fraisier et al., 1998; Pearson et al., 1990), but were never tested in clinical trials. The same is true for transdominant forms of the HIV-1 proteins Gag (Trono et al., 1989) and Vif (Morgan et al., 1990; Vallanti et al., 2005).

Cellular proteins required for virus replication have also been targeted by dominant-negative mutants. Membrane expression of chemokine receptor 5 (CCR5), which acts as a co-receptor for HIV-1, has been blocked by transdominant negative CCR5 variants upon retroviral expression in human T cells (Luis Abad et al., 2003). Even though inhibition of virus replication was observed in the gene-modified cells, this concept was not pursued further. A truncated soluble form of the cell surface receptor CD4 (sCD4) has been described to protect T cells from entry of laboratory-adapted strains of HIV-1, however, inhibition was less efficient for primary virus isolates (Daar & Ho, 1991; Morgan et al., 1994; Morgan et al., 1990). In a clinical phase I study recombinant soluble CD4 was administered by continuous intravenous infusion to paediatric AIDS patients. Although the therapy was well tolerated, evidence of *in vivo* antiviral activity was not observed and consequently, sCD4 has never been investigated in gene therapy clinical trials (Husson et al., 1992).

Nevertheless, gene therapeutic strategies targeting early steps in the viral life cycle are expected to be the most promising therapeutics for HIV/AIDS, as discussed below. Protein-based inhibitors targeting the virus entry process are thought to be especially powerful tools as they can prevent infection of the cell. Our group has previously developed a membrane-anchored gp41-derived HIV-1 fusion inhibitor, maC46. This protein is expressed on the surface of T cells after transduction with retroviral or lentiviral vectors (Egelhofer et al., 2004; Hermann et al., 2009b; Perez et al., 2005). The protein binds to the HIV-1 gp41 heptad repeat 1 region thereby interfering with six-helix bundle formation during the viral and cellular membrane fusion process. MaC46 expressing T cells are almost completely protected from HIV-1 entry and have a strong selective survival advantage compared to unmodified cells *in vitro* and in mouse models of HIV-1 infection (Egelhofer et al., 2004; Hermann et al., 2009a; Kimpel et al., 2010). Likewise, maC46 has been shown to be one of the most potent anti-HIV gene products currently available (Kimpel et al., 2010). However, in a clinical trial with 10 HIV-1-infected patients with advanced disease and HAART failure, infusion of autologous CD4+ T cells genetically modified to express maC46 did not achieve sustained success. Although a significant rise in overall CD4+ T cell counts was observed in this study, the gene-protected cells did not accumulate over time and consequently, viral loads were not affected (van Lunzen et al., 2007). Recently, we described a secreted version of the fusion inhibitory C46 molecule. This '*in vivo* secreted antiviral entry inhibitor' (iSAVE) showed promising anti-HIV activity *in vitro* and has the potential to confer an overall antiviral effect *in vivo* despite low levels of gene marking (Egerer et al., 2011).

A different protein-based approach for HIV-1 gene therapy uses antibodies that bind and inactivate proteins and enzymes required for virus replication. Antibodies can be expressed within gene-modified cells as single-chain fragments (scFv), so-called intrabodies, or they can be secreted into the supernatant as neutralizing antibodies. Various intrabodies against HIV-1 proteins including Tat, Vif, Reverse Transcriptase and Integrase have been shown to inhibit virus replication in gene-modified cells *in vitro* (Goncalves et al., 2002; Kitamura et al., 1999; Levy-Mintz et al., 1996; Mhashilkar et al., 1995; Shaheen et al., 1996). Moreover, intrabodies against the viral co-receptors CXCR4 and CCR5 have been designed that retain these proteins in the ER (BouHamdan et al., 2001; Cordelier et al., 2004; Swan et al., 2006). Although these approaches efficiently inhibited HIV-1 replication in cell culture systems, intrabody techniques have not been further evaluated *in vivo*. The secreted version of the broadly neutralizing anti-gp41 monoclonal antibody 2F5 has been analyzed in a humanized mouse model of HIV-1 infection (Sanhadji et al., 2000). In this study, gene-modified cell lines expressing the antibody were implanted as neo-organs into immunodeficient mice repopulated with human CD4+ T cells. The neo-organs engrafted in the peritoneum and permitted continuous secretion of the antibody. Upon infection of the mice with HIV-1, viral loads were greatly reduced compared to control animals. However, due to safety problems, the implantation of neo-organs is not an option for treatment of patients. Recently, Joseph and colleagues reported the secretion of therapeutic concentrations of the broadly neutralizing anti-gp120 antibody 2G12 in humanized mice. Here, immunodeficient mice were transplanted with human hematopoietic stem cells that had previously been modified with a lentiviral vector encoding 2G12. The transduced stem cells differentiated into human progeny cells that secreted the functional antibody into the serum. This genetic immunization clearly reduced viral burden upon HIV-1 infection (Joseph et al., 2010). Another strategy described by Sarkar et al. involves the expression of a modified version of the Cre recombinase (termed Tre) in HIV-1 infected cells. This recombinase has been engineered in a directed evolution approach to recombine a sequence present in the HIV-1 LTRs resulting in site-specific excision of the integrated provirus from an HIV-1 infected host cell genome (Sarkar et al., 2007). Even though proof-of-concept was provided *in vitro*, this approach is far from clinical application as the Tre recombinase is specific for one exclusive LTR sequence and does not recognize the LTRs of other virus strains.

Finally, zinc finger nucleases (ZFNs) are a novel tool in protein-based HIV-1 gene therapy. ZFNs are artificial fusion proteins composed of a DNA-binding and a DNA-cleavage domain. They can be engineered to bind any desired genome sequence and induce double-strand breaks in the targeted DNA. Repair of the damaged DNA is associated with the introduction of high-frequency deletions and insertions at the site of cleavage. Individuals with a naturally occurring 32 bp deletion mutant of the CCR5 receptor (CCR5Δ32) are perfectly healthy, but resistant to infection with R5-tropic strains of HIV-1 (Huang et al., 1996; Samson et al., 1996). Consequently, disruption of the CCR5 locus using ZFNs is not expected to alter immune functions, making it an ideal target for ZFN-based gene therapy. CCR5-specific ZFNs have been studied *in vitro* and in animal models and were shown to render the treated cells resistant to HIV-1 infection (Holt et al., 2010; Perez et al., 2008). Currently three clinical trials are recruiting patients to test this promising approach *in vivo* (www.ClinicalTrials.gov; identifier: NCT01044654, NCT01252641 and NCT00842634).

3.2 Antiviral RNAs

Antiviral RNAs for intracellular immunization can be grouped into four major categories: RNA interference (RNAi), ribozymes, anti-sense RNAs and RNA decoys. Several RNAi-based gene therapy regimens for treatment of HIV-1 infection have proven to be effective in blocking viral replication by selective degradation of either viral RNAs or mRNAs of host factors that are essential for HIV-1 replication. Basically all HIV-1 RNAs have been successfully downregulated by RNAi *in vitro* (Chang et al., 2005; Coburn & Cullen, 2002; Jacque et al., 2002; N. S. Lee et al., 2002; Novina et al., 2002). However, systemic delivery of siRNAs to the relevant cell types *in vivo* is difficult. Kumar and colleagues administered antiviral siRNAs conjugated to a T cell-specific single-chain antibody that undergoes internalization upon binding to T cell surface receptors to humanized mice. This approach allowed targeted delivery of the siRNAs to T cells, which resulted in effective virus inhibition and preserved CD4+ T cell numbers (Kumar et al., 2008). An alternative to the regular injection of exogenous siRNAs is the expression of shRNAs directly in the HIV-1 target cells, but achieving stable transgene expression in the gene-modified cells is a challenge. Yet, constant endogenous expression would be required to obtain efficient suppression of HIV-1 replication and prevent viral escape mutants. At the same time, expression levels have to be tightly regulated in order to avoid cellular toxicity, as saturation of the cellular small RNA-processing pathway due to overexpression of shRNAs can lead to downregulation of cellular microRNAs (miRNAs) and cause severe toxicity (Grimm et al., 2006). Insertion of shRNAs into a natural miRNA backbone has been shown to reduce such toxic effects (McBride et al., 2008).

The high mutation rate of HIV-1 is an additional challenge in developing RNAi-based therapeutics, as a single point mutation within the targeted HIV-1 RNA sequence can abolish function of small RNAs and escape mutants emerge rapidly (Boden et al., 2003; Das et al., 2004; Sabariegos et al., 2006). This problem can be partly overcome by using a combination of small RNAs targeting several conserved regions of the viral genome and ideally expressed from a single therapeutic vector (ter Brake et al., 2006). Alternatively, cellular genes required for virus replication can be targeted, including CD4, CXCR4, CCR5, nuclear factor κB, or LEDGF/p75, which all have been shown to be susceptible to RNAi silencing, thereby blocking viral entry or replication (Anderson & Akkina, 2005; Cordelier et al., 2003; Novina et al., 2002; Surabhi & Gaynor, 2002; Vandekerckhove et al., 2006). The CCR5 receptor is a particularly promising target, as disruption of the CCR5 gene does not alter immune functions (Huang et al., 1996; Samson et al., 1996). A highly potent and non-cytotoxic siRNA directed against CCR5 has been developed by the group of Irvin Chen. Stable long-term expression of the siRNA and silencing of the CCR5 gene was observed after transplantation of gene-modified CD34+ hematopoietic progenitor cells in non-human primates. Gene-modified cells isolated from the animals were resistant to simian immunodeficiency virus infection *ex vivo* (An et al., 2007; Liang et al., 2010). The only RNAi approach that has been examined in patients so far is a tat/rev specific short hairpin RNA, which was tested in combination with a ribozyme targeting CCR5 and a TAR decoy in four patients receiving CD34+ hematopoietic progenitor cell transplantation due to AIDS-related lymphoma. In this recently reported clinical trial, stable, but low-level expression of the antiviral RNAs from gene-modified cells was observed for up to 24 months; however, there were no major effects on viral load (DiGiusto et al., 2010).

Ribozymes are anti-sense RNA molecules with enzymatic activity that have been designed to target and site-specifically cleave essential viral RNAs or cellular mRNAs leading to gene silencing. Many ribozyme-based strategies for treatment of HIV-1 infection have been developed and show promising antiviral activity *in vitro* (Hotchkiss et al., 2004; Sarver et al., 1990; Zhou et al., 1994). Three ribozymes directed against HIV-1 tat/vrp (Amado et al., 2004; Macpherson et al., 2005; Mitsuyasu et al., 2009), HIV-1 rev/tat (Michienzi et al., 2003) and the viral U5 leader region (Wong-Staal et al., 1998) have already been tested in separate clinical trials. The gene transfer was proven to be safe in all studies, but none showed significant antiviral efficacy. As mentioned above, a CCR5-specific ribozyme has recently been analyzed in the clinic in combination with two other types of anti-HIV RNAs, but did not have a major influence on HIV-1 replication (DiGiusto et al., 2010).

Antisense RNAs are short or long single-stranded RNA molecules binding to complementary HIV-1 mRNAs resulting in the formation of non-functional duplexes. Antisense molecules directed against the HIV-1 trans-activation response element (TAR) and the viral envelope RNA have been developed (Humeau et al., 2004; Lu et al., 2004; Vickers et al., 1991). The conditionally replicating lentiviral vector VRX496™ encodes a long antisense gene against the HIV-1 envelope. In clinical trials patients received autologous CD4+ T cells transduced with VRX496™. A stabilization of viral load and slightly increased CD4+ T cell counts were observed, the significance of these results, however, remains unclear (Levine et al., 2006).

In contrast to the antiviral RNA molecules described above, RNA decoys do not attack the HIV-1 RNA. Instead, these small RNA fragments, which are derived from cis-acting elements in the viral genome, competitively bind and sequester viral proteins, thereby interfering with HIV-1 replication. Anti-HIV decoys are mainly based on the HIV-1 regulatory sequences TAR and Rev-responsive-element (RRE), which are bound by the two HIV-1 regulatory proteins Tat and Rev, respectively. The TAR element is a sequence contained in the 5' region of all HIV-1 mRNAs, which forms a stable stem-loop structure (Baudin et al., 1993; Muesing et al., 1987). Binding of the HIV-1 Tat (trans-activator) protein to the TAR element mediates increased viral gene expression (Keen et al., 1996); moreover, the TAR region is required for initiation of reverse transcription (Harrich et al., 1996). Disruption of the Tat/TAR interaction by TAR decoy RNA was shown to effectively prevent HIV-1 replication *in vitro* (Sullenger et al., 1990, 1991). A combination of three antiviral RNAs including a TAR decoy was successfully tested in humanized mouse models of HIV-1 infection (Anderson et al., 2007) and, as mentioned above, was shown to be safe in a clinical trial, although only minor effects on HIV-1 infection could be observed (DiGiusto et al., 2010). Interaction of the viral Rev protein with the RRE is critically required for transport of the unspliced genomic viral mRNA to the cytoplasm (Olsen et al., 1990). RRE decoys provide strong inhibition of HIV-1 replication by blocking the nuclear export of genomic HIV-1 RNA (T. C. Lee et al., 1992; Michienzi et al., 2006). Genetic modification of CD34+ hematopoietic stem cells by retroviral transfer of an RRE decoy gene followed by infusion of the gene-modified cells, was shown to be safe in a clinical trial with paediatric AIDS patients. However, transduction and engraftment levels were very low and no antiviral effect was observed (Kohn et al., 1999).

3.3 The mode of action: Classification of antiviral genes

The impact of gene-modified cells on systemic HIV-1 kinetics depends critically on the stage of the viral replication cycle at which the inhibition occurs. The antiviral genes can accordingly be grouped into three classes, depending on their effect on the viral life cycle (von Laer et al., 2006). Class I genes inhibit the first steps of the replication cycle prior to integration of the proviral DNA into the host cell genome and thus prevent infection of the cell. Hence, class I includes genes encoding entry inhibitors, as well as inhibitors of reverse transcription and integration. Class II genes have no effect on early steps of the viral replication cycle, but prevent the expression of viral RNA or proteins. Thus, they inhibit the production of infectious virus progeny and the viral cytopathic effect, however, integration of the proviral genome into the host cell chromosomes is not hindered. Cells expressing a class II gene and infected with HIV-1 resemble latently infected cells and according to computer simulations accumulate with time, counteracting the antiviral effect (von Laer et al., 2006). Furthermore, reverse transcription, which can give rise to resistant virus variants, is not inhibited by class II genes. Class III genes interfere with late steps in the viral life cycle such as virion assembly and budding. Consequently, they neither protect the infected cell from recognition by the immune system, as viral protein production is not inhibited, nor from the viral cytopathic effect. Therefore, class III genes alone are not expected to have an overall antiviral effect unless high percentages of cells are genetically modified.

Mathematical modelling predicts that only genes inhibiting early steps in the viral replication cycle provide a selective advantage strong enough to allow for the selection and accumulation of the gene modified cells (Lund et al., 1997; von Laer et al., 2006). Consequently, class I genes are the most promising candidates for successful intracellular immunization strategies. The group of Warner Greene recently found that in *ex vivo* cultures of human tonsils infected with HIV-1 the vast majority of CD4+ T cells died due to non-productive abortive infection. In these non-permissive cells DNA reverse transcription intermediates elicited proapoptotic responses resulting in release of proinflammatory cytokines and caspase-mediated cell death (Doitsh et al., 2010). Inhibition of HIV-1 entry or early steps of reverse transcription could protect the cells from these fatal effects, indicating that very early inhibitors are even more favorable, as they can prevent the massive 'bystander" killing observed in HIV-1 infection. However, combination of several antiviral genes, targeting different steps in the viral life cycle might synergize most efficiently and could be the only way to achieve sustained suppression of HIV-1 replication.

3.4 Selective survival advantage and bystander effect

The major drawback of intracellular immunization approaches is the huge number of HIV-1 target cells in the human body (> 10^{11}) that cannot be genetically modified with the available technologies. The frequencies of gene-modified CD4+ T cells achieved in vivo, whether by T cell or stem cell targeting, have been disappointingly low, in the range of 0,01% to 1%, or less (Amado et al., 2004; Levine et al., 2006; Macpherson et al., 2005; Morgan et al., 2005; van Lunzen et al., 2007). A significant impact of these few genetically HIV-resistant cells is neither expected on overall HIV-1 infection dynamics nor on immune reconstitution. However, if the gene-protected cells are able to proliferate and preferentially survive compared with unmodified cells, they could accumulate with time and progressively repopulate the immune system (Lund et al., 1997; von Laer et al., 2006). A number of gene products that have been developed could theoretically mediate such a selective survival advantage of the transduced cells as they have been shown to efficiently suppress virus replication and protect the cells from the viral cytopathic effect in vitro. However, selective accumulation of gene-protected cells has never been observed in clinical trials so far. In a comparative study, we recently evaluated three intracellular immunization strategies that had previously been used in the clinic, with respect to antiviral activity and survival advantage (Kimpel et al., 2010): (1) the viral entry inhibitor maC46 (class I gene); (2) an HIV-1 tat/rev-specific small hairpin (sh) RNA (class II gene); and (3) an RNA antisense gene specific for the HIV-1 envelope (class II gene). We found robust inhibition of HIV-1 replication with the fusion inhibitor maC46 and the antisense envelope inhibitor. Interestingly, and importantly, a survival advantage was merely demonstrated for cells expressing the maC46 fusion inhibitor both in vitro and in vivo in a humanized xenotransplant mouse model (Kimpel et al., 2010). This finding confirms in silico predictions stating that only class I genes can confer a sufficient selective advantage to allow preferential survival and accumulation of gene-protected, non-infected cells in vivo (von Laer et al., 2006). However, even this highly active fusion inhibitor failed to show a clear accumulation of gene-protected cells to therapeutic levels in a previous clinical trial in 10 AIDS patients (van Lunzen et al., 2007). These data show that efficient engraftment and proliferation of the gene-protected cells remain a major challenge in gene therapy for HIV-1 infection.
Yet, such a strong selection and accumulation may not be required for a secreted antiviral gene product. Secreted antiviral proteins or peptides are expected to produce a bystander effect on unmodified neighboring cells, thereby suppressing virus replication and protecting the overall T cell pool even at low levels of gene modification. Such a bystander effect can only be conferred by antiviral proteins, but not by RNAs, as secretion is limited to proteins and peptides. However, the number of reports on secreted antiviral proteins in HIV-1 gene therapy is still very limited. Examples are neutralizing antibodies (Sanhadji et al., 2000), truncated soluble CD4 (Morgan et al., 1994; Morgan et al., 1990) and interferon β (Gay et al., 2004). We have recently reported the generation of an in vivo secreted antiviral entry inhibitor (iSAVE), which exerted a strong bystander effect in cell culture (Egerer et al., 2011). Lymphatic tissue is the major site of HIV-1 replication and thus T or B cells could be an ideal target cell for gene therapy approaches based on secreted gene products. Secretion of

antiviral proteins directly in the lymphoid tissues is likely to lead to high and stable local peptide concentrations and to substantially suppress virus replication. On the other hand, secreted antiviral gene products no longer depend on expression in HIV-1 target cells, but instead several other cell types could serve as producer cells in the body. This facilitates the development of direct *in vivo* gene transfer approaches (e.g. by the use of AAV-vectors), making gene therapy less complex and practicable also for treatment of patients in the developing world. Furthermore, such strategies have the potential for application as a gene transfer vaccine in a prophylactic setting. In this regard, a secreted antiviral gene product could for instance be used as a genetic topical microbicide that aims at the prevention of HIV-1 mucosal transmission. High-level secretion of the antiviral molecules from gene-modified target cells in the vagina or rectum has the potential to confer local sterilizing immunity, thus preventing HIV-1 genital transmission.

3.5 Immunogenicity of the antiviral gene product
Gene therapeutic strategies based on the expression of antiviral proteins are limited by the potential immunogenicity of the antiviral gene product, which can severely impair survival of the transduced cells. Antiviral RNAs have an advantage here, as they generally lack immunogenicity. Also, natural or only slightly altered variants of human proteins are not expected to mount significant immune responses. However, many antiviral proteins are non-self and bear the risk of eliciting a cellular immune response. Thus, to prevent selective deletion of the gene-modified cells by transgene-specific CTLs, it is necessary to minimize or eliminate immunogenicity of the antiviral gene product. The fusion of a Glycine-Alanine repeat derived from the Epstein-Barr virus nuclear antigen 1 (EBNA-1) to immunogenic proteins, such as transdominant HIV-1 Gag, has been shown to significantly reduce immunogenicity and prolong survival of transduced cells *in vivo* (Hammer et al., 2008). The Glycine-Alanine repeat protects the fusion protein from proteasomal degradation and prevents subsequent presentation of potentially immunogenic peptides on MHC class I molecules (Levitskaya et al., 1997). This frustrates the induction of CTLs directed against the transgene product and conceals it from CTL-mediated immune attack.
Another possibility to facilitate immune-evasion, which is feasible for small antiviral peptides only, is the generation of peptides which are devoid of MHC class I epitopes. Our group recently developed antiviral C peptides with potentially reduced immunogenicity, by mutating *in silico*-predicted immunodominant CTL epitopes within the peptide sequence. The mutated peptides retained excellent anti-HIV activity, while no immune responses could be detected in ELIspot assays (unpublished data).

3.6 The target cell for intracellular immunization strategies
Target cells for intracellular immunization are usually cells that can become infected with HIV-1 (mainly CD4+ T cells) or their progenitors (hematopoietic stem cells). For gene therapeutic approaches based on secreted antiviral molecules, the modification of non-HIV-target cells is also feasible. So far, mature T cells and hematopoietic stem cells have been used in clinical trials. Advantages and disadvantages of both cell types are summarized in Table 1. Both have in common that they are relatively easy to obtain, and there are protocols for efficient *ex vivo* cultivation and transduction available. Gene modification of HSC has greater therapeutic potential, as it could restore a normal T cell repertoire, allow regeneration of HIV-specific T-helper cells and also protect monocytes/macrophages. However, current stem-cell based therapies are associated with greater risks and toxicity.

Target cell	T cell	HSC
Easy to obtain	++	+
Conditioning required	-	+
Cell dose	$>10^{10}$	10^8-10^9
Regeneration of T cell repertoire	-	+
Protection of all HIV-1 target cells	-	+
Insertional mutagenesis	Limited	+

Table 1. The target cell: T cells versus hematopoietic stem cells (HSC).

4. Vector systems for gene transfer

The choice of the vector system may have a major impact on the efficacy of HIV-1 gene therapy approaches. There is no ideal vector suitable for all purposes, but the pros and cons have to be balanced for each application. Table 2 summarizes advantages and disadvantages of several vector systems commonly used for gene transfer.

Vector type	Application	Titer	Packaging capacity	Inte-gration	Immuno-genicity	Clinical trials
Adenoviral	ex vivo + in vivo	10^{13} VP/ml	up to 36 kb	-	++	+
AAV	in vivo	10^{13} VP/ml	3-5 kb	only with Rep	+	+
Gamma-retroviral	ex vivo	10^5-10^7 TU/ml	8-10 kb	+	-	+
Lentiviral	ex vivo	10^7 TU/ml (10^9-10^{10} TU/ml)*	up to 10 kb	+	-	+
SV-40	ex vivo	10^{12} VP/ml	up to 5 kb	+	-	-
Foamyviral	ex vivo	10^5-10^6 TU/ml (10^7 TU/ml)*	>9 kb	+	-	-

Table 2. Vector systems for gene transfer in HIV-1 gene therapy.
AAV, Adeno-Associated Virus; kb, kilo bases; SV-40, Simian Virus-40; TU, transducing units; VP, vector particles; * after concentration.

Basic questions to be asked are, whether *ex vivo* or *in vivo* gene transfer is preferred and if long-term expression of the gene product is required. To our knowledge, a vector system that allows efficient direct *in vivo* gene transfer specifically into CD4+ T cells or HSC has not been developed so far. Therefore, approaches based on modification of these cell types (arming of T cells with TCRs or CARs, most intracellular immunizations) always rely on *ex vivo* gene transfer. In contrast, genes encoding secreted antiviral molecules may also be delivered to distinct production sites (e.g. liver, muscle) directly *in vivo* using adenovirus (Ad) or adeno-associated virus (AAV)-derived vectors. The second basic question deals with the long-term-expression of the transferred antiviral gene. Strategies involving arming of T cells with antigen-specific receptors and intracellular immunization require stable and long-lasting production of the antiviral molecules in proliferating cells (T cells or HSC). Consequently, for such approaches, integrating vectors are favorable. These include SV-40 vectors and vectors derived from retroviruses. Stable expression of secreted gene products from slowly dividing cells like liver or muscle cells may also be achieved using non-integrating vectors like adenoviral or AAV vectors.

4.1 Non-integrating viral vectors

The only vectors systems that currently allow direct *in vivo* gene transfer are non-integrating viral vectors. As their genome is not stably incorporated into the host cell chromosomes, these vectors have an improved safety profile compared to integrating vectors. For a direct *in vivo* application of integrating vectors, efficient systems for targeted vector delivery would be required, which are not yet available for use in man. Despite the lack of integration, non-integrating vector systems still allow sustained long-term transgene expression, if cells or tissues with a slow turnover are targeted, where the vector genome can stably persist. Moreover, non-integrating vectors can also be used to deliver zinc finger nucleases, which require only transient expression, to diving cells. A number of non-integrating viral vectors have been evaluated for gene transfer. Currently, adenoviral vectors and vectors derived from the adeno-associated virus are in the focus of interest. Accordingly, Ad vectors are currently used in the above mentioned clinical trials to deliver CCR5-specific zinc finger nucleases to T cells *ex vivo*.

Recombinant adenoviral vectors have been utilized as a gene transfer and vaccine platform for a long time. Ad vectors provide a huge packaging capacity (36 kb), allowing the transfer also of multiple therapeutic genes. Moreover, high-titer production is possible, facilitating direct *in vivo* application with high transduction efficacies. The major obstacle of adenoviral vectors is pre-existing immunity in the general human population. Vector-mediated immune responses cause rapid clearance of Ad vectors, moreover, severe side effects have been observed. This can be partly overcome by using engineered adenovirus serotypes (Dharmapuri et al., 2009). Moreover, production of Ad vectors is prone to contamination with replication competent adenovirus, which complicates clinical grade vector production.

AAV is a non-pathogenic virus that belongs to the family of Parvoviridae. AAV-derived vectors have recently gained particular interest as gene transfer vehicles due to their apathogenicity and very low immunogenicity. Moreover, they can be used for direct *in vivo* gene delivery to both dividing and non-dividing cells. AAV can infect a variety of cell types *in vivo* and different serotypes of AAV have been shown to have varying preferences in their target cell type of choice (Chao et al., 2000; Halbert et al., 2000). However, AAV variants with a preference for T cells or hematopoietic stem cells have not been described. In the absence of the viral Rep protein, AAV vectors do not integrate into the host cell genome, but are maintained in episomal form in the nucleus. This allows very stable transgene expression without causing genotoxicity. The major disadvantage of AAV vectors is their small packaging capacity. In addition, vector production used to be laborious in the past and large-scale manufacturing for clinical trials was complicated. However, novel production systems facilitate faster and simpler high-titer production of AAV vectors in scaleable processes (Clement et al., 2009; Lock et al., 2010).

4.2 Integrating viral vectors

Vectors derived from gamma-retroviruses (mostly murine leukaemia virus) and lentiviruses (HIV-1) have been used in numerous clinical trials, including *ex vivo* gene transfer trials for HIV-1 infection (DiGiusto et al., 2010; van Lunzen et al., 2007). Replication incompetent viral vectors are made from these viruses by deletion of all genes encoding enzymes and structural proteins (Gag, Pol, Env) from the viral genome. These genes have to be added *in trans* to produce infectious, but replication incompetent, vector particles. The tropism of the vector particles can be altered by modification of the envelope glycoprotein or by pseudotyping with the envelope protein from a different virus (Frecha et al., 2008; Funke et al., 2008). A major difference between gamma-retroviral and lentiviral vectors is that lentiviruses can infect dividing as well as non-dividing cells. In contrast, gamma-retroviruses can only transduce dividing cells, as they rely on the collapse of the nuclear membrane during mitosis to enter the nucleus (Roe et al., 1993). Lentiviral transduction protocols therefore usually require a shorter period of pre-activation of the cells. As prolonged *in vitro* culture is associated with differentiation and a loss of *in vivo* repopulation potential, especially for HSC, lentiviral vectors have an advantage here. However, large-scale production of lentiviral vectors is more difficult than gamma-retroviral vector production due to a lack of stable packaging cell lines.

Both, gamma-retroviral and lentiviral vectors integrate randomly into the host cell genome. While gamma-retroviruses usually integrate near transcriptional start sites, lentiviruses have a preference for transcribed regions (Mitchell et al., 2004). As a consequence, transduction with these vectors is always associated with a risk of transformation due to insertional mutagenesis. Indeed, severe side effects caused by vector integration have been reported in gene therapy clinical trials (Hacein-Bey-Abina et al., 2008; Howe et al., 2008). Experiments in animal models showed that vector genotoxicity is higher for transduction of hematopoietic stem cells than for mature T cells (Newrzela et al., 2008) and lower for self inactivating (SIN) vectors compared to conventional long terminal repeat (LTR)-driven vectors (Modlich et al., 2009). SIN vectors have deletions in the promotor and enhancer elements of the 3'LTR, thereby reducing the genotoxic risks, as transactivation of neighboring protooncogenes is less likely. In these vectors, expression of the transgene cassette is driven from an internal promoter.

Foamyviruses also belong to the family of retroviruses. Foamyviral vectors are generated by deleting enzymes and structural genes from the viral genome and adding these *in trans* during vector production (Rethwilm, 2007). Foamyvirus-derived vectors efficiently transduce resting cells, which makes them an ideal tool to transduce hematopoietic stem cells *ex vivo* (Hirata et al., 1996; Leurs et al., 2003). However, just like SV-40 vectors, foamyviral vectors have not yet been tested in clinical trials.

Simian virus-40 (SV-40) belongs to the family of Polyomaviridae. It has been one of the first viruses used as a gene transfer vehicle (Gething & Sambrook, 1981). For the construction of gene transfer vectors, all coding sequences except the origin of replication and the packaging signal can be deleted from wild type SV-40 (Strayer et al., 2002). The resulting vectors efficiently transduce hematopoietic stem cells and lymphocytes *in vitro*, but have never been tested in clinical trials (Strayer et al., 2005).

4.3 Targeted integration

Past clinical trials have shown that random integration of a transgene delivered by an integrating vector bears the risk of severe side effects due to insertional mutagenesis.

Targeted integration of transgenes into the host cell genome is therefore expected to massively increase safety. The CCR5 locus is considered to be a safe harbor for transgene integration, as a naturally occurring deletion of 32 bp in the coding sequence for CCR5 causes no clinical symptoms. Moreover, this deletion is associated with a reduced susceptibility for HIV-1 infection (Huang et al., 1996; Samson et al., 1996). Therefore, targeted integration of an anti-HIV transgene into the CCR5 locus could even provide an additional antiviral effect, due to disruption of the CCR5 gene. Zinc finger nucleases binding to CCR5 have been used *in vitro* and in animal models to destroy the CCR5 locus, rendering the treated cells resistant to HIV-1 infection (Holt et al., 2010; Perez et al., 2008). A combination of this approach with targeted integration of antiviral genes holds especially great promise. For such a strategy a donor DNA encoding the desired antiviral gene and containing sequences homologous to the target site has to be present in the cells during the repair of ZFN-induced double-strand breaks by cellular enzymes. This results in the incorporation of the foreign DNA into the targeted region of the host genome by non-homologous end joining mediated by the cellular DNA repair machinery (Cathomen & Joung, 2008). Such approaches require only transient expression of the zinc finger nuclease and the transgene to achieve stable integration into the host cell genome, which allows use of non-integrating vector systems for gene transfer.

As an alternative to zinc finger nucleases, AAV vectors that contain the viral Rep protein in *cis* or in *trans* can also be used for targeted integration, as in the presence of Rep, AAV vectors target their genome preferentially to a locus on the human chromosome 19, termed AAVS1, without causing any apparent adverse effects (Surosky et al., 1997). As the CCR5 locus, AAVS1 is thus considered a safe harbor for vector integration.

5. Conclusions

Gene therapeutic approaches for the treatment and possibly prevention of HIV-1 infection hold considerable promise. Although the final breakthrough has not yet been achieved in clinical trials, there has been substantial progress over the last years and future developments might leverage this technology. The major reason for the limited efficacy seen in all HIV-1 gene therapy clinical trials up to now has been the insufficient level of gene modification. It will therefore be particularly important to develop optimized therapeutic regimen and gene transfer technologies that allow therapeutically effective engraftment levels of functional, gene modified cells. Efficient protection of CD4+ T cells could possibly be achieved by using a combination of antiviral genes targeting different steps of the viral life cycle, conferring a substantial *in vivo* selective survival advantage and ideally also a therapeutic bystander effect on unmodified cells. This review describes the potent gene therapeutic tools that have been developed in the past years and it will be exciting to see if these can be integrated into an effective treatment regimen in the near future.

6. References

Amado, R. G.; Mitsuyasu, R. T.; Rosenblatt, J. D.; Ngok, F. K.; Bakker, A.; Cole, S.; Chorn, N.; Lin, L. S.; Bristol, G.; Boyd, M. P.; MacPherson, J. L.; Fanning, G. C.; Todd, A. V.; Ely, J. A.; Zack, J. A. & Symonds, G. P. (2004). Anti-human immunodeficiency virus hematopoietic progenitor cell-delivered ribozyme in a phase I study: myeloid and lymphoid reconstitution in human immunodeficiency virus type-1-infected patients, *Hum Gene Ther*, Vol.15, No.3, pp. 251-262

An, D. S.; Donahue, R. E.; Kamata, M.; Poon, B.; Metzger, M.; Mao, S. H.; Bonifacino, A.; Krouse, A. E.; Darlix, J. L.; Baltimore, D.; Qin, F. X. & Chen, I. S. (2007). Stable reduction of CCR5 by RNAi through hematopoietic stem cell transplant in non-human primates, *Proc Natl Acad Sci U S A*, Vol.104, No.32, pp. 13110-13115

Anderson, J. & Akkina, R. (2005). CXCR4 and CCR5 shRNA transgenic CD34+ cell derived macrophages are functionally normal and resist HIV-1 infection, *Retrovirology*, Vol.2, pp. 53

Anderson, J.; Li, M. J.; Palmer, B.; Remling, L.; Li, S.; Yam, P.; Yee, J. K.; Rossi, J.; Zaia, J. & Akkina, R. (2007). Safety and efficacy of a lentiviral vector containing three anti-HIV genes--CCR5 ribozyme, tat-rev siRNA, and TAR decoy--in SCID-hu mouse-derived T cells, *Mol Ther*, Vol.15, No.6, pp. 1182-1188

Baltimore, D. (1988). Gene therapy. Intracellular immunization, *Nature*, Vol.335, No.6189, pp. 395-396

Baudin, F.; Marquet, R.; Isel, C.; Darlix, J. L.; Ehresmann, B. & Ehresmann, C. (1993). Functional sites in the 5' region of human immunodeficiency virus type 1 RNA form defined structural domains, *J Mol Biol*, Vol.229, No.2, pp. 382-397

Boden, D.; Pusch, O.; Lee, F.; Tucker, L. & Ramratnam, B. (2003). Human immunodeficiency virus type 1 escape from RNA interference, *J Virol*, Vol.77, No.21, pp. 11531-11535

Borrow, P.; Lewicki, H.; Hahn, B. H.; Shaw, G. M. & Oldstone, M. B. (1994). Virus-specific CD8+ cytotoxic T-lymphocyte activity associated with control of viremia in primary human immunodeficiency virus type 1 infection, *J Virol*, Vol.68, No.9, pp. 6103-6110

BouHamdan, M.; Strayer, D. S.; Wei, D.; Mukhtar, M.; Duan, L. X.; Hoxie, J. & Pomerantz, R. J. (2001). Inhibition of HIV-1 infection by down-regulation of the CXCR4 co-receptor using an intracellular single chain variable fragment against CXCR4, *Gene Ther*, Vol.8, No.5, pp. 408-418

Brinkman, K.; Smeitink, J. A.; Romijn, J. A. & Reiss, P. (1999). Mitochondrial toxicity induced by nucleoside-analogue reverse-transcriptase inhibitors is a key factor in the pathogenesis of antiretroviral-therapy-related lipodystrophy, *Lancet*, Vol.354, No.9184, pp. 1112-1115

Brodie, S. J.; Lewinsohn, D. A.; Patterson, B. K.; Jiyamapa, D.; Krieger, J.; Corey, L.; Greenberg, P. D. & Riddell, S. R. (1999). In vivo migration and function of transferred HIV-1-specific cytotoxic T cells, *Nat Med*, Vol.5, No.1, pp. 34-41

Brodie, S. J.; Patterson, B. K.; Lewinsohn, D. A.; Diem, K.; Spach, D.; Greenberg, P. D.; Riddell, S. R. & Corey, L. (2000). HIV-specific cytotoxic T lymphocytes traffic to lymph nodes and localize at sites of HIV replication and cell death, *J Clin Invest*, Vol.105, No.10, pp. 1407-1417

Cathomen, T. & Joung, J. K. (2008). Zinc-finger nucleases: the next generation emerges, *Mol Ther*, Vol.16, No.7, pp. 1200-1207

Chang, L. J.; Liu, X. & He, J. (2005). Lentiviral siRNAs targeting multiple highly conserved RNA sequences of human immunodeficiency virus type 1, *Gene Ther*, Vol.12, No.14, pp. 1133-1144

Chao, H.; Liu, Y.; Rabinowitz, J.; Li, C.; Samulski, R. J. & Walsh, C. E. (2000). Several log increase in therapeutic transgene delivery by distinct adeno-associated viral serotype vectors, *Mol Ther*, Vol.2, No.6, pp. 619-623

Clement, N.; Knop, D. R. & Byrne, B. J. (2009). Large-scale adeno-associated viral vector production using a herpesvirus-based system enables manufacturing for clinical studies, *Hum Gene Ther*, Vol.20, No.8, pp. 796-806

Coburn, G. A. & Cullen, B. R. (2002). Potent and specific inhibition of human immunodeficiency virus type 1 replication by RNA interference, *J Virol*, Vol.76, No.18, pp. 9225-9231

Cordelier, P.; Morse, B. & Strayer, D. S. (2003). Targeting CCR5 with siRNAs: using recombinant SV40-derived vectors to protect macrophages and microglia from R5-tropic HIV, *Oligonucleotides*, Vol.13, No.5, pp. 281-294

Cordelier, P.; Kulkowsky, J. W.; Ko, C.; Matskevitch, A. A.; McKee, H. J.; Rossi, J. J.; Bouhamdan, M.; Pomerantz, R. J.; Kari, G. & Strayer, D. S. (2004). Protecting from R5-tropic HIV: individual and combined effectiveness of a hammerhead ribozyme and a single-chain Fv antibody that targets CCR5, *Gene Ther*, Vol.11, No.22, pp. 1627-1637

Daar, E. S. & Ho, D. D. (1991). Relative resistance of primary HIV-1 isolates to neutralization by soluble CD4, *Am J Med*, Vol.90, No.4A, pp. 22S-26S

Das, A. T.; Brummelkamp, T. R.; Westerhout, E. M.; Vink, M.; Madiredjo, M.; Bernards, R. & Berkhout, B. (2004). Human immunodeficiency virus type 1 escapes from RNA interference-mediated inhibition, *J Virol*, Vol.78, No.5, pp. 2601-2605

Deeks, S. G.; Wagner, B.; Anton, P. A.; Mitsuyasu, R. T.; Scadden, D. T.; Huang, C.; Macken, C.; Richman, D. D.; Christopherson, C.; June, C. H.; Lazar, R.; Broad, D. F.; Jalali, S. & Hege, K. M. (2002). A phase II randomized study of HIV-specific T-cell gene therapy in subjects with undetectable plasma viremia on combination antiretroviral therapy, *Mol Ther*, Vol.5, No.6, pp. 788-797

Demoustier, A.; Gubler, B.; Lambotte, O.; de Goer, M. G.; Wallon, C.; Goujard, C.; Delfraissy, J. F. & Taoufik, Y. (2002). In patients on prolonged HAART, a significant pool of HIV infected CD4 T cells are HIV-specific, *Aids*, Vol.16, No.13, pp. 1749-1754

Dharmapuri, S.; Peruzzi, D. & Aurisicchio, L. (2009). Engineered adenovirus serotypes for overcoming anti-vector immunity, *Expert Opin Biol Ther*, Vol.9, No.10, pp. 1279-1287

DiGiusto, D. L.; Krishnan, A.; Li, L.; Li, H.; Li, S.; Rao, A.; Mi, S.; Yam, P.; Stinson, S.; Kalos, M.; Alvarnas, J.; Lacey, S. F.; Yee, J. K.; Li, M.; Couture, L.; Hsu, D.; Forman, S. J.; Rossi, J. J. & Zaia, J. A. (2010). RNA-based gene therapy for HIV with lentiviral vector-modified CD34(+) cells in patients undergoing transplantation for AIDS-related lymphoma, *Sci Transl Med*, Vol.2, No.36, pp. 36ra43

Doitsh, G.; Cavrois, M.; Lassen, K. G.; Zepeda, O.; Yang, Z.; Santiago, M. L.; Hebbeler, A. M. & Greene, W. C. (2010). Abortive HIV infection mediates CD4 T cell depletion and inflammation in human lymphoid tissue, *Cell*, Vol.143, No.5, pp. 789-801

Douek, D. C.; Brenchley, J. M.; Betts, M. R.; Ambrozak, D. R.; Hill, B. J.; Okamoto, Y.; Casazza, J. P.; Kuruppu, J.; Kunstman, K.; Wolinsky, S.; Grossman, Z.; Dybul, M.; Oxenius, A.; Price, D. A.; Connors, M. & Koup, R. A. (2002). HIV preferentially infects HIV-specific CD4+ T cells, *Nature*, Vol.417, No.6884, pp. 95-98

Egelhofer, M.; Brandenburg, G.; Martinius, H.; Schult-Dietrich, P.; Melikyan, G.; Kunert, R.; Baum, C.; Choi, I.; Alexandrov, A. & von Laer, D. (2004). Inhibition of human immunodeficiency virus type 1 entry in cells expressing gp41-derived peptides, *J Virol*, Vol.78, No.2, pp. 568-575

Egerer, L.; Volk, A.; Kahle, J.; Kimpel, J.; Brauer, F.; Hermann, F. G. & von Laer, D. (2011). Secreted Antiviral Entry Inhibitory (SAVE) Peptides for Gene Therapy of HIV Infection, *Mol Ther*, advance online publication, 01.03.2011 (doi: 10.1038/mt.2001.30)

Eshhar, Z.; Waks, T.; Bendavid, A. & Schindler, D. G. (2001). Functional expression of chimeric receptor genes in human T cells, *J Immunol Methods*, Vol.248, No.1-2, pp. 67-76

Finzi, D.; Hermankova, M.; Pierson, T.; Carruth, L. M.; Buck, C.; Chaisson, R. E.; Quinn, T. C.; Chadwick, K.; Margolick, J.; Brookmeyer, R.; Gallant, J.; Markowitz, M.; Ho, D. D.; Richman, D. D. & Siliciano, R. F. (1997). Identification of a reservoir for HIV-1 in patients on highly active antiretroviral therapy, *Science*, Vol.278, No.5341, pp. 1295-1300

Fraisier, C.; Abraham, D. A.; van Oijen, M.; Cunliffe, V.; Irvine, A.; Craig, R. & Dzierzak, E. A. (1998). Inhibition of Tat-mediated transactivation and HIV replication with Tat mutant and repressor domain fusion proteins, *Gene Ther*, Vol.5, No.7, pp. 946-954

Frecha, C.; Szecsi, J.; Cosset, F. L. & Verhoeyen, E. (2008). Strategies for targeting lentiviral vectors, *Curr Gene Ther*, Vol.8, No.6, pp. 449-460

Funke, S.; Maisner, A.; Muhlebach, M. D.; Koehl, U.; Grez, M.; Cattaneo, R.; Cichutek, K. & Buchholz, C. J. (2008). Targeted cell entry of lentiviral vectors, *Mol Ther*, Vol.16, No.8, pp. 1427-1436

Gay, W.; Lauret, E.; Boson, B.; Larghero, J.; Matheux, F.; Peyramaure, S.; Rousseau, V.; Dormont, D.; De Maeyer, E. & Le Grand, R. (2004). Low autocrine interferon beta production as a gene therapy approach for AIDS: Infusion of interferon beta-engineered lymphocytes in macaques chronically infected with SIVmac251, *Retrovirology*, Vol.1, pp. 29

Gething, M. J. & Sambrook, J. (1981). Cell-surface expression of influenza haemagglutinin from a cloned DNA copy of the RNA gene, *Nature*, Vol.293, No.5834, pp. 620-625

Goncalves, J.; Silva, F.; Freitas-Vieira, A.; Santa-Marta, M.; Malho, R.; Yang, X.; Gabuzda, D. & Barbas, C., 3rd (2002). Functional neutralization of HIV-1 Vif protein by intracellular immunization inhibits reverse transcription and viral replication, *J Biol Chem*, Vol.277, No.35, pp. 32036-32045

Grimm, D.; Streetz, K. L.; Jopling, C. L.; Storm, T. A.; Pandey, K.; Davis, C. R.; Marion, P.; Salazar, F. & Kay, M. A. (2006). Fatality in mice due to oversaturation of cellular microRNA/short hairpin RNA pathways, *Nature*, Vol.441, No.7092, pp. 537-541

Hacein-Bey-Abina, S.; Garrigue, A.; Wang, G. P.; Soulier, J.; Lim, A.; Morillon, E.; Clappier, E.; Caccavelli, L.; Delabesse, E.; Beldjord, K.; Asnafi, V.; MacIntyre, E.; Dal Cortivo, L.; Radford, I.; Brousse, N.; Sigaux, F.; Moshous, D.; Hauer, J.; Borkhardt, A.; Belohradsky, B. H.; Wintergerst, U.; Velez, M. C.; Leiva, L.; Sorensen, R.; Wulffraat, N.; Blanche, S.; Bushman, F. D.; Fischer, A. & Cavazzana-Calvo, M. (2008).

Insertional oncogenesis in 4 patients after retrovirus-mediated gene therapy of SCID-X1, *J Clin Invest*, Vol.118, No.9, pp. 3132-3142

Halbert, C. L.; Rutledge, E. A.; Allen, J. M.; Russell, D. W. & Miller, A. D. (2000). Repeat transduction in the mouse lung by using adeno-associated virus vectors with different serotypes, *J Virol*, Vol.74, No.3, pp. 1524-1532

Hammer, D.; Wild, J.; Ludwig, C.; Asbach, B.; Notka, F. & Wagner, R. (2008). Fusion of Epstein-Barr virus nuclear antigen-1-derived glycine-alanine repeat to trans-dominant HIV-1 Gag increases inhibitory activities and survival of transduced cells in vivo, *Hum Gene Ther*, Vol.19, No.6, pp. 622-634

Harrich, D.; Ulich, C. & Gaynor, R. B. (1996). A critical role for the TAR element in promoting efficient human immunodeficiency virus type 1 reverse transcription, *J Virol*, Vol.70, No.6, pp. 4017-4027

Hermann, F. G.; Egerer, L.; Brauer, F.; Gerum, C.; Schwalbe, H.; Dietrich, U. & von Laer, D. (2009a). Mutations in gp120 contribute to the resistance of human immunodeficiency virus type 1 to membrane-anchored C-peptide maC46, *J Virol*, Vol.83, No.10, pp. 4844-4853

Hermann, F. G.; Martinius, H.; Egelhofer, M.; Giroglou, T.; Tonn, T.; Roth, S. D.; Zahn, R.; Schult-Dietrich, P.; Alexandrov, A.; Dietrich, U.; Baum, C. & von Laer, D. (2009b). Protein scaffold and expression level determine antiviral activity of membrane-anchored antiviral peptides, *Hum Gene Ther*, Vol.20, No.4, pp. 325-336

Heslop, H. E.; Ng, C. Y.; Li, C.; Smith, C. A.; Loftin, S. K.; Krance, R. A.; Brenner, M. K. & Rooney, C. M. (1996). Long-term restoration of immunity against Epstein-Barr virus infection by adoptive transfer of gene-modified virus-specific T lymphocytes, *Nat Med*, Vol.2, No.5, pp. 551-555

Hirata, R. K.; Miller, A. D.; Andrews, R. G. & Russell, D. W. (1996). Transduction of hematopoietic cells by foamy virus vectors, *Blood*, Vol.88, No.9, pp. 3654-3661

Holt, N.; Wang, J.; Kim, K.; Friedman, G.; Wang, X.; Taupin, V.; Crooks, G. M.; Kohn, D. B.; Gregory, P. D.; Holmes, M. C. & Cannon, P. M. (2010). Human hematopoietic stem/progenitor cells modified by zinc-finger nucleases targeted to CCR5 control HIV-1 in vivo, *Nat Biotechnol*, Vol.28, No.8, pp. 839-847

Hotchkiss, G.; Maijgren-Steffensson, C. & Ahrlund-Richter, L. (2004). Efficacy and mode of action of hammerhead and hairpin ribozymes against various HIV-1 target sites, *Mol Ther*, Vol.10, No.1, pp. 172-180

Howe, S. J.; Mansour, M. R.; Schwarzwaelder, K.; Bartholomae, C.; Hubank, M.; Kempski, H.; Brugman, M. H.; Pike-Overzet, K.; Chatters, S. J.; de Ridder, D.; Gilmour, K. C.; Adams, S.; Thornhill, S. I.; Parsley, K. L.; Staal, F. J.; Gale, R. E.; Linch, D. C.; Bayford, J.; Brown, L.; Quaye, M.; Kinnon, C.; Ancliff, P.; Webb, D. K.; Schmidt, M.; von Kalle, C.; Gaspar, H. B. & Thrasher, A. J. (2008). Insertional mutagenesis combined with acquired somatic mutations causes leukemogenesis following gene therapy of SCID-X1 patients, *J Clin Invest*, Vol.118, No.9, pp. 3143-3150

Huang, Y.; Paxton, W. A.; Wolinsky, S. M.; Neumann, A. U.; Zhang, L.; He, T.; Kang, S.; Ceradini, D.; Jin, Z.; Yazdanbakhsh, K.; Kunstman, K.; Erickson, D.; Dragon, E.; Landau, N. R.; Phair, J.; Ho, D. D. & Koup, R. A. (1996). The role of a mutant CCR5 allele in HIV-1 transmission and disease progression, *Nat Med*, Vol.2, No.11, pp. 1240-1243

Hufert, F. T.; van Lunzen, J.; Janossy, G.; Bertram, S.; Schmitz, J.; Haller, O.; Racz, P. & von Laer, D. (1997). Germinal centre CD4+ T cells are an important site of HIV replication in vivo, *Aids*, Vol.11, No.7, pp. 849-857

Humeau, L. M.; Binder, G. K.; Lu, X.; Slepushkin, V.; Merling, R.; Echeagaray, P.; Pereira, M.; Slepushkina, T.; Barnett, S.; Dropulic, L. K.; Carroll, R.; Levine, B. L.; June, C. H. & Dropulic, B. (2004). Efficient lentiviral vector-mediated control of HIV-1 replication in CD4 lymphocytes from diverse HIV+ infected patients grouped according to CD4 count and viral load, *Mol Ther*, Vol.9, No.6, pp. 902-913

Husson, R. N.; Chung, Y.; Mordenti, J.; Butler, K. M.; Chen, S.; Duliege, A. M.; Brouwers, P.; Jarosinski, P.; Mueller, B. U.; Ammann, A. & et al. (1992). Phase I study of continuous-infusion soluble CD4 as a single agent and in combination with oral dideoxyinosine therapy in children with symptomatic human immunodeficiency virus infection, *J Pediatr*, Vol.121, No.4, pp. 627-633

Jacque, J. M.; Triques, K. & Stevenson, M. (2002). Modulation of HIV-1 replication by RNA interference, *Nature*, Vol.418, No.6896, pp. 435-438

Joseph, A.; Zheng, J. H.; Follenzi, A.; Dilorenzo, T.; Sango, K.; Hyman, J.; Chen, K.; Piechocka-Trocha, A.; Brander, C.; Hooijberg, E.; Vignali, D. A.; Walker, B. D. & Goldstein, H. (2008). Lentiviral vectors encoding human immunodeficiency virus type 1 (HIV-1)-specific T-cell receptor genes efficiently convert peripheral blood CD8 T lymphocytes into cytotoxic T lymphocytes with potent in vitro and in vivo HIV-1-specific inhibitory activity, *J Virol*, Vol.82, No.6, pp. 3078-3089

Joseph, A.; Zheng, J. H.; Chen, K.; Dutta, M.; Chen, C.; Stiegler, G.; Kunert, R.; Follenzi, A. & Goldstein, H. (2010). Inhibition of in vivo HIV infection in humanized mice by gene therapy of human hematopoietic stem cells with a lentiviral vector encoding a broadly neutralizing anti-HIV antibody, *J Virol*, Vol.84, No.13, pp. 6645-6653

Keen, N. J.; Gait, M. J. & Karn, J. (1996). Human immunodeficiency virus type-1 Tat is an integral component of the activated transcription-elongation complex, *Proc Natl Acad Sci U S A*, Vol.93, No.6, pp. 2505-2510

Kemball, C. C.; Pack, C. D.; Guay, H. M.; Li, Z. N.; Steinhauer, D. A.; Szomolanyi-Tsuda, E. & Lukacher, A. E. (2007). The antiviral CD8+ T cell response is differentially dependent on CD4+ T cell help over the course of persistent infection, *J Immunol*, Vol.179, No.2, pp. 1113-1121

Kimpel, J.; Braun, S. E.; Qiu, G.; Wong, F. E.; Conolle, M.; Schmitz, J. E.; Brendel, C.; Humeau, L. M.; Dropulic, B.; Rossi, J. J.; Berger, A.; von Laer, D. & Johnson, R. P. (2010). Survival of the fittest: positive selection of CD4+ T cells expressing a membrane-bound fusion inhibitor following HIV-1 infection, *PLoS One*, Vol.5, No.8, pp. e12357

Kitamura, Y.; Ishikawa, T.; Okui, N.; Kobayashi, N.; Kanda, T.; Shimada, T.; Miyake, K. & Yoshiike, K. (1999). Inhibition of replication of HIV-1 at both early and late stages of the viral life cycle by single-chain antibody against viral integrase, *J Acquir Immune Defic Syndr Hum Retrovirol*, Vol.20, No.2, pp. 105-114

Kohn, D. B.; Bauer, G.; Rice, C. R.; Rothschild, J. C.; Carbonaro, D. A.; Valdez, P.; Hao, Q.; Zhou, C.; Bahner, I.; Kearns, K.; Brody, K.; Fox, S.; Haden, E.; Wilson, K.; Salata, C.; Dolan, C.; Wetter, C.; Aguilar-Cordova, E. & Church, J. (1999). A clinical trial of retroviral-mediated transfer of a rev-responsive element decoy gene into CD34(+) cells from the bone marrow of human immunodeficiency virus-1-infected children, *Blood*, Vol.94, No.1, pp. 368-371

Kumar, P.; Ban, H. S.; Kim, S. S.; Wu, H.; Pearson, T.; Greiner, D. L.; Laouar, A.; Yao, J.; Haridas, V.; Habiro, K.; Yang, Y. G.; Jeong, J. H.; Lee, K. Y.; Kim, Y. H.; Kim, S. W.; Peipp, M.; Fey, G. H.; Manjunath, N.; Shultz, L. D.; Lee, S. K. & Shankar, P. (2008). T cell-specific siRNA delivery suppresses HIV-1 infection in humanized mice, *Cell*, Vol.134, No.4, pp. 577-586

Lee, N. S.; Dohjima, T.; Bauer, G.; Li, H.; Li, M. J.; Ehsani, A.; Salvaterra, P. & Rossi, J. (2002). Expression of small interfering RNAs targeted against HIV-1 rev transcripts in human cells, *Nat Biotechnol*, Vol.20, No.5, pp. 500-505

Lee, T. C.; Sullenger, B. A.; Gallardo, H. F.; Ungers, G. E. & Gilboa, E. (1992). Overexpression of RRE-derived sequences inhibits HIV-1 replication in CEM cells, *New Biol*, Vol.4, No.1, pp. 66-74

Leurs, C.; Jansen, M.; Pollok, K. E.; Heinkelein, M.; Schmidt, M.; Wissler, M.; Lindemann, D.; Von Kalle, C.; Rethwilm, A.; Williams, D. A. & Hanenberg, H. (2003). Comparison of three retroviral vector systems for transduction of nonobese diabetic/severe combined immunodeficiency mice repopulating human CD34+ cord blood cells, *Hum Gene Ther*, Vol.14, No.6, pp. 509-519

Levine, B. L.; Humeau, L. M.; Boyer, J.; MacGregor, R. R.; Rebello, T.; Lu, X.; Binder, G. K.; Slepushkin, V.; Lemiale, F.; Mascola, J. R.; Bushman, F. D.; Dropulic, B. & June, C. H. (2006). Gene transfer in humans using a conditionally replicating lentiviral vector, *Proc Natl Acad Sci U S A*, Vol.103, No.46, pp. 17372-17377

Levitskaya, J.; Sharipo, A.; Leonchiks, A.; Ciechanover, A. & Masucci, M. G. (1997). Inhibition of ubiquitin/proteasome-dependent protein degradation by the Gly-Ala repeat domain of the Epstein-Barr virus nuclear antigen 1, *Proc Natl Acad Sci U S A*, Vol.94, No.23, pp. 12616-12621

Levy-Mintz, P.; Duan, L.; Zhang, H.; Hu, B.; Dornadula, G.; Zhu, M.; Kulkosky, J.; Bizub-Bender, D.; Skalka, A. M. & Pomerantz, R. J. (1996). Intracellular expression of single-chain variable fragments to inhibit early stages of the viral life cycle by targeting human immunodeficiency virus type 1 integrase, *J Virol*, Vol.70, No.12, pp. 8821-8832

Liang, M.; Kamata, M.; Chen, K. N.; Pariente, N.; An, D. S. & Chen, I. S. (2010). Inhibition of HIV-1 infection by a unique short hairpin RNA to chemokine receptor 5 delivered into macrophages through hematopoietic progenitor cell transduction, *J Gene Med*, Vol.12, No.3, pp. 255-265

Lock, M.; Alvira, M.; Vandenberghe, L. H.; Samanta, A.; Toelen, J.; Debyser, Z. & Wilson, J. M. (2010). Rapid, simple, and versatile manufacturing of recombinant adeno-associated viral vectors at scale, *Hum Gene Ther*, Vol.21, No.10, pp. 1259-1271

Lu, X.; Yu, Q.; Binder, G. K.; Chen, Z.; Slepushkina, T.; Rossi, J. & Dropulic, B. (2004). Antisense-mediated inhibition of human immunodeficiency virus (HIV) replication by use of an HIV type 1-based vector results in severely attenuated mutants incapable of developing resistance, *J Virol*, Vol.78, No.13, pp. 7079-7088

uis Abad, J.; Gonzalez, M. A.; del Real, G.; Mira, E.; Manes, S.; Serrano, F. & Bernad, A. (2003). Novel interfering bifunctional molecules against the CCR5 coreceptor are efficient inhibitors of HIV-1 infection, *Mol Ther*, Vol.8, No.3, pp. 475-484

und, O.; Lund, O. S.; Gram, G.; Nielsen, S. D.; Schonning, K.; Nielsen, J. O.; Hansen, J. E. & Mosekilde, E. (1997). Gene therapy of T helper cells in HIV infection: mathematical model of the criteria for clinical effect, *Bull Math Biol*, Vol.59, No.4, pp. 725-745

Macpherson, J. L.; Boyd, M. P.; Arndt, A. J.; Todd, A. V.; Fanning, G. C.; Ely, J. A.; Elliott, F.; Knop, A.; Raponi, M.; Murray, J.; Gerlach, W.; Sun, L. Q.; Penny, R.; Symonds, G. P.; Carr, A. & Cooper, D. A. (2005). Long-term survival and concomitant gene expression of ribozyme-transduced CD4+ T-lymphocytes in HIV-infected patients, *J Gene Med*, Vol.7, No.5, pp. 552-564

Malim, M. H.; Bohnlein, S.; Hauber, J. & Cullen, B. R. (1989). Functional dissection of the HIV-1 Rev trans-activator--derivation of a trans-dominant repressor of Rev function, *Cell*, Vol.58, No.1, pp. 205-214

Matloubian, M.; Concepcion, R. J. & Ahmed, R. (1994). CD4+ T cells are required to sustain CD8+ cytotoxic T-cell responses during chronic viral infection, *J Virol*, Vol.68, No.12, pp. 8056-8063

McBride, J. L.; Boudreau, R. L.; Harper, S. Q.; Staber, P. D.; Monteys, A. M.; Martins, I.; Gilmore, B. L.; Burstein, H.; Peluso, R. W.; Polisky, B.; Carter, B. J. & Davidson, B. L. (2008). Artificial miRNAs mitigate shRNA-mediated toxicity in the brain: implications for the therapeutic development of RNAi, *Proc Natl Acad Sci U S A*, Vol.105, No.15, pp. 5868-5873

Mhashilkar, A. M.; Bagley, J.; Chen, S. Y.; Szilvay, A. M.; Helland, D. G. & Marasco, W. A. (1995). Inhibition of HIV-1 Tat-mediated LTR transactivation and HIV-1 infection by anti-Tat single chain intrabodies, *Embo J*, Vol.14, No.7, pp. 1542-1551

Michienzi, A.; Castanotto, D.; Lee, N.; Li, S.; Zaia, J. A. & Rossi, J. J. (2003). RNA-mediated inhibition of HIV in a gene therapy setting, *Ann N Y Acad Sci*, Vol.1002, pp. 63-71

Michienzi, A.; De Angelis, F. G.; Bozzoni, I. & Rossi, J. J. (2006). A nucleolar localizing Rev binding element inhibits HIV replication, *AIDS Res Ther*, Vol.3, pp. 13

Mitchell, R. S.; Beitzel, B. F.; Schroder, A. R.; Shinn, P.; Chen, H.; Berry, C. C.; Ecker, J. R. & Bushman, F. D. (2004). Retroviral DNA integration: ASLV, HIV, and MLV show distinct target site preferences, *PLoS Biol*, Vol.2, No.8, pp. E234

Mitsuyasu, R. T.; Anton, P. A.; Deeks, S. G.; Scadden, D. T.; Connick, E.; Downs, M. T.; Bakker, A.; Roberts, M. R.; June, C. H.; Jalali, S.; Lin, A. A.; Pennathur-Das, R. & Hege, K. M. (2000). Prolonged survival and tissue trafficking following adoptive transfer of CD4zeta gene-modified autologous CD4(+) and CD8(+) T cells in human immunodeficiency virus-infected subjects, *Blood*, Vol.96, No.3, pp. 785-793

Mitsuyasu, R. T.; Merigan, T. C.; Carr, A.; Zack, J. A.; Winters, M. A.; Workman, C.; Bloch, M.; Lalezari, J.; Becker, S.; Thornton, L.; Akil, B.; Khanlou, H.; Finlayson, R.; McFarlane, R.; Smith, D. E.; Garsia, R.; Ma, D.; Law, M.; Murray, J. M.; von Kalle, C.; Ely, J. A.; Patino, S. M.; Knop, A. E.; Wong, P.; Todd, A. V.; Haughton, M.; Fuery, C.; Macpherson, J. L.; Symonds, G. P.; Evans, L. A.; Pond, S. M. & Cooper, D.

A. (2009). Phase 2 gene therapy trial of an anti-HIV ribozyme in autologous CD34+ cells, *Nat Med*, Vol.15, No.3, pp. 285-292

Modlich, U.; Navarro, S.; Zychlinski, D.; Maetzig, T.; Knoess, S.; Brugman, M. H.; Schambach, A.; Charrier, S.; Galy, A.; Thrasher, A. J.; Bueren, J. & Baum, C. (2009). Insertional transformation of hematopoietic cells by self-inactivating lentiviral and gammaretroviral vectors, *Mol Ther*, Vol.17, No.11, pp. 1919-1928

Morgan, R. A.; Looney, D. J.; Muenchau, D. D.; Wong-Staal, F.; Gallo, R. C. & Anderson, W. F. (1990). Retroviral vectors expressing soluble CD4: a potential gene therapy for AIDS, *AIDS Res Hum Retroviruses*, Vol.6, No.2, pp. 183-191

Morgan, R. A.; Baler-Bitterlich, G.; Ragheb, J. A.; Wong-Staal, F.; Gallo, R. C. & Anderson, W. F. (1994). Further evaluation of soluble CD4 as an anti-HIV type 1 gene therapy: demonstration of protection of primary human peripheral blood lymphocytes from infection by HIV type 1, *AIDS Res Hum Retroviruses*, Vol.10, No.11, pp. 1507-1515

Morgan, R. A.; Walker, R.; Carter, C. S.; Natarajan, V.; Tavel, J. A.; Bechtel, C.; Herpin, B.; Muul, L.; Zheng, Z.; Jagannatha, S.; Bunnell, B. A.; Fellowes, V.; Metcalf, J. A.; Stevens, R.; Baseler, M.; Leitman, S. F.; Read, E. J.; Blaese, R. M. & Lane, H. C. (2005). Preferential survival of CD4+ T lymphocytes engineered with anti-human immunodeficiency virus (HIV) genes in HIV-infected individuals, *Hum Gene Ther*, Vol.16, No.9, pp. 1065-1074

Morgan, R. A.; Dudley, M. E.; Wunderlich, J. R.; Hughes, M. S.; Yang, J. C.; Sherry, R. M.; Royal, R. E.; Topalian, S. L.; Kammula, U. S.; Restifo, N. P.; Zheng, Z.; Nahvi, A.; de Vries, C. R.; Rogers-Freezer, L. J.; Mavroukakis, S. A. & Rosenberg, S. A. (2006). Cancer regression in patients after transfer of genetically engineered lymphocytes, *Science*, Vol.314, No.5796, pp. 126-129

Muesing, M. A.; Smith, D. H. & Capon, D. J. (1987). Regulation of mRNA accumulation by a human immunodeficiency virus trans-activator protein, *Cell*, Vol.48, No.4, pp. 691-701

Newrzela, S.; Cornils, K.; Li, Z.; Baum, C.; Brugman, M. H.; Hartmann, M.; Meyer, J.; Hartmann, S.; Hansmann, M. L.; Fehse, B. & von Laer, D. (2008). Resistance of mature T cells to oncogene transformation, *Blood*, Vol.112, No.6, pp. 2278-2286

Novina, C. D.; Murray, M. F.; Dykxhoorn, D. M.; Beresford, P. J.; Riess, J.; Lee, S. K.; Collman, R. G.; Lieberman, J.; Shankar, P. & Sharp, P. A. (2002). siRNA-directed inhibition of HIV-1 infection, *Nat Med*, Vol.8, No.7, pp. 681-686

Olsen, H. S.; Nelbock, P.; Cochrane, A. W. & Rosen, C. A. (1990). Secondary structure is the major determinant for interaction of HIV rev protein with RNA, *Science*, Vol.247, No.4944, pp. 845-848

Pearson, L.; Garcia, J.; Wu, F.; Modesti, N.; Nelson, J. & Gaynor, R. (1990). A transdominant tat mutant that inhibits tat-induced gene expression from the human immunodeficiency virus long terminal repeat, *Proc Natl Acad Sci U S A*, Vol.87, No.13, pp. 5079-5083

Perez, E. E.; Riley, J. L.; Carroll, R. G.; von Laer, D. & June, C. H. (2005). Suppression of HIV-1 infection in primary CD4 T cells transduced with a self-inactivating lentiviral vector encoding a membrane expressed gp41-derived fusion inhibitor, *Clin Immunol*, Vol.115, No.1, pp. 26-32

erez, E. E.; Wang, J.; Miller, J. C.; Jouvenot, Y.; Kim, K. A.; Liu, O.; Wang, N.; Lee, G.; Bartsevich, V. V.; Lee, Y. L.; Guschin, D. Y.; Rupniewski, I.; Waite, A. J.; Carpenito, C.; Carroll, R. G.; Orange, J. S.; Urnov, F. D.; Rebar, E. J.; Ando, D.; Gregory, P. D.; Riley, J. L.; Holmes, M. C. & June, C. H. (2008). Establishment of HIV-1 resistance in CD4+ T cells by genome editing using zinc-finger nucleases, *Nat Biotechnol*, Vol.26, No.7, pp. 808-816

hillips, R. E.; Rowland-Jones, S.; Nixon, D. F.; Gotch, F. M.; Edwards, J. P.; Ogunlesi, A. O.; Elvin, J. G.; Rothbard, J. A.; Bangham, C. R.; Rizza, C. R. & et al. (1991). Human immunodeficiency virus genetic variation that can escape cytotoxic T cell recognition, *Nature*, Vol.354, No.6353, pp. 453-459

odsakoff, G. M.; Engel, B. C.; Carbonaro, D. A.; Choi, C.; Smogorzewska, E. M.; Bauer, G.; Selander, D.; Csik, S.; Wilson, K.; Betts, M. R.; Koup, R. A.; Nabel, G. J.; Bishop, K.; King, S.; Schmidt, M.; von Kalle, C.; Church, J. A. & Kohn, D. B. (2005). Selective survival of peripheral blood lymphocytes in children with HIV-1 following delivery of an anti-HIV gene to bone marrow CD34(+) cells, *Mol Ther*, Vol.12, No.1, pp. 77-86

.anga, U.; Woffendin, C.; Verma, S.; Xu, L.; June, C. H.; Bishop, D. K. & Nabel, G. J. (1998). Enhanced T cell engraftment after retroviral delivery of an antiviral gene in HIV-infected individuals, *Proc Natl Acad Sci U S A*, Vol.95, No.3, pp. 1201-1206

ethwilm, A. (2007). Foamy virus vectors: an awaited alternative to gammaretro- and lentiviral vectors, *Curr Gene Ther*, Vol.7, No.4, pp. 261-271

.inaldo, C.; Huang, X. L.; Fan, Z. F.; Ding, M.; Beltz, L.; Logar, A.; Panicali, D.; Mazzara, G.; Liebmann, J.; Cottrill, M. & et al. (1995). High levels of anti-human immunodeficiency virus type 1 (HIV-1) memory cytotoxic T-lymphocyte activity and low viral load are associated with lack of disease in HIV-1-infected long-term nonprogressors, *J Virol*, Vol.69, No.9, pp. 5838-5842

.oberts, M. R.; Qin, L.; Zhang, D.; Smith, D. H.; Tran, A. C.; Dull, T. J.; Groopman, J. E.; Capon, D. J.; Byrn, R. A. & Finer, M. H. (1994). Targeting of human immunodeficiency virus-infected cells by CD8+ T lymphocytes armed with universal T-cell receptors, *Blood*, Vol.84, No.9, pp. 2878-2889

.oe, T.; Reynolds, T. C.; Yu, G. & Brown, P. O. (1993). Integration of murine leukemia virus DNA depends on mitosis, *Embo J*, Vol.12, No.5, pp. 2099-2108

abariegos, R.; Gimenez-Barcons, M.; Tapia, N.; Clotet, B. & Martinez, M. A. (2006). Sequence homology required by human immunodeficiency virus type 1 to escape from short interfering RNAs, *J Virol*, Vol.80, No.2, pp. 571-577

amson, M.; Libert, F.; Doranz, B. J.; Rucker, J.; Liesnard, C.; Farber, C. M.; Saragosti, S.; Lapoumeroulie, C.; Cognaux, J.; Forceille, C.; Muyldermans, G.; Verhofstede, C.; Burtonboy, G.; Georges, M.; Imai, T.; Rana, S.; Yi, Y.; Smyth, R. J.; Collman, R. G.; Doms, R. W.; Vassart, G. & Parmentier, M. (1996). Resistance to HIV-1 infection in caucasian individuals bearing mutant alleles of the CCR-5 chemokine receptor gene, *Nature*, Vol.382, No.6593, pp. 722-725

anhadji, K.; Grave, L.; Touraine, J. L.; Leissner, P.; Rouzioux, C.; Firouzi, R.; Kehrli, L.; Tardy, J. C. & Mehtali, M. (2000). Gene transfer of anti-gp41 antibody and CD4 immunoadhesin strongly reduces the HIV-1 load in humanized severe combined immunodeficient mice, *Aids*, Vol.14, No.18, pp. 2813-2822

Sarkar, I.; Hauber, I.; Hauber, J. & Buchholz, F. (2007). HIV-1 proviral DNA excision using an evolved recombinase, *Science*, Vol.316, No.5833, pp. 1912-1915

Sarver, N.; Cantin, E. M.; Chang, P. S.; Zaia, J. A.; Ladne, P. A.; Stephens, D. A. & Rossi, J. J (1990). Ribozymes as potential anti-HIV-1 therapeutic agents, *Science*, Vol.247 No.4947, pp. 1222-1225

Schmitz, J. E.; Kuroda, M. J.; Santra, S.; Sasseville, V. G.; Simon, M. A.; Lifton, M. A.; Racz, P. Tenner-Racz, K.; Dalesandro, M.; Scallon, B. J.; Ghrayeb, J.; Forman, M. A. Montefiori, D. C.; Rieber, E. P.; Letvin, N. L. & Reimann, K. A. (1999). Control of viremia in simian immunodeficiency virus infection by CD8+ lymphocytes, *Science* Vol.283, No.5403, pp. 857-860

Shaheen, F.; Duan, L.; Zhu, M.; Bagasra, O. & Pomerantz, R. J. (1996). Targeting human immunodeficiency virus type 1 reverse transcriptase by intracellular expression of single-chain variable fragments to inhibit early stages of the viral life cycle, *J Virol* Vol.70, No.6, pp. 3392-3400

Shankar, P.; Russo, M.; Harnisch, B.; Patterson, M.; Skolnik, P. & Lieberman, J. (2000) Impaired function of circulating HIV-specific CD8(+) T cells in chronic human immunodeficiency virus infection, *Blood*, Vol.96, No.9, pp. 3094-3101

Sommermeyer, D.; Neudorfer, J.; Weinhold, M.; Leisegang, M.; Engels, B.; Noessner, E. Heemskerk, M. H.; Charo, J.; Schendel, D. J.; Blankenstein, T.; Bernhard, H. & Uckert, W. (2006). Designer T cells by T cell receptor replacement, *Eur J Immunol* Vol.36, No.11, pp. 3052-3059

Strayer, D. S.; Zern, M. A. & Chowdhury, J. R. (2002). What can SV40-derived vectors do for gene therapy?, *Curr Opin Mol Ther*, Vol.4, No.4, pp. 313-323

Strayer, D. S.; Akkina, R.; Bunnell, B. A.; Dropulic, B.; Planelles, V.; Pomerantz, R. J.; Rossi, J J. & Zaia, J. A. (2005). Current status of gene therapy strategies to treat HIV/AIDS *Mol Ther*, Vol.11, No.6, pp. 823-842

Streeck, H.; Jolin, J. S.; Qi, Y.; Yassine-Diab, B.; Johnson, R. C.; Kwon, D. S.; Addo, M. M. Brumme, C.; Routy, J. P.; Little, S.; Jessen, H. K.; Kelleher, A. D.; Hecht, F. M. Sekaly, R. P.; Rosenberg, E. S.; Walker, B. D.; Carrington, M. & Altfeld, M. (2009) Human immunodeficiency virus type 1-specific CD8+ T-cell responses during primary infection are major determinants of the viral set point and loss of CD4+ T cells, *J Virol*, Vol.83, No.15, pp. 7641-7648

Sullenger, B. A.; Gallardo, H. F.; Ungers, G. E. & Gilboa, E. (1990). Overexpression of TAR sequences renders cells resistant to human immunodeficiency virus replication, *Cell*, Vol.63, No.3, pp. 601-608

Sullenger, B. A.; Gallardo, H. F.; Ungers, G. E. & Gilboa, E. (1991). Analysis of trans-acting response decoy RNA-mediated inhibition of human immunodeficiency virus type 1 transactivation, *J Virol*, Vol.65, No.12, pp. 6811-6816

Surabhi, R. M. & Gaynor, R. B. (2002). RNA interference directed against viral and cellular targets inhibits human immunodeficiency Virus Type 1 replication, *J Virol*, Vol.76, No.24, pp. 12963-12973

Burosky, R. T.; Urabe, M.; Godwin, S. G.; McQuiston, S. A.; Kurtzman, G. J.; Ozawa, K. & Natsoulis, G. (1997). Adeno-associated virus Rep proteins target DNA sequences to a unique locus in the human genome, *J Virol*, Vol.71, No.10, pp. 7951-7959

Swan, C. H.; Buhler, B.; Steinberger, P.; Tschan, M. P.; Barbas, C. F., 3rd & Torbett, B. E. (2006). T-cell protection and enrichment through lentiviral CCR5 intrabody gene delivery, *Gene Ther*, Vol.13, No.20, pp. 1480-1492

ter Brake, O.; Konstantinova, P.; Ceylan, M. & Berkhout, B. (2006). Silencing of HIV-1 with RNA interference: a multiple shRNA approach, *Mol Ther*, Vol.14, No.6, pp. 883-892

Trimble, L. A. & Lieberman, J. (1998). Circulating CD8 T lymphocytes in human immunodeficiency virus-infected individuals have impaired function and downmodulate CD3 zeta, the signaling chain of the T-cell receptor complex, *Blood*, Vol.91, No.2, pp. 585-594

Trono, D.; Feinberg, M. B. & Baltimore, D. (1989). HIV-1 Gag mutants can dominantly interfere with the replication of the wild-type virus, *Cell*, Vol.59, No.1, pp. 113-120

Vallanti, G.; Lupo, R.; Federico, M.; Mavilio, F. & Bovolenta, C. (2005). T Lymphocytes transduced with a lentiviral vector expressing F12-Vif are protected from HIV-1 infection in an APOBEC3G-independent manner, *Mol Ther*, Vol.12, No.4, pp. 697-706

van Lunzen, J.; Glaunsinger, T.; Stahmer, I.; von Baehr, V.; Baum, C.; Schilz, A.; Kuehlcke, K.; Naundorf, S.; Martinius, H.; Hermann, F.; Giroglou, T.; Newrzela, S.; Muller, I.; Brauer, F.; Brandenburg, G.; Alexandrov, A. & von Laer, D. (2007). Transfer of autologous gene-modified T cells in HIV-infected patients with advanced immunodeficiency and drug-resistant virus, *Mol Ther*, Vol.15, No.5, pp. 1024-1033

Vandekerckhove, L.; Christ, F.; Van Maele, B.; De Rijck, J.; Gijsbers, R.; Van den Haute, C.; Witvrouw, M. & Debyser, Z. (2006). Transient and stable knockdown of the integrase cofactor LEDGF/p75 reveals its role in the replication cycle of human immunodeficiency virus, *J Virol*, Vol.80, No.4, pp. 1886-1896

Varela-Rohena, A.; Molloy, P. E.; Dunn, S. M.; Li, Y.; Suhoski, M. M.; Carroll, R. G.; Milicic, A.; Mahon, T.; Sutton, D. H.; Laugel, B.; Moysey, R.; Cameron, B. J.; Vuidepot, A.; Purbhoo, M. A.; Cole, D. K.; Phillips, R. E.; June, C. H.; Jakobsen, B. K.; Sewell, A. K. & Riley, J. L. (2008). Control of HIV-1 immune escape by CD8 T cells expressing enhanced T-cell receptor, *Nat Med*, Vol.14, No.12, pp. 1390-1395

Vickers, T.; Baker, B. F.; Cook, P. D.; Zounes, M.; Buckheit, R. W., Jr.; Germany, J. & Ecker, D. J. (1991). Inhibition of HIV-LTR gene expression by oligonucleotides targeted to the TAR element, *Nucleic Acids Res*, Vol.19, No.12, pp. 3359-3368

Vigouroux, C.; Gharakhanian, S.; Salhi, Y.; Nguyen, T. H.; Chevenne, D.; Capeau, J. & Rozenbaum, W. (1999). Diabetes, insulin resistance and dyslipidaemia in lipodystrophic HIV-infected patients on highly active antiretroviral therapy (HAART), *Diabetes Metab*, Vol.25, No.3, pp. 225-232

von Laer, D.; Hasselmann, S. & Hasselmann, K. (2006). Impact of gene-modified T cells on HIV infection dynamics, *J Theor Biol*, Vol.238, No.1, pp. 60-77

Walker, R. E.; Bechtel, C. M.; Natarajan, V.; Baseler, M.; Hege, K. M.; Metcalf, J. A.; Stevens, R.; Hazen, A.; Blaese, R. M.; Chen, C. C.; Leitman, S. F.; Palensky, J.; Wittes, J.; Davey, R. T., Jr.; Falloon, J.; Polis, M. A.; Kovacs, J. A.; Broad, D. F.; Levine, B. L.;

Roberts, M. R.; Masur, H. & Lane, H. C. (2000). Long-term in vivo survival of receptor-modified syngeneic T cells in patients with human immunodeficiency virus infection, *Blood*, Vol.96, No.2, pp. 467-474

Walter, E. A.; Greenberg, P. D.; Gilbert, M. J.; Finch, R. J.; Watanabe, K. S.; Thomas, E. D. & Riddell, S. R. (1995). Reconstitution of cellular immunity against cytomegalovirus in recipients of allogeneic bone marrow by transfer of T-cell clones from the donor, *N Engl J Med*, Vol.333, No.16, pp. 1038-1044

Woffendin, C.; Ranga, U.; Yang, Z.; Xu, L. & Nabel, G. J. (1996). Expression of a protective gene-prolongs survival of T cells in human immunodeficiency virus-infected patients, *Proc Natl Acad Sci U S A*, Vol.93, No.7, pp. 2889-2894

Wong-Staal, F.; Poeschla, E. M. & Looney, D. J. (1998). A controlled, Phase 1 clinical trial to evaluate the safety and effects in HIV-1 infected humans of autologous lymphocytes transduced with a ribozyme that cleaves HIV-1 RNA, *Hum Gene Ther*, Vol.9, No.16, pp. 2407-2425

Zhou, C.; Bahner, I. C.; Larson, G. P.; Zaia, J. A.; Rossi, J. J. & Kohn, E. B. (1994). Inhibition of HIV-1 in human T-lymphocytes by retrovirally transduced anti-tat and rev hammerhead ribozymes, *Gene*, Vol.149, No.1, pp. 33-39

6

Crippling of HIV at Multiple Stages with Recombinant Adeno-Associated Viral Mediated RNA Interference

Ramesh B. Batchu[1,2] et al.*
Laboratory of Surgical Oncology & Developmental Therapeutics, Department of Surgery,
Wayne State University, Detroit, MI
[2]John D. Dingell VA Medical Center, Detroit, MI
USA

1. Introduction

Acquired immunodeficiency syndrome (AIDS) is a disease caused by the infection of human immunodeficiency virus-1 (HIV-1) that primarily impairs immune function by reducing the CD4 T-lymphocyte count. More than two decades after the first clinical evidence of AIDS was reported, AIDS continues to be a major public health problem worldwide with millions of people infected and new infections rising in an alarming rate in third world countries especially in Asia and sub-Saharan Africa.(1, 2) AIDS has become one of the most devastating diseases that the scientific community has ever faced, struggling till today to come up with a therapeutic strategy that successfully controls the disease. AIDS is now the leading cause of death in sub-Saharan Africa, and is presently the fourth biggest killer worldwide. AIDS-related deaths totaled over 5 million by 2009 reaching a cumulative death toll of over 30 million since the beginning of the epidemic. More than 75 million people have been infected with HIV-1, and roughly 2.7 million new HIV-1 infections were diagnosed in 2009(3) even though this rate has decreased from one decade ago.

To date, there is no effective treatment and the number of individuals infected with HIV-1 is growing dramatically in the eastern part of the world. Considering its infection rate, it is imperative to devise newer strategies to control progression of the disease. Although newer approaches such as highly active antiretroviral therapy (HAART) have proven to be effective in prolonging life, other constraints associated with their use underscores the need for development of other effective therapies. Protease inhibitors appear to be successful at controlling the viral replication immediately following budding of immature virus particle, but the development of drug resistant viral mutants and toxicity after prolonged therapy contributes to their failure.(4) HAART has considerable toxicity and its inability to

*Oksana V. Gruzdyn[1], Aamer M. Qazi[1,2], Assaad Y. Semaan[1], Shelly M. Seward[1], Christopher P. Steffes[1], David L. Bouwman[1], Donald W. Weaver[1] and Scott A. Gruber[2]
[1]Laboratory of Surgical Oncology & Developmental Therapeutics, Department of Surgery, Wayne State University, Detroit, MI, USA
[2]John D. Dingell VA Medical Center, Detroit, MI, USA

effectively act on virus in secondary lymphoid tissue is a significant drawback. Vast majority of people with AIDS live in poorer countries. HAART is expensive and unreachable to low and middle-income countries.(5) Many of these places do not have access to HAART, or if they do, supply can be intermittent. The finding that infections with drug-resistant HIV-1 are increasing further underscores the need to develop inhibitors of HIV-1 that are effective, affordable and universally accessible.

With the discovery of RNA interference (RNA*i*) phenomenon, that operates in mammalian cells and is highly effective in selective gene silencing, new, potent, small interfering RNA (siRNA) molecules have become available to add to control HIV-1. By analyzing the challenges of HIV-1 drug development, we review novel and multi-faceted therapies by simultaneously targeting multiple regions of HIV-1 so as to effectively cripple of the virus. The targets include essential cellular genes to avoid viral escape through mutations; multiple regions at various phases of the viral life cycle for a synergistic effect; and anti-sense approach as well to avoid viral escape strategies of HIV-1 against RNA*i*. Current challenges facing the advancement of RNA*i* therapy are its safety and inefficient delivery *in vivo*. Self-complimentary recombinant adeno-associated viral (rAAV-sc) vectors can overcome shortcomings associated with RNA*i*-mediated gene silence therapy.(6) AAV vectors are safe and clinically proven. New generation vectors with mutant capsids circumvent pitfalls of ubiquitin-proteasome mediated degradation leading to high-efficiency transduction at low doses ideally suited to be part of a new arsenal for in vivo RNA*i* delivery to fight HIV-1.(7) Unlike present drugs in the clinical trial or R&D stage, the multi-targeted AAV mediated RNA*i* approach not only kills the virus but also prevents the development of escape strategies and emergence of resistant viruses by simultaneous attack at multiple targets employing multiple technologies.

2. Traditional AIDS therapies

Anti-retroviral drugs such as nucleoside reverse transcriptase inhibitors and non-nucleoside inhibitors are first generation drugs successful in reducing the viral burden.(8-13) Although they prolong life in selected patients, these agents have significant side effects and generate drug resistant viral mutants. Protease inhibitors appear to be most effective at blocking HIV-1 replication, substantially reducing AIDS-related hospital admissions and death rates.(14)

Present-day therapy uses a combination of nucleoside analogues and protease inhibitors known as HAART.(15) HAART has been shown to be effective in controlling the spread of the virus by reducing the plasma viral load to undetectable levels and to some extent depleting the pool of virus in lymphoid tissues. In the past decade, HAART has become more effective with the introduction of several protease inhibitors, but the treatment is expensive and unavailable in poor countries.(5, 15) Approximately 30 million HIV-1 positive people of whom the vast majority live in low- and middle-income countries do not have access to proper treatment. This underscores the need for the development of inexpensive, yet effective drugs that can reach the majority of patients. Despite the apparent success of HAART therapy, the capacity of HIV-1 to establish latent infection of CD4+ T cells allows viral particles to persist in tissues. Some studies indicated that the therapy does not completely eliminate viral replication in secondary lymphoid tissues. HIV-1 was routinely isolated from lymphoid organs of patients even after years of therapy due to continued replication.(16) Moreover, the initiation of HAART even as early as days after the onset of AIDS symptoms, could not prevent the establishment of a pool of latently-infected T lymphocytes.(17)These observations clearly indicate that traditional combinatorial therapies with protease inhibitors and nucleoside analogs for HIV-1, though effective in selected patients in prolonging life, unfortunately generate drug resistant viral mutants, unacceptable levels of drug toxicity, and are ineffective against virus in secondary lymphoid tissue.

3. Newer approaches to therapy

Introduction of molecules that are able to dominantly interfere with intracellular replication of HIV-1 is known as "intracellular immunization". Intracellular immunization by gene therapy strategies offers a promising alternative approach for controlling and managing HIV-1 disease. These include protein-based approaches such as trans-dominant strategies to inhibit HIV-1: toxins, zinc finger nucleases and single-chain antibodies.(18) Protein-based strategies have been the single largest area of anti-HIV-1 gene transfer trials in humans in the recent past.(19) Other RNA-based intracellular immunization approaches include the use of ribozymes and decoys. These second generation ribozymes are RNA molecules that cleave viral transcripts such as *tat*, *rev*, and *gag* at specific sequences targeting HIV-1 at critical stages, and have been shown to reduce HIV-1 levels *in vitro*.(20-22) RNA decoys are RNA homologues, such as TAR and RRE that bind viral proteins and compete with native ligands necessary for replication. They were also shown to inhibit HIV-1 *in vitro*.(20, 23, 24) In comparison with protein-based strategies, RNA-based approaches may have the advantage of not being immunogenic. Both viral or host cellular factors can be targeted, the latter potentially mitigating the possibility of escape mutants, but nevertheless, these trans-dominant approaches had shown initial promise but fell short of practical utility in providing adequate protection. DNA-based vaccines have shown partial success.(23, 25, 26) Anti-sense molecules were shown by several groups to inhibit HIV-1 *in vitro* when targeted towards critical HIV-1 genes such as *tat*, *rev*, and integrase, but the need for large amounts for *in vivo* studies apart from the problems associated with stability contributed to their failure to enter the clinic.(27)

4. RNA interference (RNA*i*): A natural way of gene silencing

Diseases, for which a foreign gene can be identified as the cause, such as in the case of viral infections, are potentially treatable by blocking its expression that will cripple the causative agent. Over the last decade, small non-coding RNA molecules such as short interfering RNA (siRNA), micro RNA (miRNA) and piwi RNA (*pi*RNA), collectively known as RNA interference (RNA*i*), emerged as critical regulators in mammalian gene expression and hold the promise of selectively inhibiting expression of disease-causing genes.(28, 29) RNA*i* is an evolutionarily conserved mechanism of gene inhibition or silencing first described in Caenorhabditis elegans and was shown to produce sequence-specific gene silencing.(30) In 1999, it was recognized as the natural cellular process to destroy unwanted foreign genes such as those causing viral infections(31). In 2001, for the first time, *the use of synthetic siRNA to silence genes in mammalian cells was demonstrated, and was referred to* as 'Biotech's billion dollar break through.(32) In short, RNA*i* has the potential to revolutionize the treatment approach to various diseases. Over the years, it has become clear that RNA*i* is a highly conserved molecular mechanism used by eukaryotic organisms to control gene expression during development and to defend their genomes against invaders, such as transposons and RNA viruses. siRNAs are primarily exogenous in origin, derived directly from the virus or transposon. siRNAs are 21 to 23 double-stranded RNA molecules that recognize the cognate mRNA with complementary sequence and cleave by naturally occurring cellular mechanisms.(31) *In vivo* silencing occurs after the formation of long double-stranded RNAs that are processed into short interfering RNAs (siRNAs) by an enzyme called Dicer, forming a ribonucleo-protein complex called RNA induced silencing complex (RISC). In the RISC, the anti-sense strand of the siRNA serves as a guide for the degradation of the homologous RNA target. In recent years, siRNA has emerged as a method of choice for specific and efficient gene silencing.

Since discovery of their mechanism, chemically synthesized siRNA molecules are being used to target abnormally elevated genes in many diseases. Since siRNA is a natural biological mechanism against viruses, it can elicit specific intracellular antiviral resistance that may provide a therapeutic strategy against human viruses. siRNAs have been shown to inhibit viral replication or block gene expression in cell culture systems for several viruses. In one study, pre-treatment of cells siRNAs specific to the poliovirus genome promoted the clearance of the virus from most of the infected cells.(33) Shlomai et al observed significant reduction in hepatitis B virus (HBV) by siRNA-producing vectors.(34) A number of groups have demonstrated that siRNAs interfere with hepatitis C virus (HCV) gene expression and replication.(35-39) Over 90% of human cervical cancers are positive for human papilloma virus (HPV) and siRNA-mediated silencing of E6 and E7, the viral genes necessary for the HPV life cycle, completely inhibited them in mammalian cells.(40)

5. Targeting HIV-1 with RNA*i*

Since siRNA can elicit specific knockdown of transcripts and they have been successfully used against human viruses, this ancient defense mechanism can be recruited as a weapon in the fight against HIV-1. Several laboratories have shown that the introduction of siRNAs specific for HIV-1 transcripts has shown viral RNA degradation and inhibition of replication. (41-43) Stable and modified promoters for the expression of siRNA molecules have further shown to increase the potency of HIV *in vitro*.(44) The successful silencing of HIV-1 replication by several investigators through siRNA-mediated targeted knockdown of viral proteins made RNA interference a weapon of choice against HIV-1. (41, 45, 46)

HIV-1 has a total of 15 proteins encoded by 9 genes.(47) Essentially, these can be grouped into four potential target sets for siRNA knockdown. The first potential target for gene silencing is the viral genomic RNA upon viral entry. Jacque et al demonstrated siRNA-mediated destruction of incoming HIV-1(48), although other studies of RNA*i* inhibition of retroviral infection suggested that incoming genomic RNA may not be the best target for siRNAs.(49) Once viral DNA is integrated, the viral mRNA transcripts as well as the un-spliced genomic RNA can be potential target. Early transcripts of HIV-1 such as *rev, nef* and *tat* are an important second group of targets for gene silencing with RNA*i* because they not only regulate the subsequent expression of the structural genes, *gag, pol*, and *env* but also the synthesis of full length viral genomic RNA. siRNA targeting the *nef* gene has been demonstrated to provide efficient silencing in a transient-transfection system.(50) There have been efficient demonstrations of silencing of the expression of various regulatory genes in a transient-transfection system.(44, 51, 52) siRNAs targeted to the TAR regulatory region and nef of the HIV-1 genome have also been shown to be effective at silencing the level of virus replication and inhibiting reverse transcription intermediates.(53, 54) After regulatory genes, structural genes also represent a potential target group.(55-57) It was found that inhibition was more significant when the siRNA were present before the viral infection. This is because the vulnerability of genomic HIV RNA for RNA*i*-mediated knockdown is much greater immediately after viral entry into the cytoplasm due to the availability of target transcripts.

A crucial finding was that a high degree of specificity of the RNA*i* for the sequence of its target was required. Even one base pair change dramatically lowers the potency of RNA*i*-mediated inhibition.(58)This becomes important, given the high error rate of HIV-1 reverse transcriptase that leads to the emergence of RNA*i* escape mutants. The HIV-1 virus often becomes resistant to RNAi therapy as a result of the appearance of mutant variants. Because of these mutations, although siRNA directed against various HIV-1 genes shows initial success, the virus may soon escape inhibition within weeks. (44) Silencing evasion can also result from loss of target sequences within viral genomes, owing to the high viral mutation rates. In lymphocytes, for example, the effects of anti-HIV-1 siRNAs were progressively dampened by the emergence of viral quasi species that harbor mutations within the siRNA target sequence.(59) RNA*i*-mediated inhibition with single target has not yet been shown to protect cells against HIV-1 in long-term. RNA*i* could become a realistic therapeutic option, however, if used in a combined fashion while targeting multiple genes to prevent the emergence of mutant viruses. Simultaneous attacks by siRNA on various targets will minimize the escape of the resistant virus.

6. Cellular targets of HIV for RNA*i*

An essential cellular HIV receptor or co-receptor target may have more appeal than viral targets, which are prone to mutations. Cellular mRNAs that encode critical proteins involved in HIV-1 replication may circumvent pitfalls associated with viral escape mechanisms. Targeting cellular genes that are an essential part of the HIV-1 life cycle could therefore be advantageous. CD4 is the primary cellular receptor for HIV-1 entry on T lymphocytes. In addition to the CD4 primary receptor, the cellular chemokine receptors CCR5 and CXCR4, which function as co-receptors for HIV-1, have provided new therapeutic targets and a better understanding of the progression of viral infection. Several investigators targeted cellular proteins necessary for the HIV-1 life cycle by siRNAs and produced decreased levels of virus production.(60, 61) Preliminary observations from various laboratories have demonstrated that siRNAs specific for CD4 receptor do indeed inhibit HIV-1 replication.(62, 63) After transfection of cultured T cells with siRNA against the mRNA for CD4, HIV production, after exposure of the cells to the virus, decreased substantially. (64) CCR5, an HIV-1 co-receptor for the M-tropic HIV-1 variant, providing an attractive cellular target for siRNAs since homozygous deletions of CCR5 effectively confer protection from HIV-1 without any serious deleterious effects in immune function.(65) At least one group has taken advantage of this target for RNA*i*-mediated gene silencing, demonstrating that in vitro knockdown of CCR5 by siRNAs provided marked protection from HIV-1 infection.(63)

Although suppression of the primary receptor CD4 may be restricted by its normal role in the immune system, CCR5 seems dispensable for normal life.(66) Unfortunately, not all HIV-1 strains require CCR5, and the inhibition of CCR5 may result in the selection of HIV-1 variants that use CXCR4 as a co-receptor. It is critical to identify this particular aspect by studying strain variants.

7. Escape strategies of HIV-1 from siRNA

One of the hallmarks of RNA*i* is its sequence-specific knockdown of the target transcript, but unfortunately, it also presents a way out for HIV-1, since single nucleotide substitutions in the target region can drastically decrease the efficiency of the knockdown. HIV-1 has a high mutation rate, and this is one of the reasons why RNA*i* gene silencing has not yet been shown to protect cells against HIV-1 in long-term virus replication assays although they were successful in the short term. For example, the effects of anti-HIV-1 siRNAs in lymphocytes were progressively dampened by the emergence of viral mutant genes *tat* and *nef* through nucleotide substitution or deletions within the siRNA target sequences.(44, 59) HIV-1 can also escape from RNA*i*-mediated inhibition through mutations that alter the local RNA secondary structure.(67) This emergence of escape mutants occurs even without necessarily changing the encoded protein after prolonged culturing. In order to circumvent the emergence of resistant viruses, targeting of conserved sequences and the simultaneous use of multiple siRNAs have been suggested. Further strategies to prevent this siRNA escape strategy by HIV-1 suggested the use of anti-sense for *tat* and *nef* genes. Unlike siRNA, the anti-sense approach is not a natural phenomenon occurring in the cells and no escape strategies have been developed by HIV-1. By the combination of gene knockout by two approaches, an effective and complete suppression of HIV-1 can be achieved.

8. Multi-targeted knockdown of HIV-1 genes

Although targeting a single HIV-1 sequence can result in strong inhibition of viral replication, it is likely followed by viral escape. Thus far, studies establishing the utility of siRNAs in suppressing HIV-1 infection failed in the long run because of the high mutation rate of HIV-1 replication. There are considerable challenges in achieving this long-term inhibition, preventing the transient success achieved from translating into clinical advantage. Therefore, approaches that not only target different stages of the viral life cycle but also simultaneously target specific sets of cellular genes that are needed for viral entry should be explored. In fact, it has been clearly demonstrated that the introduction of multiple siRNAs specific for HIV-1 could lead to viral RNA degradation and replication during different stages of the viral life cycle.(59) This multi-frontal RNA*i*-mediated attack on HIV-1 potentially inhibits the mutation escape mechanism. There have been several successful demonstrations of inhibition of HIV-1 replication using siRNA targeting distinct steps of the viral life cycle. HIV RNA in the post entry complex was successfully degraded abolishing the integration of proviral DNA when siRNAs targeted more than one region.(43) Dual-specific short hairpin siRNA constructs containing an intervening bridge, targeted against both receptors were demonstrated to successfully inhibit HIV-1 replication, thus demonstrating the practical utility of an siRNA multi-frontal attack on HIV-1.(60)

It has been previously established that if the length of siRNA exceeds 30 bp, there is an induction of nonspecific antiviral interferon responses.(33) Contrary to this belief, it was shown recently that this phenomenon might not be applicable to all sequences. Chang et al. generated 38 bp siRNAs that can induce targeted gene silencing of more than one gene without nonspecific antiviral responses. This structural flexibility of gene silencing with siRNAs needs to be further explored in order to achieve complete inhibition of HIV-1 by targeting simultaneously several regions.(68) By targeting two separate regions to knockout transcription of the gene *rev*, the highest degree of inhibition of viral replication was achieved.(69)

These newer drug designs had shown initial promise, but fell short of practical utility in providing adequate protection in every case. Since no effective therapy is currently available for prevention, new and innovative therapies are urgently needed to control, prevent and eradicate HIV-1 disease. With this backdrop of HIV-1 drug development research, we propose to develop a cocktail of HIV-1 drug analogous to the current clinical use of combinations of antiviral drugs that target the reverse transcriptase and protease enzymes. These combinatorial approaches attacking multiple targets were designed essentially to prevent escape strategies observed by HIV-1 by various labs. Analogous to the current clinical practice of HAART therapy, RNA*i* approaches should also be administered in a combined fashion to prevent HIV-1 escape strategies.

9. Limitations and hurdles of *in vivo* delivery of RNA*i*

Although RNA*i* mediated inhibition through siRNAs to knockdown HIV-1 genes in the laboratory has been successful, transfection of these purchased siRNA from commercial sources is impractical and has little value for translational work. siRNA is highly labile and often requires exceptionally high levels to achieve gene silencing *in vivo*. Further, the gene-silencing effect of siRNA is directly dependent on the number of molecules available in the cells, underscoring the need for development of plasmid vectors for the continuous synthesis of siRNA inside the cell. Current challenges facing the *in vivo* application of siRNA are the maintenance of duplex stability to avoid endonuclease degradation, need for improved delivery and the need to minimize immunological responses.(70) Though successful *in vivo* application of siRNA was demonstrated in liver through high-pressure tail vein injection in a murine model, its applicability to humans is limited.(71, 72) The quantity of siRNA necessary for efficient silencing is incompatible with scale-up to larger preclinical models.(73) Liposomal packaging(74) and chemical modification of the RNA and polyethylene glycol (PEG)(75) conjugated methods give stability to siRNA molecules, but still require large amounts of RNA*i* and are financially non-viable techniques. Hydrodynamic transfection of siRNA has been successful in targeting organs in mice, but this approach is not practical for clinical use. (76, 77)
One way to address this problem is to construct a siRNA sequence for insertion in a vector for intracellular expression of siRNA. Here the siRNA cassette is driven by RNA polymerase III promoter such as U6 that express sense and antisense strands separated by short "hairpin" RNAs (shRNAs) that are cleaved by the dicer to produce siRNA. In some cases both the sense and anti-sense siRNA strands are transcribed separately, which then hybridize *in vivo* to make the siRNA. Expression from a DNA plasmid or a viral vector such as shRNA enhances stability and safe delivery of siRNA apart from providing continuous production *in vivo*. It has been demonstrated that the transfection of human cells with plasmid encoding shRNA against HIV-1 *rev* drastically inhibited viral replication over a period of several days. Further, the highest degree of inhibition of viral replication was achieved by simultaneously targeting two distinct sites within *rev*.(51, 69)
Selection of highly accessible targets within the HIV-1 RNA genome should be determined first with antisense DNA oligonucleotide arrays before designing shRNA.(78, 79) There is recent evidence that the efficacy of siRNAs is similarly influenced by secondary structure in the target transcript.(80). These selection criteria should be used in the design of the siRNA molecule in order to get optimal inhibition.

10. Efficient delivery and expression of shRNA by viral vectors

One of the important limitations of siRNA-mediated drug delivery is the vehicle to carry the inhibitory molecules to the target cells. Viral vectors are generally more efficient vehicles for shRNA *in vivo* than nonviral vectors.(81) Adenovirus, retro- or lentivirus, and AAV have been successfully used for this purpose. Retroviral/lentiviral vectors can potentially generate insertional mutagenesis, while adenoviral vectors trigger unacceptable levels of immune responses with concerns of safety.(82) shRNA can be packaged as recombinant viral vectors for better delivery in the whole organism. Retroviral vectors are successfully used for shRNA delivery, derived from moloney murine leukemia virus (MMLV). Lentiviral vectors are derived from HIV itself and can infect all the cells without the need for receptor interaction. Studies with lentiviral vectors silencing CCR5 have been performed but showed that the down regulating effect of CCR5 alone was insufficient. However, combinatorial constructs targeted to both CXCR4 and CCR5 and have shown better efficacy.(61) Retroviral/lentiviral vectors randomly integrate into the genome, generate insertional mutagenesis, and are derived from pathogenic viruses.

Dual-specific short hairpin siRNA constructs containing an intervening spacer, targeting receptor and co-receptor, demonstrated the practical utility of shRNA constructs synthesized as a single transcript. Since the shRNA design will permit tandem assembly of multiple motifs, it is now possible to introduce promising multivalent siRNA constructs into viral vectors for *in vivo* gene therapeutic applications. Based on this rationale, recent work with synthetic siRNAs demonstrated that down regulating either CXCR4 or CCR5 will protect cells from X4 or R5 HIV-1 strains, respectively, at the level of viral entry.(83) As mentioned earlier, CCR5 is a co-receptor, necessary for cellular entry by HIV-1 (R5 tropic viral strain), but is dispensable for normal human physiology. Owing to its crucial role in HIV-1 infection, the CCR5 co-receptor has been the subject of many therapeutic approaches, including RNAi-mediated gene silence therapy. siRNA targeting was shown to be effective; however, complete knockdown remained an elusive goal. In one study, transgenic macrophages expressing high levels of CCR5 were used for testing the efficacy of lentiviral vectors carrying CCR5 shRNA. Lentiviral delivery of longer (28-mer) shRNA were shown to be very effective in gene knockdown.(84) Thus, anti-CCR5 shRNA viral delivery is a promising candidate for clinical application.

We have tested retroviral vectors for gene therapy(85, 86); however, retroviral-mediated gene therapy is limited by a variety of practical and theoretical concerns, such as the immunogenicity of viral capsid proteins and insertional mutagenesis, which limit their utility for clinical purposes.(87)

Adenoviral vectors have also been successfully used for the delivery of shRNA(88) but they are well known to trigger unacceptable levels of immune responsiveness due to their large size and thereby limit repeat administration. Stability and efficiency is not the concern with viral vectors, but safety is a primary concern.

11. Recombinant Adeno-Associated Virus (rAAV) – Ideal RNAi gene silence therapy vectors

AAV belongs to the parvovirus family and is the only viral vector not known to be associated with any human disease(89) and the smallest vector suitable for RNAi-mediated gene silencing. Due to the safety(90), efficacy and potency provided by rAAV vectors, they make better alternative to the more commonly-used retroviral, lentiviral and adenovirus based vectors for gene therapy. rAAV vectors are easy to propagate and have many characteristics that make them a better choice for somatic gene therapy with RNAi-mediated gene silencing.(91, 92) rAAV vectors have long been established to transduce a wide variety of tissues.(93-95) First generation rAAV vectors were single stranded, but the development of self-complimentary (double stranded) rAAV vectors helped to avoid delay in trans-gene expression.(96) Multiple administration of the rAAV vectors is possible to overcome neutralization by the antibody produced following the initial administration due to the availability of multiple serotypes with significantly higher trans-gene expression levels than that of prototype single stranded-vectors.(97) rAAV-based vectors have the potential for stable long-term trans-gene expression. rAAV is naturally gutless vector, which do not express any viral genes or cause a cytotoxic cellular immune response in the host. Furthermore, rAAV vectors show only a modest frequency of integration into host genome, thus avoiding insertional mutagenesis.(89) Overall, rAAV vectors fulfill the requirements for an ideal *in vivo* RNAi delivery vehicle.

12. Capsid mutant rAAV for enhanced transduction

One of the shortcomings of the traditional rAAV vectorology is low transduction efficiency, which requires large doses of vectors to achieve the desired effect. This is due to the phosphorylation of AAV capsids at tyrosine residues in the cell, which leads to a ubiquitin-proteasome-mediated destruction of the majority of rAAV particles and a decrease in transduction efficiency.(98) Gene therapy with these traditional rAAV vectors necessitates the delivery of undesirably high doses of the virus in order to achieve therapeutic benefit.(99) Recent advances have lead to the generation of rAAV vectors with mutant capsids protecting them from ubiquitin-proteasome-mediated degradation in the cytosol, eventually leading to an increase in DNA transduction efficiency.(7) We acquired these next generation rAAV vectors from Dr. Srivastava's laboratory consisting of a variant of rAAV-2/8 with a mutated capsid making the vector resistant to degradation in the cytosol.(7) By using triple-capsid mutant, pACG2-3M (Y444F, Y500F & Y730F)(7), along with the self-complimentary rAAV vector, we achieved a significant enhancement in rAAV2-sc green fluorescent protein (GFP) mediated transduction (Fig-1). With pseudo-typed rAAV vectors and capsid mutations, even greater *in vivo* transduction efficiency has been demonstrated.(7)

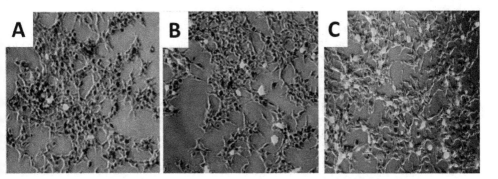

Fig. 1. HEK-293 cells transduced with various preparations of rAAV-GFP showing transduction efficiency based on green fluorescence intensity. A. Wild type rAAV-GFP; B. rAAV double stranded-GFP; C. rAAV-Capsid mutant.

13. rAAV vectors for siRNA delivery *in vivo* as short hairpin RNA (shRNA)

An ideal vector system for RNA*i* expression should be efficient and allow stable expression of the shRNA cassette without causing insertional mutagenesis or undesired immune responses. AAV is a small virus of 4.7 kb and relatively simple in its organization, comprising only two genes *Rep* and *Cap*. AAV vectors are extremely efficient tools for gene delivery *in vitro* and *in vivo*, as demonstrated by a number of laboratories. rAAV vectors have been shown to efficiently transduce hematopoietic cells.(100-102) Moreover, rAAV only retain inverted terminal repeats but do not express any viral genes and thus are gutless by design and definition more over it has not been associated with any human pathogenic, making it the vector of choice for human gene therapy. Because of their efficient transcription and inability to recombine with HIV-1, rAAV vectors represent a promising form of anti-retroviral gene therapy.(100)

One of the first studies using rAAV vector to deliver shRNA by Tomar et al. provided initial proof of principle that rAAV vector particles can be engineered to express shRNA.(88) They showed efficient knockdown of p53 and caspase 8 proteins. Subsequent studies by several investigators further demonstrated the usefulness of the rAAV vectors to express the shRNA cassette.(103-106) rAAV vectors have also been successfully used for a variety of gene silence experiments.(103-105) Use of rAAV vector encoding an anti-sense RNA against HIV-1 has been well documented by various labs.(23, 27, 100, 107) We studied the effect of anti-sense p53 gene transduction in a multiple myeloma cell line, ARH77, using AAV vector, where we delivered p53 cDNA in an anti-sense orientation.(108) *In vivo* studies in mice showed persistent knockdown of the target tyrosine hydroxylase in a Parkinson's disease model. They further demonstrated that reduction in the target elicited behavioral defects in the treated mice and created a phenotype reminiscent of rodent models of Parkinson's disease.

rAAV-mediated transduction is very efficient, particularly when compared with passive entry of simple siRNA or plasmid DNA.(109-111) rAAV siRNA delivery has been recently tested by several groups and shown to be highly efficient. Specific and efficient inhibition of HIV-1 replication was demonstrated in cultures.(91, 112) Together, this underscores the great promise of pseudo-typing shRNA-expressing AAV vectors to achieve targeted and controlled siRNA induction *in vivo*. Although the targeting of a single HIV-1 sequence can result in strong inhibition of viral replication, it is likely to be followed by viral escape. In fact, in most *in vitro* tests, siRNA did not stand the test of long-term protection against HIV-1. To overcome this escape strategy by HIV-1, we have a multi-pronged attack on HIV-1. First, HIV-1 is targeted at multiple genes for inhibition. Second, HIV-1 entry is inhibited by targeting siRNA to its cellular receptor CCR5 that is resistant to mutation. Third, we are introducing an anti-sense approach to knockdown HIV-1 *tat*, shown to be responsible for siRNA escape. Synthetic bi-specific or combinatorial constructs targeting both CXCR4 and CCR5 receptors have shown to confer resistance to HIV-1 infection much stronger than that conferred by targeting each one alone, giving a clear indication that multiple targeting is better than a single target.(22, 43, 61, 113)

14. Conclusion

Gene silencing therapy has the potential to inhibit HIV-1 replication and increase patient quality of life as an additional therapeutic class, and may serve as an adjuvant to current HAART treatment. This review gives a brief introduction regarding the emergence of RNAi, the hurdles to overcome to proceed to the next stage, and possible solutions. Although RNAi molecules can be introduced into cells as double stranded or expressed from a plasmid to inhibit abnormally elevated genes, transfection of these purchased molecules from commercial sources is impractical and has little value for translational work. The main difficulty thus far in extending the power of RNA interference (RNAi) to clinical practice has been the development of safe vectors coding for shRNAs to achieve persistent knockdown *in vivo*. rAAV vectors are different from other vectors, since the only gene expressed from recombinant vector is the trans-gene itself, naturally gutless by design and thus avoiding any cytotoxic cellular immune responses in the host. Furthermore, rAAV vectors show only a modest frequency of integration into the host genome, thus avoiding insertional mutagenesis, which has been a stumbling block for the clinical use of retroviral or lentiviral vectors. Development of self-complimentary (also known as double stranded) vectors to avoid delay in trans-gene expression(96, 114) and packaging with capsid mutants(115) to increase transduction efficiency has further contributed to rAAV vectorology. Recent advances in our understanding of RNAi make rAAV an especially attractive candidate for anti-HIV-1 gene therapy, and rAAV-based RNAi approaches can be combined with other therapeutic modalities to make a combinatorial therapy akin to HAART.

15. Acknowledgments

This work has been conducted at the John D Dingell VA Medical Center, Detroit, MI 48201 and Karmanos Cancer Institute, Detroit, MI 48201. Ariel J. Harden helped with manuscript corrections.

16. References

[1] C.J. Liand C.J. Li. Therapeutic biology: checkpoint pathway activation therapy, HIV Tat, and transkingdom RNA interference. Journal of Cellular Physiology. 209:695-700 (2006).

[2] Q.E. Yang. Eradication of HIV in infected patients: some potential approaches. Medical Science Monitor. 10:RA155-165 (2004).

[3] J. Ambrosioni, A. Calmy, and B. Hirschel. HIV treatment for prevention. Journal of the International AIDS Society. 14:28 (2011).

[4] M. Harringtonand J. Hidalgo. HIV TREATMENT FAILURE: A REVIEW OF CURRENT CLINICAL RESEARCH, Vol. 1, 2010.

[5] T. Gonzalo, M.G. Goñi, and M.Á. Muñoz-Fernández. Socio-economic impact of antiretroviral treatment in HIV patients. An economic review of cost savings after introduction of HAART. AIDS Reviews. 11:79-90 (2009).

[6] C. Muellerand T. Flotte. Clinical gene therapy using recombinant adeno-associated virus vectors. Gene Therapy. 15:858-863 (2008).

[7] L. Zhong, B. Li, C.S. Mah, L. Govindasamy, M. Agbandje-McKenna, M. Cooper, R.W. Herzog, I. Zolotukhin, K.H. Warrington, and K.A. Weigel-Van Aken. Next generation of adeno-associated virus 2 vectors: point mutations in tyrosines lead to high-efficiency transduction at lower doses. Proceedings of the National Academy of Sciences. 105:7827 (2008).

[8] S. Beckerand L. Thornton. Fosamprenavir: advancing HIV protease inhibitor treatment options. Expert Opinion on Pharmacotherapy. 5:1995-2005 (2004).

[9] M. Boffito, D. Maitland, Y. Samarasinghe, and A. Pozniak. The pharmacokinetics of HIV protease inhibitor combinations. Current Opinion in Infectious Diseases. 18:1-7 (2005).

[10] B.A. Boyle, R.A. Elion, G.J. Moyle, and C.J. Cohen. Considerations in selecting protease inhibitor therapy. AIDS Reviews. 6:218-225 (2004).

[11] R. Hazra, F.M. Balis, A.N. Tullio, E. DeCarlo, C.J. Worrell, S.M. Steinberg, J.F. Flaherty, K. Yale, M. Poblenz, B.P. Kearney, L. Zhong, D.F. Coakley, S. Blanche, J.L. Bresson, J.A. Zuckerman, and S.L. Zeichner. Single-dose and steady-state pharmacokinetics of tenofovir disoproxil fumarate in human immunodeficiency virus-infected children. Antimicrobial Agents & Chemotherapy. 48:124-129 (2004).

[12] B.L. Musial, J.K. Chojnacki, and C.I. Coleman. Atazanavir: a new protease inhibitor to treat HIV infection.[erratum appears in Am J Health Syst Pharm. 2004 Nov 1;61(21):2243]. American Journal of Health-System Pharmacy. 61:1365-1374 (2004).

[13] A. Winstonand M. Boffito. The management of HIV-1 protease inhibitor pharmacokinetic interactions. Journal of Antimicrobial Chemotherapy. 56:1-5 (2005).

[14] P. Braitstein, M. Brinkhof, F. Dabis, M. Schechter, A. Boulle, P. Miotti, R. Wood, C. Laurent, E. Sprinz, and C. Seyler. Mortality of HIV-1-infected patients in the first year of antiretroviral therapy: comparison between low-income and high-income countries. Lancet. 367:817 (2006).

[15] K.M. Johnston, A.R. Levy, V.D. Lima, R.S. Hogg, M.W. Tyndall, P. Gustafson, A. Briggs, and J.S. Montaner. Expanding access to HAART: a cost-effective approach for treating and preventing HIV. AIDS. 24:1929 (2010).

[16] D. Finzi, M. Hermankova, T. Pierson, L.M. Carruth, C. Buck, R.E. Chaisson, T.C. Quinn, K. Chadwick, J. Margolick, R. Brookmeyer, J. Gallant, M. Markowitz, D.D. Ho, D.D. Richman, and R.F. Siliciano. Identification of a reservoir for HIV-1 in patients on highly active antiretroviral therapy.[see comment]. Science. 278:1295-1300 (1997).

[17] J. Uy, C. Armon, K. Buchacz, K. Wood, and J.T. Brooks. Initiation of HAART at higher CD4 cell counts is associated with a lower frequency of antiretroviral drug resistance mutations at virologic failure. JAIDS Journal of Acquired Immune Deficiency Syndromes. 51:450 (2009).

[18] G.P. Symonds, H.A. Johnstone, M.L. Millington, M.P. Boyd, B.P. Burke, and L.R. Breton. The use of cell-delivered gene therapy for the treatment of HIV/AIDS. Immunologic Research:1-15 (2010).

[19] M. Giacca. Gene therapy to induce cellular resistance to HIV-1 infection: lessons from clinical trials. Advances in Pharmacology. 56:297-325 (2008).

[20] R. Akkina, A. Banerjea, J. Bai, J. Anderson, M.J. Li, and J. Rossi. siRNAs, ribozymes and RNA decoys in modeling stem cell-based gene therapy for HIV/AIDS. Anticancer Research. 23:1997-2005 (2003).

[21] J. Bai, S. Gorantla, N. Banda, L. Cagnon, J. Rossi, and R. Akkina. Characterization of anti-CCR5 ribozyme-transduced CD34+ hematopoietic progenitor cells in vitro and in a SCID-hu mouse model in vivo. Molecular Therapy: the Journal of the American Society of Gene Therapy. 1:244-254 (2000).

[22] Y. Feng, M. Leavitt, R. Tritz, E. Duarte, D. Kang, M. Mamounas, P. Gilles, F. Wong-Staal, S. Kennedy, J. Merson, M. Yu, and J.R. Barber. Inhibition of CCR5-dependent HIV-1 infection by hairpin ribozyme gene therapy against CC-chemokine receptor 5. Virology. 276:271-278 (2000).

[23] S.F. Ding, R. Lombardi, R. Nazari, and S. Joshi. A combination anti-HIV-1 gene therapy approach using a single transcription unit that expresses antisense, decoy, and sense RNAs, and trans-dominant negative mutant Gag and Env proteins. Frontiers in Bioscience. 7:a15-28 (2002).

[24] A. Michienzi, S. Li, J.A. Zaia, and J.J. Rossi. A nucleolar TAR decoy inhibitor of HIV-1 replication. Proceedings of the National Academy of Sciences of the United States of America. 99:14047-14052 (2002).

[25] M.L. Bonyhadi, K. Moss, A. Voytovich, J. Auten, C. Kalfoglou, I. Plavec, S. Forestell, L. Su, E. Bohnlein, and H. Kaneshima. RevM10-expressing T cells derived in vivo from transduced human hematopoietic stem-progenitor cells inhibit human immunodeficiency virus replication. Journal of Virology. 71:4707-4716 (1997).

[26] M.H. Malim, W.W. Freimuth, J. Liu, T.J. Boyle, H.K. Lyerly, B.R. Cullen, and G.J. Nabel. Stable expression of transdominant Rev protein in human T cells inhibits human immunodeficiency virus replication. Journal of Experimental Medicine. 176:1197-1201 (1992).

[27] J. Goodchild, S. Agrawal, M.P. Civeira, P.S. Sarin, D. Sun, and P.C. Zamecnik. Inhibition of human immunodeficiency virus replication by antisense oligodeoxynucleotides.[erratum appears in Proc Natl Acad Sci U S A 1989 Mar;86(5):1504]. Proceedings of the National Academy of Sciences of the United States of America. 85:5507-5511 (1988).

[28] M.T. McManusand P.A. Sharp. Gene silencing in mammals by small interfering RNAs. Nature Reviews Genetics. 3:737-747 (2002).

[29] N.J. Caplen, S. Parrish, F. Imani, A. Fire, and R.A. Morgan. Specific inhibition of gene expression by small double-stranded RNAs in invertebrate and vertebrate systems. Proceedings of the National Academy of Sciences of the United States of America. 98:9742-9747 (2001).

[30] A. Fire, S. Xu, M.K. Montgomery, S.A. Kostas, S.E. Driver, and C.C. Mello. Potent and specific genetic interference by double-stranded RNA in Caenorhabditis elegans.[see comment]. Nature. 391:806-811 (1998).

[31] A.J. Hamiltonand D.C. Baulcombe. A species of small antisense RNA in posttranscriptional gene silencing in plants.[comment]. Science. 286:950-952 (1999).

[32] D. Stipp. Biotech's Billion Dollar Breakthrough. Fortune (2003).

[33] L. Gitlin, S. Karelsky, and R. Andino. Short interfering RNA confers intracellular antiviral immunity in human cells.[see comment]. Nature. 418:430-434 (2002).

[34] A. Shlomaiand Y. Shaul. Inhibition of hepatitis B virus expression and replication by RNA interference. Hepatology. 37:764-770 (2003).

[35] T. Hugleand A. Cerny. Current therapy and new molecular approaches to antiviral treatment and prevention of hepatitis C. Reviews in Medical Virology. 13:361-371 (2003).

[36] C. Martinand-Mari, B. Lebleu, and I. Robbins. Oligonucleotide-based strategies to inhibit human hepatitis C virus. Oligonucleotides. 13:539-548 (2003).

[37] G. Randalland C.M. Rice. Interfering with hepatitis C virus RNA replication. Virus Research. 102:19-25 (2004).

[38] P.D. Zamoreand N. Aronin. siRNAs knock down hepatitis.[comment]. Nature Medicine. 9:266-267 (2003).

[39] J.A. Wilson, S. Jayasena, A. Khvorova, S. Sabatinos, I.G. Rodrigue-Gervais, S. Arya, F. Sarangi, M. Harris-Brandts, S. Beaulieu, and C.D. Richardson. RNA interference blocks gene expression and RNA synthesis from hepatitis C replicons propagated

in human liver cells. Proceedings of the National Academy of Sciences of the United States of America. 100:2783-2788 (2003).

[40] M. Jiangand J. Milner. Selective silencing of viral gene expression in HPV-positive human cervical carcinoma cells treated with siRNA, a primer of RNA interference. Oncogene. 21:6041-6048 (2002).

[41] B. Berkhout. RNA interference as an antiviral approach: targeting HIV-1. Current Opinion in Molecular Therapeutics. 6:141-145 (2004).

[42] C. Chakrabortyand C. Chakraborty. Potentiality of small interfering RNAs (siRNA) as recent therapeutic targets for gene-silencing. Current Drug Targets. 8:469-482 (2007).

[43] M.A. Martinez, B. Clotet, and J.A. Este. RNA interference of HIV replication. Trends in Immunology. 23:559-561 (2002).

[44] A.T. Das, T.R. Brummelkamp, E.M. Westerhout, M. Vink, M. Madiredjo, R. Bernards, and B. Berkhout. Human immunodeficiency virus type 1 escapes from RNA interference-mediated inhibition. Journal of Virology. 78:2601-2605 (2004).

[45] J. Capodici, K. Kariko, and D. Weissman. Inhibition of HIV-1 infection by small interfering RNA-mediated RNA interference. Journal of Immunology. 169:5196-5201 (2002).

[46] J.M. Jacque, K. Triques, and M. Stevenson. Modulation of HIV-1 replication by RNA interference. Cell. 15:20.

[47] B.M. Peterlinand D. Trono. Hide, shield and strike back: how HIV-infected cells avoid immune eradication. Nature Reviews Immunology. 3:97-107 (2003).

[48] J.M. Jacque, K. Triques, and M. Stevenson. Modulation of HIV-1 replication by RNA interference.[see comment]. Nature. 418:435-438 (2002).

[49] W.Y. Hu, F.D. Bushman, and A.C. Siva. RNA interference against retroviruses. Virus Research. 102:59-64 (2004).

[50] R. Kretschmer-Kazemi Farand G. Sczakiel. The activity of siRNA in mammalian cells is related to structural target accessibility: a comparison with antisense oligonucleotides. Nucleic Acids Research. 31:4417-4424 (2003).

[51] N.S. Lee, T. Dohjima, G. Bauer, H. Li, M.J. Li, A. Ehsani, P. Salvaterra, and J. Rossi. Expression of small interfering RNAs targeted against HIV-1 rev transcripts in human cells.[see comment]. Nature Biotechnology. 20:500-505 (2002).

[52] R.M. Surabhiand R.B. Gaynor. RNA interference directed against viral and cellular targets inhibits human immunodeficiency Virus Type 1 replication. Journal of Virology. 76:12963-12973 (2002).

[53] C.D. Novina, M.F. Murray, D.M. Dykxhoorn, P.J. Beresford, J. Riess, S.K. Lee, R.G. Collman, J. Lieberman, P. Shankar, and P.A. Sharp. siRNA-directed inhibition of HIV-1 infection.[see comment]. Nature Medicine. 8:681-686 (2002).

[54] H. Takaku. Gene silencing of HIV-1 by RNA interference. Antiviral Chemistry & Chemotherapy. 15:57-65 (2004).

[55] E. Song, P. Zhu, S.K. Lee, D. Chowdhury, S. Kussman, D.M. Dykxhoorn, Y. Feng, D. Palliser, D.B. Weiner, P. Shankar, W.A. Marasco, and J. Lieberman. Antibody mediated in vivo delivery of small interfering RNAs via cell-surface receptors.[see comment]. Nature Biotechnology. 23:709-717 (2005).

[56] W. Han, M. Wind-Rotolo, R.L. Kirkman, and C.D. Morrow. Inhibition of human immunodeficiency virus type 1 replication by siRNA targeted to the highly conserved primer binding site. Virology. 330:221-232 (2004).

57] W.S. Park, M. Hayafune, N. Miyano-Kurosaki, and H. Takaku. Specific HIV-1 env gene silencing by small interfering RNAs in human peripheral blood mononuclear cells. Gene Therapy. 10:2046-2050 (2003).

58] L. Scherer, J. Rossi, and M. Weinberg. Progress and prospects: RNA-based therapies for treatment of HIV infection. Gene Therapy. 14:1057-1064 (2007).

59] D. Boden, O. Pusch, F. Lee, L. Tucker, and B. Ramratnam. Human immunodeficiency virus type 1 escape from RNA interference. Journal of Virology. 77:11531-11535 (2003).

60] J. Anderson, A. Banerjea, and R. Akkina. Bispecific short hairpin siRNA constructs targeted to CD4, CXCR4, and CCR5 confer HIV-1 resistance. Oligonucleotides. 13:303-312 (2003).

61] X.F. Qin, D.S. An, I.S. Chen, and D. Baltimore. Inhibiting HIV-1 infection in human T cells by lentiviral-mediated delivery of small interfering RNA against CCR5. Proceedings of the National Academy of Sciences of the United States of America. 100:183-188 (2003).

62] C.D. Novina, M.F. Murray, D.M. Dykxhoorn, P.J. Beresford, J. Riess, S.K. Lee, R.G. Collman, J. Lieberman, P. Shankar, and P.A. Sharp. siRNA-directed inhibition of HIV-1 infection. Nature Medicine. 8:681-686 (2002).

63] M.A. Martìnez, A. GutiÈrrez, M. Armand-UgÛn, J. Blanco, M. Parera, J. GÛmez, B. Clotet, and J.A. EstÈ. Suppression of chemokine receptor expression by RNA interference allows for inhibition of HIV-1 replication. AIDS. 16:2385 (2002).

64] M.A. Martinez, B. Clotet, and J.A. Este. RNA interference of HIV replication. Trends in Immunology. 23:559-561 (2002).

65] J. Rucker, M. Samson, B.J. Doranz, F. Libert, J.F. Berson, Y. Yi, R.J. Smyth, R.G. Collman, C.C. Broder, and G. Vassart. Regions in [beta]-chemokine receptors CCR5 and CCR2b that determine HIV-1 cofactor specificity. Cell. 87:437-446 (1996).

66] Q.H. Liu, D.A. Williams, C. McManus, F. Baribaud, R.W. Doms, D. Schols, E. De Clercq, M.I. Kotlikoff, R.G. Collman, and B.D. Freedman. HIV-1 gp120 and chemokines activate ion channels in primary macrophages through CCR5 and CXCR4 stimulation. Proceedings of the National Academy of Sciences of the United States of America. 97:4832 (2000).

67] E.M. Westerhout, M. Ooms, M. Vink, A.T. Das, and B. Berkhout. HIV-1 can escape from RNA interference by evolving an alternative structure in its RNA genome. Nucleic Acids Research. 33:796 (2005).

68] C.I. Chang, H.S. Kang, C. Ban, S. Kim, and D. Lee. Dual-target gene silencing by using long, synthetic siRNA duplexes without triggering antiviral responses. Molecules and cells. 27:689-695 (2009).

69] K.V. Morrisand J.J. Rossi. Anti-HIV-1 gene expressing lentiviral vectors as an adjunctive therapy for HIV-1 infection. Current HIV Research. 2:185-191 (2004).

70] Y. Higuchi, S. Kawakami, and M. Hashida. Strategies for in vivo delivery of siRNAs: recent progress. Biodrugs. 24:195-205 (2010).

71] D.L. Lewis, J.E. Hagstrom, A.G. Loomis, J.A. Wolff, and H. Herweijer. Efficient delivery of siRNA for inhibition of gene expression in postnatal mice. Nature Genetics. 32:107-108 (2002).

72] A. McCaffrey, L. Meuse, T. Pham, D. Conklin, G. Hannon, and M. Kay. Gene expression: RNA interference in adult mice. Nature. 418:38-39 (2002).

[73] T. Zimmermann, A. Lee, A. Akinc, B. Bramlage, D. Bumcrot, M. Fedoruk, J. Harborth, J. Heyes, L. Jeffs, and M. John. RNAi-mediated gene silencing in non-human primates. Nature. 441:111-114 (2006).

[74] J. Yano, K. Hirabayashi, S.-I. Nakagawa, T. Yamaguchi, M. Nogawa, I. Kashimori, H. Naito, H. Kitagawa, K. Ishiyama, T. Ohgi, and T. Irimura. Antitumor activity of small interfering RNA/cationic liposome complex in mouse models of cancer. Clinical Cancer Research. 10:7721-7726 (2004).

[75] S.H. Kim, J.H. Jeong, S.H. Lee, S.W. Kim, and T.G. Park. PEG conjugated VEGF siRNA for anti-angiogenic gene therapy. Journal of Controlled Release. 116:123-129 (2006).

[76] A. Inoue, S.Y. Sawata, and K. Taira. Molecular design and delivery of siRNA. Journal of Drug Targeting. 14:448-455 (2006).

[77] Z. Parooand D.R. Corey. Challenges for RNAi in vivo. Trends in Biotechnology. 22:390-394 (2004).

[78] B. Berkhout, M. Ooms, N. Beerens, H. Huthoff, E. Southern, and K. Verhoef. In vitro evidence that the untranslated leader of the HIV-1 genome is an RNA checkpoint that regulates multiple functions through conformational changes. Journal of Biological Chemistry. 277:19967-19975 (2002).

[79] M. Ooms, K. Verhoef, E. Southern, H. Huthoff, and B. Berkhout. Probing alternative foldings of the HIV-1 leader RNA by antisense oligonucleotide scanning arrays. Nucleic Acids Research. 32:819-827 (2004).

[80] E.A. Bohula, A.J. Salisbury, M. Sohail, M.P. Playford, J. Riedemann, E.M. Southern, and V.M. Macaulay. The efficacy of small interfering RNAs targeted to the type 1 insulin-like growth factor receptor (IGF1R) is influenced by secondary structure in the IGF1R transcript. Journal of Biological Chemistry. 278:15991-15997 (2003).

[81] D. Bouard, N. Alazard-Dany, and F. Cosset. Viral vectors: from virology to transgene expression. British Journal of Pharmacology. 157:153-165 (2009).

[82] K. Park, W.J. Kim, Y.H. Cho, Y.I. Lee, H. Lee, S. Jeong, E.S. Cho, S.I. Chang, S.K. Moon, B.S. Kang, Y.J. Kim, S.H. Cho, K. Park, W.-J. Kim, Y.-H. Cho, Y.-I. Lee, H. Lee, S. Jeong, E.-S. Cho, S.-I. Chang, S.-K. Moon, B.-S. Kang, Y.-J. Kim, and S.-H. Cho. Cancer gene therapy using adeno-associated virus vectors. Frontiers in Bioscience. 13:2653-2659 (2008).

[83] J. Andersonand R. Akkina. HIV-1 resistance conferred by siRNA cosuppression of CXCR 4 and CCR 5 coreceptors by a bispecific lentiviral vector. AIDS Research and Therapy. 2:1 (2005).

[84] J. Andersonand R. Akkina. Complete knockdown of CCR5 by lentiviral vector-expressed siRNAs and protection of transgenic macrophages against HIV-1 infection. Gene Therapy. 14:1287-1297 (2007).

[85] Batchu RB, Moreno AM, Szmania S, Gupta SK, Zhan F, Rosen N, Kozlowski M, Spencer T, Spagnoli GC, Shaughnessy J, Barlogie B, Tricot G, and V.R. F. High-Level Expression of Cancer/Testis Antigen NY-ESO-1 and Human Granulocyte-Macrophage Colony-Stimulating Factor in Dendritic Cells with a Bicistronic Retroviral Vector. Human Gene Therapy. 14:1333-1345 (2003).

[86] L. Ding, S. Lu, R. Batchu, R.S. Iii, and N. Munshi. Bone marrow stromal cells as a vehicle for gene transfer. Gene Ther. 6:1611-1616. (1999).

[87] I.M. Vermaand N. Somia. Gene therapy -- promises, problems and prospects. Nature. 389:239-242 (1997).

[88] R.S. Tomar, H. Matta, and P.M. Chaudhary. Use of adeno-associated viral vector for delivery of small interfering RNA. Oncogene. 22:5712-5715 (2003).

[89] K.I. Bernsand C. Giraud. Biology of adeno-associated virus. Current Topics in Microbiology & Immunology. 218:1-23 (1996).

[90] L. Tenenbaum, E. Lehtonen, and P.E. Monahan. Evaluation of risks related to the use of adeno-associated virus-based vectors. Current Gene Therapy. 3:545-565 (2003).

[91] M. Hallekand C.M. Wendtner. Recombinant adeno-associated virus (rAAV) vectors for somatic gene therapy: recent advances and potential clinical applications. Cytokines & Molecular Therapy. 2:69-79 (1996).

[92] A. Handa, S. Muramatsu, J. Qiu, H. Mizukami, and K.E. Brown. Adeno-associated virus (AAV)-3-based vectors transduce haematopoietic cells not susceptible to transduction with AAV-2-based vectors.[see comment]. Journal of General Virology. 81:2077-2084 (2000).

[93] T.R. Flotte, S.A. Afione, C. Conrad, S.A. McGrath, R. Solow, H. Oka, P.L. Zeitlin, W.B. Guggino, and B.J. Carter. Stable in vivo expression of the cystic fibrosis transmembrane conductance regulator with an adeno-associated virus vector. Proceedings of the National Academy of Sciences of the United States of America. 90:10613-10617 (1993).

[94] R.O. Snyder, C.H. Miao, G.A. Patijn, S.K. Spratt, O. Danos, D. Nagy, A.M. Gown, B. Winther, L. Meuse, L.K. Cohen, A.R. Thompson, and M.A. Kay. Persistent and therapeutic concentrations of human factor IX in mice after hepatic gene transfer of recombinant AAV vectors. Nat Genet. 16:270-276. (1997).

[95] X. Xiao, J. Li, and R.J. Samulski. Efficient long-term gene transfer into muscle tissue of immunocompetent mice by adeno-associated virus vector. Journal of Virology. 70:8098-8108 (1996).

[96] D. McCarty, P. Monahan, and R. Samulski. Self-complementary recombinant adeno-associated virus(scAAV) vectors promote efficient transduction independently of DNA synthesis. Gene therapy(Basingstoke). 8:1248-1254 (2001).

[97] H. Nakai, S. Yant, T. Storm, S. Fuess, L. Meuse, and M. Kay. Extrachromosomal recombinant adeno-associated virus vector genomes are primarily responsible for stable liver transduction in vivo. Journal of Virology. 75:6969-6976 (2001).

[98] W. Ding, L. Zhang, Z. Yan, and J. Engelhardt. Intracellular trafficking of adeno-associated viral vectors. Gene Therapy. 12:873-880 (2005).

[99] J. Hansen, K. Qing, and A. Srivastava. Adeno-associated virus type 2-mediated gene transfer: altered endocytic processing enhances transduction efficiency in murine fibroblasts. Journal of Virology. 75:4080-4090 (2001).

[100] S. Chatterjee, P.R. Johnson, and K.K. Wong, Jr. Dual-target inhibition of HIV-1 in vitro by means of an adeno-associated virus antisense vector. Science. 258:1485-1488 (1992).

[101] A. Srivastava. Obstacles to human hematopoietic stem cell transduction by recombinant adeno-associated virus 2 vectors. Journal of Cellular Biochemistry - Supplement. 38:39-45 (2002).

[102] V.F. Van Tendeloo, P. Ponsaerts, F. Lardon, G. Nijs, M. Lenjou, C. Van Broeckhoven, D.R. Van Bockstaele, and Z.N. Berneman. Highly efficient gene delivery by mRNA electroporation in human hematopoietic cells: superiority to lipofection and passive pulsing of mRNA and to electroporation of plasmid cDNA for tumor antigen loading of dendritic cells. Blood. 98:49-56 (2001).

[103] M.D. Moore, M.J. McGarvey, R.A. Russell, B.R. Cullen, and M.O. McClure. Stable inhibition of hepatitis B virus proteins by small interfering RNA expressed from viral vectors. Journal of Gene Medicine. 7:918-925 (2005).

[104] O. Pinkenburg, J. Platz, C. Beisswenger, C. Vogelmeier, and R. Bals. Inhibition of NF-kappaB mediated inflammation by siRNA expressed by recombinant adeno-associated virus. Journal of Virological Methods. 120:119-122 (2004).

[105. H. Xia, Q. Mao, S.L. Eliason, S.Q. Harper, I.H. Martins, H.T. Orr, H.L. Paulson, L. Yang, R.M. Kotin, and B.L. Davidson. RNAi suppresses polyglutamine-induced neurodegeneration in a model of spinocerebellar ataxia.[see comment]. Nature Medicine. 10:816-820 (2004).

[106] D. Boden, O. Pusch, F. Lee, L. Tucker, P.R. Shank, and B. Ramratnam. Promoter choice affects the potency of HIV-1 specific RNA interference. Nucleic Acids Research. 31:5033-5038 (2003).

[107] A. Horster, B. Teichmann, R. Hormes, D. Grimm, J. Kleinschmidt, and G. Sczakiel. Recombinant AAV-2 harboring gfp-antisense/ribozyme fusion sequences monitor transduction, gene expression, and show anti-HIV-1 efficacy. Gene Ther. 6:1231-1238. (1999).

[108] R. Iyer, L. Ding, R.B. Batchu, S. Naugler, M.A. Shammas, and N.C. Munshi. Antisense p53 transduction leads to overexpression of bcl-2 and dexamethasone resistance in multiple myeloma. Leukemia Research. 27:73-78 (2003).

[109] M.L. Aitken, R.B. Moss, D.A. Waltz, M.E. Dovey, M.R. Tonelli, S.C. McNamara, R.L. Gibson, B.W. Ramsey, B.J. Carter, and T.C. Reynolds. A phase I study of aerosolized administration of tgAAVCF to cystic fibrosis subjects with mild lung disease. Human Gene Therapy. 12:1907-1916 (2001).

[110] S.C. Jung, I.P. Han, A. Limaye, R. Xu, M.P. Gelderman, P. Zerfas, K. Tirumalai, G.J. Murray, M.J. During, R.O. Brady, and P. Qasba. Adeno-associated viral vector-mediated gene transfer results in long-term enzymatic and functional correction in multiple organs of Fabry mice. Proceedings of the National Academy of Sciences of the United States of America. 98:2676-2681 (2001).

[111] M.Y. Mastakov, K. Baer, R. Xu, H. Fitzsimons, and M.J. During. Combined injection of rAAV with mannitol enhances gene expression in the rat brain. Molecular Therapy: the Journal of the American Society of Gene Therapy. 3:225-232 (2001).

[112] D. Boden, O. Pusch, F. Lee, L. Tucker, B. Ramratnam, D. Boden, O. Pusch, F. Lee, L. Tucker, and B. Ramratnam. Efficient gene transfer of HIV-1-specific short hairpin RNA into human lymphocytic cells using recombinant adeno-associated virus vectors. Molecular Therapy: the Journal of the American Society of Gene Therapy. 9:396-402 (2004).

[113] E. Song, S.K. Lee, D.M. Dykxhoorn, C. Novina, D. Zhang, K. Crawford, J. Cerny, P.A. Sharp, J. Lieberman, N. Manjunath, and P. Shankar. Sustained small interfering RNA-mediated human immunodeficiency virus type 1 inhibition in primary macrophages. Journal of Virology. 77:7174-7181 (2003).

[114] D. Xu, D. McCarty, A. Fernandes, M. Fisher, R.J. Samulski, and R.L. Juliano. Delivery of MDR1 small interfering RNA by self-complementary recombinant adeno-associated virus vector. Molecular Therapy: the Journal of the American Society of Gene Therapy. 11:523-530 (2005).

[115] L. Zhong, B. Li, G. Jayandharan, C.S. Mah, L. Govindasamy, M. Agbandje-McKenna, R.W. Herzog, K.A. Weigel-Van Aken, J.A. Hobbs, S. Zolotukhin, N. Muzyczka, A. Srivastava, L. Zhong, B. Li, G. Jayandharan, C.S. Mah, L. Govindasamy, M. Agbandje-McKenna, R.W. Herzog, K.A. Weigel-Van Aken, J.A. Hobbs, S. Zolotukhin, N. Muzyczka, and A. Srivastava. Tyrosine-phosphorylation of AAV2 vectors and its consequences on viral intracellular trafficking and transgene expression. Virology. 381:194-202 (2008).

7

HIV-Screening Strategies for the Discovery of Novel HIV-Inhibitors

María José Abad, Luis Miguel Bedoya and Paulina Bermejo
Department of Pharmacology, Faculty of Pharmacy, University Complutense,
Ciudad Universitaria s/n, 28040, Madrid
Spain

Introduction

nce acquired immunodeficiency syndrome (AIDS) was recognized 27 years ago, 25 million eople have died of human immunodeficiency virus (HIV)-related causes. On a global scale, though the HIV epidemic has stabilized since 2000, unacceptably high levels of new HIV fection and AIDS death still occur each year. In 2007, there were an estimated 33 million 0-36 million) people living with HIV, and 2 million (1.8-2.3 million) people died due to IDS, compared with an estimated 1.7 million (1.5-2.3 million) in 2001.

here are two main types of HIV: type 1 (HIV-1) and type 2 (HIV-2) (Buonaguro et al., 2007). IV-1 is the most prevalent in the worldwide pandemic. HIV-2 is present mainly in West frica, where it was discovered in 1986, and infects about one million people worldwide. IV-2 is slowly but continuously spreading throughout Europe, Asia and the Americas, and as reached a significant prevalence in countries such as Portugal and India. After more an 20 years of research, HIV remains a difficult target for a vaccine; thus the treatment of IDS continues to focus on the search for chemical anti-HIV agents.

working knowledge of the HIV replication cycle is essential for understanding the echanism of action of antiviral drugs. The HIV is an enveloped virus that contains two ppies of viral genomic RNA in its core. In addition to the copies of RNA, the viral core also ontains the enzymes required for HIV replication. The first step in the HIV replication cycle the interaction between the envelope proteins of the virus (gp120) and specific host-cell irface receptors (e.g. the T-cell receptor CD4 on the cellular membrane) of the host cell. In le second step, the virus binds to the chemokine coreceptors CXC-chemokine receptor 4 ːXCR4) and CC-chemokine receptor 5 (CCR5). This induces a conformational change in p120 that opens up a high affinity binding site located within the third variable loop (V3) ıd surrounding surfaces for the chemokine coreceptors CXCR4 and CCR5. This gives rise) further conformational rearrangements of gp120 that expose the transmembrane lycoprotein gp41, and the heptad repeat (HR) regions of the three subunits of gp41, HR1 ıd HR2, fold into a six-helical bundle. This ultimately results in the "fusion" of the viral ıvelope and the cytoplasmic membrane. Fusion creates a pore through which the viral ıpsid enters the cells.

IV encodes three enzymes required for replication: HIV-1 reverse transcriptase (RT), HIV-ıtegrase (IN) and HIV-protease (PT). Following entry into the cell, the viral RT enzyme ıtalyzes the conversion of viral RNA into DNA. This viral DNA enters the nucleus and becomes inserted into the chromosomal DNA of the host cell (integration). This process is facilitated by the viral enzyme IN. Expression of the viral genes leads to production of precursor viral proteins. These proteins and viral RNA are assembled at the cell surface into new viral particles and leave the host cell by a process called budding. During the budding process, they acquire the outer layer and envelope. At this stage, the PT enzyme cleaves the precursor viral proteins into their mature products. If this final phase of the replication cycle does not take place, the released viral particles are non-infectious and not competent to initiate the replication cycle in other susceptible cells.

Once HIV has entered the cell, it must disarm and hijack the intracellular machinery for its own benefit. Normal cell functionality of viral hosts is altered by invading virus proteins to the benefit of the virus. Viral proteins are known to compete with the host proteins, thus disrupting the normal host protein-protein interaction network. HIV-1 encodes the regulatory proteins, Tat and Rev, and four accessory proteins: viral infectivity factor (Vif) viral protein R (Vpr), viral protein U (Vpu) and negative factor (Nef) (Romani & Engelbrecht, 2009, Romani et al., 2010). The regulatory proteins are essential for virus replication by controlling HIV gene expression in host cells. In contrast, accessory proteins are often dispensable for virus replication *in vitro*. The Vif directly binds to and inactivate cellular deoxycytidine deaminase APOBEC3G, a natural antiviral factor that promotes G- to A-hypermutation of viral DNA during reverse transcription. The Vpu has been shown to down-regulate the CD4 receptor, and is also required for effective release of newly formed viral particles.

Anti-HIV drugs are classified into different groups according to their activity on the replicative cycle of HIV. These are virus-cell adsorption, virus-cell fusion, uncoating, reverse transcription, integration, DNA replication, transcription, translation, budding (assembly/release) and maturation. There are currently 25 compounds approved for the treatment of HIV, and most of these are nucleoside reverse transcriptase inhibitors (NRTIs) non-nucleoside reverse transcriptase inhibitors (NNRTIs) or protease inhibitors (PIs) (Warnke & Barreto, 2007, Zhan et al., 2009) (Table 1). Highly active antiretroviral therapy (HAART), which combines several such drugs (typically three or four), has dramatically improved patients' lives. The therapeutic effects are limited, however, by adverse effect and toxicities caused by long-term use and the emergence of drug resistance.

GENERIC NAME	ADVERSE REACTIONS
Entry inhibitors	
Maraviroc (UK-427)	Upper respiratory tract infection, cough, pyrexia
Fusion inhibitors	
Enfuvirtide (T20)	Pruritus, pain, discomfort
Reverse transcriptase inhibitors	
Nucleoside inhibitors	
Abacavir (ABC)	Diarrhea, nausea, headache
Didanosine (ddI)	Rash, abdominal pain, peripheral neuropathy
Emtricitabine (FTC)	Hyperpigmentation of skin, rash, diarrhea
Stavudine (d4T)	Rash, nausea, lipoatrophy
Lamivudine (3TC)	Decrease in appetite, headache, fatigue
Tenofovir (DF)	Diarrhea, nausea osteopenia
Zalcitabine (ddC)	Hepatic steatosis, peripheral neuropathy

GENERIC NAME	ADVERSE REACTIONS
Zidovudine (AZT)	Headache, anorexia, leukopenia
Non-nucleoside inhibitors	
Delavirdine (DLV)	Rash
Efavirenz (EFV)	Dizziness, hallucinations, insomnio
Etravirine (THC125)	Rash
Nevirapine (NVP)	Rash, hepatotoxicity
Integrase inhibitors	
Raltegravir (MK-0518)	Diarrhea, injection-site reactions, headache
Protease inhibitors	
Amprenavir (AMP)	Stomach upset, diarrhea, nausea
Atazanavir (ATZ)	Rash, elevated bilirubin, depression
Darunavir (TMC-114)	Rash, hypertriglyceridemia, diarrhea
Fosamprenavir (GW-433908)	Stomach upset, diarrhea, nausea
Indinavir (IDV)	Kidney stones, vomiting, headache
Lopinavir (ABT-378)	Diarrhea, headache, fatigue
Nelfinavir (NFV)	Diarrhea, nausea, rash
Ritonavir (RTV)	Stomach upset, vomiting, taste disturbance
Saquinavir (SQV)	Stomach upset, headache, abdominal pain
Tripanavir (TPV)	Hypercholesterolemia, diarrhea, nausea

Table 1. Approved antiretroviral drugs for the treatment of HIV infection

The multiple steps of the HIV replication cycle present novel therapeutic targets other than the viral enzyme RT and PT for drug developement. Continued efforts have been made to discover new inhibitors that target not only RT and PT but also other viral targets, achievements that have been reviewed comprehensively in the literature. Several recent novel target inhibitors were discovered using virus-based screening approaches (Table 2). Alternatively, PIs, the next generation of NNRTIs, CCR5 antagonist and IN inhibitors were identified by structure-based drug design, receptor pharmacology and biochemical screening approaches (Westby et al., 2005, Menéndez-Arias & Tözser, 2008, Greene et al., 2008, Liang, 2008, Pang et al., 2009, Marchand et al., 2009, Tan et al., 2010). Historical precedent therefore suggests that diverse screening strategies should be employed for the discovery of new HIV-1 agents. In this review we present a brief overview of various HIV-1 screening strategies and highlight novel approaches and/or significant advances in HIV-1 screening technology.

2. HIV-1 Entry

As mentioned above, HIV cellular entry is a multistep process that requires the interaction of a viral envelope glycoprotein (gp120) and a host receptor (CD4), followed by binding to a coreceptor (CCR5 and CXCR4). The proteins involved in the entry process have become attractive targets for drug design, and HIV-1 replication screens have successfully identified compounds with antiviral activity that act at each of these three steps of HIV entry (Grande et al., 2008, Wang & Duan, 2009).

The chemokine receptors CCR5 and CXCR4, membrane proteins belonging to the G-protein coupled receptor super-family, have been identified as essential coreceptors for HIV entry into the cells, and molecules that inhibit HIV entry by targeting CCR5 and CXCR4 have been

Attachment inhibitors CD4 binding peptides Aminoglycoside-arginine conjugates Poly-arginine aminoglycoside conjugates Cyclotriazadisulfonamide Sulfated polysaccharides
CCR5 antagonists 3-(4-benzylpiperidin-1-yl)-N-phenylpropylamine derivatives 1-(3,3-diphenylpropyl)-piperidinyl amides Ureas 1,3,4-trisubstituted pyrrolidines 1-amino-2-phenyl-4-(piperidin-1-yl) butane analogs Prostatin (12-deoxyphorbol ester)
CXCR4 inhibitors Prostatin (12-deoxyphorbol ester) Bicyclams Non-cyclam polynitrogenated compounds Cyclic penta- and tetrapeptides Diketopiperazine mimetics Tetrahydroquinolines Thiazolylisothiourea derivatives Benzodiazepines Alkylamine analogs Non-peptide derivatives
Fusion inhibitors Fusion inhibitors peptides Pyrrole derivatives
Reverse transcriptase inhibitors Nevirapine analogs Efavirenz analogs Tetrahydroimidazo-[4,5,1-jk][1,4]-benzodiazepinone derivatives Tetrazole thioacetinilide derivatives Calanolide A
Integrase inhibitors β-diketo acids GS-9137 Chalcones
Protease inhibitors Cyclic urea derivatives Peptidomimetic protease inhibitors

Table 2. Selected novel target inhibitors with potential application for the treatment of HIV infection

in rapid development as antiviral agents. Additionally, the envelope glycoprotein gp120 exists in its native form as a homopolymeric trimer, held on the outer surface of the virion by non-covalent interactions with a fusion glycoprotein gp41 trimer. The crystal structure of gp120 core bound to CD4 reveals specific targets for developing anti-HIV drugs.

High-throughput screening technologies designed to identify compounds that inhibit binding of natural ligands to their cognate G-protein-coupled receptor have been used successfully by the pharmaceutical industry for many years. The disadvantage of this approach is the dependence upon a radiolabeled ligand, which involved a high cost and arouses significant environmental concern when screening large chemical libraries. It is therefore unlikely that radiolabeled ligand binding assays will be widely used in the future. More recently, assays have been developed which identify compounds that inhibit receptor function rather than ligand binding (and thus avoid the need for radiolabeled chemokines). HIV is an enveloped virus, and its envelope proteins complex (Env) controls the key process of viral entry. Env is a complex composed of a transmembrane gp41 subunit and a noncovalently-associated surface gp120 subunit. Infection is initiated by the binding of the virion gp120 Env protein to the CD4 molecule present on some T-cells, macrophages and microglial cells. The interaction induces a conformational change that promotes secondary gp120 binding to the coreceptor CCR5 and CXCR4. Both coreceptors are members of the chemokine receptor family, but CCR5 is the coreceptor for HIV-1 strains that infect macrophages (M-tropic or R5 strains), while CXCR4 is the coreceptor for HIV-1 strains that infect T-cells (T-tropic or X4 strains). Ochsenbauer-Jambor et al. (2006) introduced a T-cell based receptor reporter cell line (JLTRG-RS) that expresses both HIV-1 coreceptors, CXCR4 and CCR5, and offers the convenience of using enhanced green fluorescent protein (EGFP) as a direct and quantitative marker. Unlike previous EGFP-based reporter cell lines, JLTRG-RS cells have an unusually high dynamic signal range, sufficient for plate reader detection using a 384-well format. Because EGFP can be directly and continuously quantified in cell culture, the reporter cell line requires no manipulation during assay preparation or analysis. These characteristics make the system extremely flexible, rapid and inexpensive. Due to its intrinsic flexibility, the JLTRG-RS cell-based reporter system provides a powerful tool which will considerably facilitate future screening for HIV inhibitors.

Immortalized cell lines, transfected with the HIV-1 Env gene, express gp120/gp41 on their surface and can fuse to cells co-expressing CD4 and either CCR5 and CXCR4. Screens based on this approach have been described by a number of laboratories. A cell-based enzyme-linked immunosorbent assay (ELISA) was developed using and anti-CXCR4 monoclonal antibody, 12G5, and cells expressing CD4 and CXCR5, the U373-MAGI-CXCR4 (CEM) cell line (Zhao et al., 2003). The assay was sensitive to the well-characterized CXCR4 antagonists, T22, T14012 (a downsized analog of T22) and AMD3100, which effectively inhibited 12G5 binding to CXCR4-expressing cells whereas HIV-1 entry inhibitors targeting CD4 and gp41 in addition to HIV-1 RT and PT inhibitors, did not block the binding of 12G5 to U373-MAGI-CXCR4 (CEM) cells. This suggests that the cell-based ELISA is specific, sensitive, convenient, rapid and economical.

More recently, two new T-cell-based reporter cell lines were established to measure HIV-1 infectivity (Chilba-Mizutani et al., 2007). One cell naturally expresses CD4 and CXCR4, making it susceptible to X4-tropic viruses, and the other cell line, in which a CCR5 expression vector was introduced, is susceptible to both X4- and R5-tropic viruses. Reporter cells were constructed by transfecting the human T-cell line HPB-Ma, which demonstrated high susceptibility to HIV-1, with genomes expressing two different luciferase reporters: HIV-1 long terminal repeat (LTR)-driven firefly luciferase and cytomegalovirus promoter-driven renilla luciferase. The cell lines were also beneficial for screening new antiretroviral agents, as false inhibition caused by the cytotoxicity of test compounds was easily detected by monitoring renilla luciferase activity.

3. HIV-1 enzyme targets

HIV-1 encodes three enzymes required for replication: HIV-1 RT, HIV-1 IN and HIV-1 PT. A number of assays have been developed for screening test compounds against thyese well-known targetrs fir drug discovery. Utilization in screening campaigns of RT or PT enzymes that contain drug resistant mutations is a common strategy for identifying next-generation HIV-1 inhibitors against these targets.

HIV-1 RT is a multifunctional enzyme involved in several essential activities for viral replication (Sarafianos et al., 2009, Herschhorn & Hiz, 2010). These activities include DNA- and RNA-dependent DNA polymerase, ribonuclease H (RNase H), strand transfer and strand displacement activities. RT has been the main target of current antiviral therapies against AIDS. NRTIs have been widely used in HAART, combined with PIs and/or NNRTIs. The high error rates characteristic of HIV-1 RT, however, are a presumed source of the viral hypermutability that contributes mainly to the emergence of resistant variants, although the significant toxicity associated with current anti-HIV drugs also results in treatment failure. These factors in combination drive pharmacologists to develop more potent and less toxic RT inhibitors against the native and drug-resistant variants, which will most certainly remain critical components of future drug regimens.

Although currently marketed agents inhibit the DNA polymerase activity of HIV-1 RT, inhibition of any of the step in the reverse transcription process would result in inhibition of viral replication. Therefore various assays suitable for testing compounds in a high-throughput screening format have been described for measuring the DNA polymerase, RNase H and DNA strand transfer activities of HIV-1 RT.

Examples of isotopic assays for measuring DNA polymerase activity include "microarray compound screening technology", and "scintillation proximity assay technology" (Xuei et al., 2003). Inhibition reverse transcription by targeting the RNase H activity of HIV-1 RT is another approach of interest, since mutations in the NNRTI allosteric domain or the RT active site are not expected to affect inhibitors that bind to the RNase H domain. Although RNase H-mediated cleavage of hybrid RNA/DNA duplex occurs either concurrently with DNA polymerization or independently, most RNase H assays target the latter. Parniak et al. (2003) described a homogeneous "fluorescence resonance energy transfer" (FRET) assay for measuring RNase H activity. The duplex substrate contains a fluorescein label on the 3'-end of the RNA, which is quenched by a Dabcyl label on the 5'-end of the DNA strand. When the substrate is cleaved by RNase H, the interaction between the fluorescein and Dabcyl is removed, resulting in an increase in the fluorescence signal.

A fluorescence polarization (FP) microplate assay for screening compounds against the RNase H activity of HIV-1 RT has also been developed (Nakayama et al., 2006). This homogeneous assay uses a hybrid 18-mer DNA/RNA duplex substrate composed of an RNA oligonucleotide labelled with 6-carboxytetramethyl rhodamine at the 3'-end, thast is annealed to a complementary unlabeled DNA strand substrate cleavage by RNase H to produce small RNA fragments (1-4 mer), resulting in a significant change in the measured FP value.

More recently, a 6-phenylpyrrolocytidine (PhpC)-based assay has been incorporated into high-throughput microplate assay format, and may form the basis for a new screen for inhibitors of HIV-1 RNase H (Wahba et al., 2010). The PhpC-containing RNA formed native-like duplex structures with complementary DNA or RNA. The PhpC-modification was found to act as a sensitive reporter group, and was non-disruptive to structure and the enzymatic activity of RNase H. A RNA/DNA hybrid possessing a single PhpC insert was an excellent substrate for

HIV-1 RT RNase, and rapidly reported cleavage of the RNA strand with a 14-fold increase in fluorescence intensity. The PhpC-based assay for RNase H was superior to the traditional molecular beacon approach in terms of responsiveness, speed and ease.

HIV-IN represents a potential target for the development of new anti-HIV chemotherapeutic agents. This viral enzyme is required for the integration of viral DNA into the host DNA, which catalyzes two reactions known as processing and strand transfer. The viral DNA is first cleaved by HIV IN at a CA dinucleotide at the 3'-end to leave the two-nucleotide overhanging. This step is known as processing. Then, the protein-DNA complex is transported into the nucleus. The host DNA is cleaved to leave a 5' overhang of five bases, and the 3'-ends of the viral DNA are convalently linked to the 5'-end of the host DNA. Finally, the 5-bases gap between the 5'-end of the viral DNA and the 3'-end of the host DNA is filled in by host cell enzymes. Since IN-negative mutants of HIV do not produce infectious virus particles, and no cellular homologue of HIV IN has been described, IN is considered to be an attractive target. However, in contrast to RT and PT, not a single IN inhibitor has yet entered the anti-HIV drug market. However, using *in vitro* assay systems and the recombinant HIV-1 IN, a variety of HIN IN inhibitors have been identified.

Most currently used assays for HIV-1 IN target the strand transfer process and follow a similar premise. HIV IN is combined with donor dsDNA, which has been immobilized onto a solid support, to form an enzyme/DNA complex. The reaction is then initiated by the addition of target dsDNA labelled in some manner, and after an incubation period, the ligated product is quantified. John et al. (2005) reported a highly efficient and sensitive high-throughput screen, HIV IN Target SRI Assay for HIV-1 IN activity, using 5' biotin-labelled DNA (5' BIO donor) and 3' digoxygenin-labelled DNA (3' DIG target). Following 3' processing of the 5' BIO donor, strand transfer proceeds with integration of the 5' BIO donor into the 3' DIG target. The assay was used to screen drugs in a high-throughput format, and the assay was also adapted to study mechanistic questions regarding the integration process. For example, using variations of the assay format, it showed a high preference of the E strand of the LTR viral DNA as a target strand compared with its complementary A strand. Wang et al. (2005) described two homogeneous time-resolved FRET-based assays for the measurement of HIV-1 IN 3'-processing and strand transfer activities. These assays have also proven their utility for the identification of mechanistically interesting and biologically active inhibitors of HIV-1 IN that hold potential for further development into potential antiviral drugs.

In addition to recombinant enzyme screens, biochemical assays have been developed that measure HIV-1 IN activity in the context of the preintegration complex (PIC), which mediates the integration of the retroviral genome into host cell DNA. The HIV PIC is a large nucleoprotein complex containing the viral CDNA and IN as well as matrix Vpr, RT and a number of host proteins including histones and members of the non-homologous end joining pathway. It is possible that screening for PIC activity, analogous to that in a true infection, may offer an expanded set of targets and yield more biologically relevant compounds. A polymerase chain reaction-based assay for integration has been reported which employs HIV-1 PICs derived from cells infected with single-cycle HIV-1 reporter viruses.

4. HIV-1 protease

In a later stage of the HIV-1 life cycle, HIV PT hydrolyzes precursor polyproteins into functional proteins that are essential for viral assembly and subsequent activity. HIV-1 Gag and Pol polypeptide precursors are cleaved by the viral encoded aspartyl protease to form the mature structural and enzymatic gene products. During virus assembly, the viral Gag polyprotein must be effectively processed and transported to the cell membrane. Cofactors such as the phospholipid phosphatidylinositol (4,5) biphosphate, the ADP ribosylation factor binding proteins or tumour susceptibility gene 101, are required for the intracellular transport and budding of HIV particles. While these are just a few examples of virus-host cell interactions, each one represents a potential new target under rigorous research with their validation being actively pursued.

The functional structure of HIV-1 PT is a homodimer containing an active site created in the cleft between the monomers as part of a four-stranded β turn. The active site region is capped by two identical β-hairpin loops (the flaps, residues 45-55 in each monomer), which undergo significant conformational changes upon substrate binding. All PIs currently licensed for the treatment of HIV infections mimic the substrate and block the active site. Another strategy is to develop compounds that bind to the subunit interface and thus block dimerization. As a result, drug discovery efforts continue to focus on the identification of new inhibitors against this validated target that are active against HIV-1 variants which are resistant to the currently available HIV-1 PIs. In line with these efforts, the assays described here may be conducted with wild-type proteins or variants that contain mutations conferring resistance to current HIV-1 PIs.

FRET assays are more commonly used for HIV-1 PT. Synthetic peptide substrates typically consist of a cleavage sequence flanked with fluorescent donor and acceptor labels. The fluorescence signal is low in the intact peptide because the donor is quenched by the nearby acceptor. Once the substrate is cleaved by HIV-1 PT, the FRET interaction is removed, and the fluorescence increases. Hamilton et al. (2003) described a biochemical detection method for peptide products of enzymatic reactions, based on the formation of PSD95/Disc-large/ZO-1 (PDZ) domain* peptide ligand complexes. The product sensor involves using masked or cryptic PDZ domain peptide ligands as enzyme substrates. The practical applicability of this PDZ-based detection method is determined by the affinity of the PDZ* peptide ligand interaction, and the efficiency of the enzyme to process the masked peptide ligand. These results showed that the Na^+/H^+ exchanger regulatory factor, which binds to the consensus sequence Thr/Ser-X-Leu-COOH, can be used to extend the flexibility in the recognition of the carboxy-terminal amino acid of the ligand, and monitor the enzymatic activity of HIV PT.

In addition to enzyme assays, a number of cell-based assays have been reported for HIV-1 PT. A green fluorescent protein (GFP)-PT chimera was developed that can be expressed in mammalian cells, causing minimal toxicity until autocatalytic cleavage occurs (Lindsten et al., 2001). The precursor is activated *in vivo* by autocatalytic cleavage, resulting in rapid elimination of PT-expressing cells. Treatment with therapeutic doses of HIV-1 PIs results in a dose-dependent accumulation of the fluorescent precursor that can be easily detected and quantified by flow cytometric and fluorimetric assays. More recently, Majerova-Uhlikova et al. (2006) described a new assay that might serve as a non-infectious, rapid, cheap and reliable alternative to the currently used phenotypic assays. These investigations showed that in the GFP-PT reporter, the HIV wild-type PT can be replaced by a drug-resistant HIV PT mutant, yielding a simple and biologically relevant tool for the quantitative analysis of drug-resistant HIV PT mutant susceptibility to HIV PTs.

5. HIV-1 replication screens

Although biochemical high-throughput screening and structure-based drug design approaches are currently preferred over holistic approaches, HIV-1 replication screens have historically been used to identify antiviral compounds. HIV-1 replication assays offer the advantage of screening for multiple targets in the context of a natural infection.

As the methodology used in the determination of the antiviral activity and the interpretation of the results have been virtually specific to each laboratory and are thus not comparable to one another, simple procedures and guidelines for evaluating antiviral and/or virucidal activities of compounds are needed. Various cell culture-based assays are currently available and can be successfully applied for the antiviral or virucidal determination of substances. Antiviral agents interfere with one or more dynamic processes during virus biosynthesis, making them candidates for clinically useful antiviral drugs; whereas virucidal substances inactivate virus infectivity extracellularly and are therefore better candidates for antiseptics, exhibiting a broad spectrum of germicidal activities.

Cost, simplicity, accuracy and reproducibility are the key factors determining the selection of the assay system, but selectivity, specificity and sensitivity also need to be taken into account. The methods commonly used for evaluation of *in vitro* antiviral activities are based on the different abilities of viruses to replicate in cultured cells. Some viruses can cause cytopathic effect (CPE) or form plaques. Others are capable of producing specialized functions or cell transformation. Virus replications in cell culture may also be monitored by the detection of viral products such as viral DNA, RNA or polypeptides. Thus, the antiviral test selected may be based on inhibition of CPE, reduction or inhibition of plaque formation. Several different HIV-1 replication assays have been described that could be adapted for medium-to-high-throughput screening. Such assays can generally be subdivided into one of three categories: reporter virus assays, reporter cell assays or cell protection assays.

In reporter virus assays, a reporter gene is introduced into the virus genome, usually in place of a viral gene not required for replication, in the target cells of interest. The concept of using HIV-1 reporter viruses to monitor HIV-1 replication was first introduced using a replication competent HIV-1 reporter virus containing the chloramphenicol acetyltransferase gene in place of HIV-1 Nef sequences. Cells are then infected with the recombinant reporter virus and virus replication is quantified by measuring the expression of the virally encoded reporter gene (Adelson et al., 2003; Dey & Berger, 2003).

For reporter cell assays, the target cells of interest are engineered to contain a reporter gene, which is activated upon viral infection. Virus replication is measured by monitoring induction of the reporter gene in the infected target cells. These assays have been used for some time to monitor HIV-1 infection and measure the activity of HIV-1 inhibitors. Kremb et al. (2010) presented a full HIV-replication system for the identification and analysis of HIV inhibitors. This technology is based on adherently growing HIV-susceptible cells, with a stable fluorescent reporter gene activated by HIV Tat and Rev. A fluorescence-based assay was designed to measure HIV infection through two parameters relating to the early and the late phases of HIV replication respectively. These results concluded that this technology is a versatile tool for the discovery and characterization of HIV inhibitors. Reporter cell assays have also been adapted to allow analysis of CCR5 as well as CXCR4 tropic HIV strains (Miyake et al., 2003).

In cell protection assays, CPE resulting from virus replication are measured by determining cell viability using a dye reduction method. These assays represent a more conventional approach to antiviral screening and have been used successfully to execute antiviral screens and identify new HIV-1 inhibitors. Although cell protection assay formats have been available for some time, they continue to be the cornerstone of many HIV-1 drug discovery programs.

6. Acknowledgements

The technical assistance of Ms. Brooke-Turner is gratefully acknowledged.

7. References

Adelson, M.E., Pacchia, A.L., Kaul, M., Rando, R.F., Ron, Y., Peltz, S.W., Dougherty, J.P. (2003). Toward the development of a virus-cell-based assay for the discovery of novel compounds against human immunodeficiency virus type 1. *Antimicrob. Agents Chemother.*, 47, 2, (February 2003), 501-508, ISSN 1098:6596

Buonaguro, L., Tornesello, M.L., Buonaguro, F.M. (2007). Human immunodeficiency virus type 1 subtype distribution in the Worlwide epidemic: pathogenetic and therapeutic implications. *J. Virol.*, 81, 19, (October 2007), 10209-10219, ISSN 0022-538X

Chilba-Mizutani, T., Mivra, H., Matsuda, M., Matsuda, Z., Yokomaku, Y., Miyauchi, K., Nishizawa, M., Yamamoto, N., Sigiura, W. (2007). Use of new T-cell-based cell lines expressing two luciferase reporters for accurately evaluating susceptibility to anti-human immunodeficiency virus type 1 drugs. *J. Clin. Microbiol.*, 45, 2, (February 2007), 477-487, ISSN 0095-1137

Dey, B., Berger, E.A. (2003). Current Protocols in Immunology, In: *Detection and Analysis of HIV*, Straber, W., 10, John Wiley & Sons, Inc., ISBN1934-368X, Sussex, England

Grande, F., Garofalo, A., Neamati, N. (2008). Small molecules anti-HIV therapeutics targeting CXCR4. *Curr. Pharm. Des.*, 14, 4, (April 2008), 385-404, ISSN 1381-6128

Greene, W.C., Debyser, Z., Ikeda, Y., Freed, E.O., Stephens, E., Yonemoto, W., Buckheit, R.W., Este, J.A., Cihlar, T. (2008). Novel targets for HIV therapy. *Antiviral Res.*, 80, 3, (December 2008), 251-265, ISSN 0166-3542

Hamilton, A.C., Inglese, J., Ferrer, M. (2003). A PDZ domain-based assay for measuring HIV protease activity: assay design considerarions. *Protein Sci.*, 12, 3, (March 2003), 458-467, ISSN 1469-896X

Herschhorn, A., Hiz, A. (2010). Retroviral reverse transcriptases. *Cell Mol. Life Sci.*, 67, 16, (August 2010), 2717-2747, ISSN 1420-682X

John, S., Fletcher, T.M., Jonsson, C.B. (2005). Development and application of a high-throughput screening assay for HIV-1 integrase enzyme activities. *J. Biomol. Screen.*, 10, 6, (September 2005), 606-614, ISSN 1087-0571

Kremb, S., Helfer, M., Heller, W., Hoffmann, D., Wolff, H., Kleinschmidt, A., Cepok, S., Hemmer, B., Durner, J., Brack-Werner, R. (2010). EASY-HIT: HIV full-replication technology for broad discovery of multiple classes of HIV inhibitors. *Antimicrob. Agents Chemother.*, 54, 12, (December 2010), 5257-5268, ISSN 1098:6596

Liang, X. (2008). CXCR4 inhibitors and mechanism of action. *Chem. Biol. Drug Des.*, 72, 2, (August 2008), 97-110, ISSN 1747-0285

Lindsten, K., Uhlikova, T., Konvalinka, J., Masucci, M.G., Dantuna, N.P. (2001). Cell-based fluorescence assay for human immunodeficiency virus type 1 protease activity. *Antimicrob. Agents Chemother.*, 45, 9, (September 2001), 2616-2622, ISSN 1098:6596

Majerova-Uhlikova, T., Dantuma, N.P., Lindstein, K., Masucci, M.G., Konvalinka, J. (2006). Non-infectious fluorimetric assay for phenotyping of drug-resistant HIV proteinase mutants. *J. Clin. Virol.*, 36, 1, (May 2006), 50-59, ISSN 1386-6532

Marchand, C., Maddali, K., Metifiot, M., Pammier, Y. (2009). HIV-1 IN inhibitors 2010 update and perspectives. *Curr. Top. Med. Chem.*, 9, 11, (November 2009), 1016-1037, ISSN 1568-0266

Menéndez-Arias, L., Tözser, J. (2008). HIV-1 protease inhibitors: effects on HIV-2 replication and resistance. *Trends Pharmacol. Sci.*, 29, 1, (January 2008), 42-49, ISSN 0165-6147

Miyake, H., Iizawa, Y., Baba, M. (2003). Novel reporter T-cell line highly susceptible to both CCR5- and CXCR4-using human immunodeficiency virus type 1 and its application to drug susceptibility tests. *J. Clin. Microbiol.*, 41, 6, (June 2003), 2515-2521, ISSN 0095-1137

Nakayama, G.R., Binghom, P., Tan, D., Maegley, K.A. (2006). A fluorescence polarization assay for screening inhibitors against the ribonuclease H activity of HIV-1 reverse transcriptase. *Anal. Biochem.*, 351, 2, (April 2006), 260-265, ISSN 0003-2697

Ochsenbauer-Jambor, C., Jones, J., Heil, M., Zammit, K.P., Kutsch, O. (2006). T-cell line for HIV drug screening using EGFP as a quantitative marker of HIV-1 replication. *Bio Techniques*, 40, 1, (January 2006), 91-100, ISSN 0736-6205

Pang, W., Tam, S.C., Zheng, Y.T. (2009). Current peptide HIV type-1 fusion inhibitors. *Antivir. Chem. Chemother.*, 20, 1, (January 2009), 1-18, ISSN 0956-3202

Parniak, M.A., Min, K.L., Budihas, S.R., Le Grice, S.F.J., Beutle, J.A. (2003). A fluorescence based high throughput screening assay for inhibitors of human immunodeficiency virus-1 reverse transcriptase-associated ribonuclease H activity. *Anal. Biochem.*, 322, 1, (November 2003), 33-39, ISSN 0003-2697

Romani, B., Engelbrecht, S. (2009). Human immunodeficiency virus type 1 Vpr: functions and molecular interactions. *J. Gen. Virol.*, 90, 8, (August 2009), 1795-1805, ISSN 0022-1317

Romani, B., Engelbrecht, S., Glashoff, R.H. (2010). Functions of Tat: the versatile protein of human immunodeficiency virus type 1. *J. Gen. Virol.*, 91, 1, (January 2010), 1-12, ISSN 0022-1317

Sarafianos, S.G., Marchand, B., Das, K., Himmel, D.M., Parniak, M.A., Hughes, S.H., Arnold, E. (2009). Structure and function of HIV-reverse transcriptase: molecular mechanism of polymerization and inhibition. *J. Mol. Biol.*, 385, 3, (January 2009), 693-713, ISSN 0022-2836

Tan, J.J., Cong, X.J., Hu, L.M., Wang, C.X., Jia, L., Liang, X.J. (2010). Therapeutic strategies underpinning the development of novel techniques for the treatment of HIV infection. *Drug Discover. Today*, 15, 5/6, (March 2010), 186-197, ISSN 1359-6446

Wahba, A.S., Esmaeili, A., Damha, M.J., Hudson, R.M. (2010). A single-label phenylpyrrolocytidine provides a molecular beacon-like response reporting HIV-1 RT RNase H activity. *Nucleic Acid Res.*, 38, 3, (January 2010), 1048-1056, ISSN 0305-1048

Wang, Y., Klock, H., Yin, H., Wolff, K., Bieza, K., Niswonger, K., Matzen, J., Gunderson, D., Hale, J., Lesley, S., Kuhen, K., Caldwell, J., Brinker, A. (2005). Homogeneous high-throughput screening assays for HIV-1 integrase 3β-processing and strand transfer activities. *J. Biomol. Screen.*, 10, 5, (August 2005), 456-462, ISSN 1087-0571

Wang, T., Duan, Y. (2009). HIV co-receptor CCR5: structure and interactions with inhibitors. *Infect. Disord. Drug Targets*, 9, 3, (March 2009), 279-288, ISSN 1871-5265

Warnke, D., Barreto, J. (2007). Antiretroviral drugs. *J. Clin. Pharmacol.*, 47, 12, (December 2007), 1570-1579, ISSN 0091-2700

Westby, M., Nakayama, G.R., Butler, S.L., Blair, W.S. (2005). Cell-based and biochemical screening approaches for the discovery of novel HIV-1 inhibitors. *Antiviral Res.*, 67, 3, (September 2005), 121-140, ISSN 0166-3542

Xuei, X., David, C.A., Middleton, T.R., Lim, B., Pithawalla, R., Chen, C.M., Tripathi, R.L., Burns, D.J., Warrior, V. (2003). Use of SAM2® biotin capture membrane in microarrayed compound screening (μARCS) format for nucleic acid polymerization assays. *J. Biomol. Screen.*, 8, 3, (June 2003), 273-282, ISSN 1087-0571

Zhan, P., Lia, X., Li, Z. (2009). Recent advances in the discovery and development of novel HIV-1 NNRTI platforms: 2006-2008 update. *Curr. Med. Chem.*, 16, 22, (July 2009), 2876-2889, ISSN 0929-8673

Zhao, Q., Lu, H., Schols, D., De Clercq, E., Jiang, S. (2003). Development of a cell-based enzyme-linked immunosorbent assay for high-throughput screening of HIV type entry inhibitors targeting the coreceptor CXCR4. *AIDS Res. Hum. Retroviruses*, 19, 11, (November 2003), 947-955, ISSN 0889-2229

Part 3

Vaccine Development

8

HIV Vaccine

Alexandre de Almeida, Telma Miyuki Oshiro,
Alessandra Pontillo and Alberto José da Silva Duarte
University of São Paulo
Brazil

1. Introduction

More than three decades after the discovery of Human Immunodeficiency Virus (HIV) as the causative agent of Acquired Immunodeficiency Syndrome (AIDS), a vaccine is still considered as the best hope for controlling the epidemic. In fact the history of medicine shows that no viral disease have ever been controlled without a vaccine. Remarkable success in the AIDS treatment has been achieved with the development of antiretroviral drugs that, by interfering with various aspects of the HIV life cycle, allowed an impressive control of infection (Fischl et al., 1987; Egger et al., 1997). The use of these drugs, however, was accompanied by new challenges related to side effects, high cost and resistance development (Carr, 2000; Hawkins, 2010; Menéndez-Arias, 2010; www.hivresourcetracking.org/treatments/vaccines).

Antiretroviral treatment cannot prevent early infection events, such as transmission to sexual partners during the post-infection peak of viremia (Wawer et al., 1999) and the massive destruction of intestinal CD4+T cells during the first weeks of infection (Brenchley et al., 2004). Furthermore drugs delivery to poor and endemic areas is often hard due to practical limitations. In resource-limited countries only 1 out 4 HIV-positive individuals has access to antiretroviral medications, and for each person who begins the therapy, there are about 6 new infections (www.who.int/entity/hiv/mediacentre/universal_access_progress_report_en.pdf). These factors made difficult to control the pandemic through antiretroviral therapy.

Others approaches could be taken in account to reduce HIV-1 infection in subjects at risk of exposure, including public health involvement (i.e.: screening of donor blood products), educational effort (i.e.: risk reduction counselling), or social imprinting (i.e.: male circumcision and behaviour modifications such as condom usage). In high seropositive communities, pre-exposure or post-exposure antiretroviral prophylaxis may reduce susceptibility to HIV infection, as well as the vertical HIV transmission from mother to child.

The creation of an HIV-1 vaccine represents an unprecedented scientific challenge and it's an absolute priority in field of HIV prevention. We must remember that vaccines are one of the most effective public health interventions ever known, but unfortunately, in HIV infection, the current perspective is that we will not have a product, even moderately effective, in the coming years.

The truth is that often in the history of vaccinology it takes a long time since the discovery of infectious agents to the licensing of an effective vaccine (Heyward et al., 1998). This is due in part to the fact that even today no one knows for sure how the immune system protects us against infections and, consequently, how to handle it for this to occur. In HIV/AIDS, the stimulation of a specific immune response is unlikely to immunize against HIV: there are no established immune correlates of protection (i.e.: humoral or cellular response), no documented cases of spontaneous recovery from AIDS or HIV infection, and no animal model that faithfully predicts HIV disease or vaccine responses in humans beyond the variability of the virus. Moreover HIV entries predominantly through mucosal surfaces, targets preferentially CD4+T cells, and rapidly establishes a persistent reservoir of latently infected cells, making difficult the study of the host/virus interaction as well as the development of an interventional strategy.

Novel approaches for an HIV vaccination need a rational vaccine design, including a better integration of emerging scientific concepts and knowledge derived from vaccinology research fields.

Models of natural resistance to HIV infection, including individuals able to control the infection (elite controllers) and some species of non-human primates, show that some level of control can be achieved (Dunham et al., 2006; Sumpter et al., 2007; Walker, 2007; Lederman et al., 2010; Poropatich & Sullivan, 2011).

The creation of an effective HIV vaccine will require continued scientific research and cooperation between academic community and biotechnology industry with the contributions of brightest scientists, long-term commitments of stable and flexible funding, trials and vaccines accessibility for developing countries. In coming years, the prospect is that several area of scientific community will be involved seeking to combine the knowledge necessary to develop new strategies, new candidates and evaluating these products.

This chapter will describe some aspects of the development of HIV vaccines, with emphasis on scientific efforts and challenges made to producing a safe and effective vaccine, strategies and methods used in the development of anti-HIV vaccines, current outlook and perspectives in this area.

2. Major challenges to get an HIV vaccine

Primary in prevention and control of infectious diseases, vaccines are a highly effective way to stimulate the immune system to fight pathogens. In the case of HIV infection, it has not yet been possible to obtain a vaccine to control infection, despite the efforts of the scientific community, the large financial investment and scientific and technological progress achieved.

Considering the natural history of infection, an HIV vaccine has the principal aim to prevent the integration of HIV genetic material into the genome of the host cell in order to prevent systemic infection and the establishment of viral reservoirs. This occurs within a few days after exposure, when HIV rapidly replicates in the lymphoid tissues, so the window of opportunity to prevent the establishment of a persistent infection is very brief. Therefore an effective HIV vaccine should be able to activate the immune system against the virus very early after the infection.

The complexity and diversity of HIV, its high capacity to evade the immune system and the missing gap in effective host immune response against the virus represent some major challenges to design an optimal vaccine. Moreover the absence of an experimental model able to mimic human infection represents another limit for pre-clinical studies.

2.1 HIV heterogeneity and cell targets

HIV presents a genome of about 10,000 base pairs, composed of three structural genes (*gag*, *pol* and *env*) beyond the six accessory genes (*vif,vpr, rev, tat,vpu* and *nef*). The *gag* gene encodes the viral core protein as the capsid, matrix and nucleocapsid, *pol* encodes the viral enzymes (reverse transcriptase, protease, ribonuclease and integrase) and *env* gene encodes the envelope glycoproteins. Some products of these genes are targets of choice for the study of vaccines.

The great genetic diversity of HIV represents a major obstacle to developing an effective vaccine. Such diversity is the result of a highly HIV replicative rate (new 10^{10} viral particles/day) and of its prone to errors retrotranscriptase (1 new nucleotide substitution/replication for a genome of approximately 10 000 bp).

The highest degree of HIV diversity is found in the envelope glycoproteins. The amino acid sequences of Env may differ by about 15% between isolates of the same clade and in more than 35% between envelopes of different clades (Gaschen et al 2002).

As a consequence of this high degree of mutational rate, HIV can counteract the selective pressure imposed by the host immune response, and it soon become able to evade an effective response. This aspect makes it difficult to identify potential HIV targets against which the immune system could be directed.

Another important point is that an effective vaccine may protect against various HIV subtypes and clades prevalent in every region of the world. HIV is classified into two types: HIV-1 and HIV-2 that have a genetic homology around 40-50%. While HIV-2 is less pathogenic and its incidence is confined to Africa, HIV-1 is the causative agent of a worldwide pandemic. HIV-1 is divided into three groups M, O and N. The groups O and N are restricted to Central Africa, while group M is responsible for the AIDS pandemic.

Within group M, HIV-1 isolates are divided into six subtypes and clades (A, B, C, D, E and G) and have distinct geographic distributions. While subtype B is prevalent in the Americas and Europe, subtype C, which accounts for more than 50% of AIDS cases worldwide, is prevalent in Southeast Asia and Africa. The difference between the amino acid sequences among viral clades differs by 20% and the variation within clades can reach over 10% in amino acid sequence. Furthermore, different subtypes may be associated with generating circulating recombinant forms (CRFs), further increasing the viral diversity.

Another major challenge that hinders the design of an effective vaccine is the HIV tropism for immune cells. HIV uses the CD4 molecule as a receptor for cell entry. This molecule, in turn, is expressed mainly by T helper lymphocytes and to a lesser degree by dendritic cells, macrophages and monocytes. Since these are strategic cells within the immune system, the immune response in HIV-infected individuals is compromised (Figure1).

Belonging to retroviruses, HIV integrates its genetic material into host cell genome. Days after infection the virus begins its haematogenous spreading from mucosal to lymphoid sites, particularly gut-associated lymphoid tissue (GALT) where a lot of CD4+ CCR5+ T memory lymphocytes are destructed (Matapallil et al., 2005).

The massive loss of CD4+ T cells compromises the host immune response during the infection. Moreover, since the HIV genome is integrated latently until cells become activated, establishing viral reservoirs that hinder the complete elimination of infection.

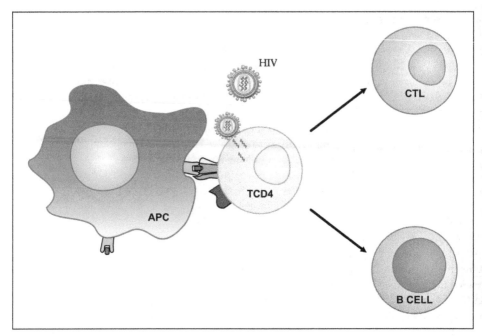

Fig. 1. HIV cell target. HIV predominantly infects CD4+ lymphocytes, which play a
fundamental role in the induction of specific immune response.
APC: Antigen-presenting cell
CTL: Cytotoxic T lymphocyte

2.2 Host/virus interaction

A key feature of the immune system is to "remember" and respond to antigens with which
they've previously met. This property, called immunological memory, is the basis of the
vaccination process. To play its role, a vaccine must therefore deliver the antigen to the
immune system in order to stimulate it and to enable the development of memory.

In this sense, a basic problem in developing an HIV vaccine is the lack of definition of the
correlates of immune protection in HIV infection, so that is not completely clear what types
of immune response should ideally be stimulated by vaccination and consequently what
measure and criteria should be used to evaluate the effectiveness of the vaccine.

Initially the first strategies implied to obtain an HIV vaccine were focused on inducing
neutralizing antibodies against the viral envelope proteins (Dolin, 1995) and from mid-1990,
studies began to focus on the activation of a cellular immune response.

Stimulation of neutralizing antibodies with broad specificity for all HIV variants would be
definitely interesting for a vaccine strategy. Evidence in nonhuman primates suggest that a
protection could be afforded if neutralizing antibodies could be present in high
concentration both in blood and mucosa at the time of first infection (Parren et al., 2001).
However, the induction of neutralizing antibodies against HIV is hampered by some
specific characteristics of the virus, such as

a.   The high epitopes mutation rate, which causes loss of recognition capacity by
       antibodies;

- The large number of subtypes of HIV that exhibit little cross-reactivity;
- The high rate of glycosylation on the viral envelope
- The existence of hidden CD4/receptor binding sites which difficult the access of the antibodies. (Figure 2)

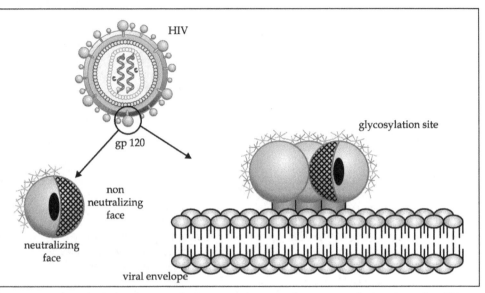

Fig. 2. Sites of antibody binding to gp120. Neutralizing and non-neutralizing sites of gp120. The sites of glycosylation of the molecule are also shown.

Considering that HIV infects CD4+ T cells, the stimulation of a cellular response is important for the destruction of infected cells by cytotoxic T lymphocytes (CTLs) before the release of new viral particles. Thus, in a context of an anti-HIV vaccine CD4+ T cells should be rapidly expanded to stimulate the right cytotoxic response against infected cells and drive memory cells to sites potentially susceptible to infection such as mucosal and lymph nodes.

Although many studies provide strong evidence that a cellular response can effectively suppress HIV (Rowland-Jones et al., 1998; Hladik et al., 2003), it remains unclear how this viral suppression occurs and how a vaccine could stimulate it. Peculiar characteristics of the virus and the nature of infection hinder the development of an appropriate cellular response, for example,

a. The reduction of the expression of MHC class I molecules mediated by the HIV Nef protein;
b. The establishment and maintenance of latent viral reservoirs in cells
c. The massive destruction of T cells specific or not for HIV, caused mainly by activation-induced apoptosis. (Cadogan & Dalgleish, 2008).

In this context, even though there are not clear evidences regarding the type of immune response to be induced by an HIV vaccine, it is reasonable to assume that elements of the immune response important to ensure a real effectiveness of an HIV vaccine may depend on both neutralizing antibody and specific cellular immunity, and besides, also on innate immunity. In a simplified view, neutralizing antibodies prevent the entry of virus into the cell by blocking the transmission and infection, while the cellular response would ac destroying HIV-infected cells before the release of new viral particles in order to control ar yet established infection.

Another interesting tips is that being mucosal the primary site of natural HIV infectior (Kozlowski & Neutra, 2003) an effective vaccine must induce anti-HIV-1 neutralizing antibodies at mucosal surfaces to prevent the infection and cytotoxic T lymphocytes (CTLs in sub-mucosal areas to kill virus-infected cells, or a combination of both. Unfortunately, the immune response within the mucosa may be associated with a high viral replication anc dissemination: HIV activates and recruits a lot of target cells and the virus uptake by dendritic cells allow its dissemination to draining lymph nodes avoiding antibody recognition. The challenge to an effective vaccine is to activate mucosal immunity at the right time. Moreover, all mucosal vaccines have to overcome tolerance, which is related with regulatory cells and depend on the nature of the antigen, the dosage, the method of delivery and on whether or not adjuvant is used.

2.3 Lack of animal models

Actually there is no animal model capable of to mimic the human HIV infection and AIDS development. The use of animal models could help the investigation of disease pathogenesis and provide information about toxicity and efficacy of drugs and vaccines to reduce risk duration and cost of a clinical trial.

Despite its relatively low cost and ease of maintenance in animal houses, the use of smal rodents as experimental models for HIV infection is not appropriate since HIV is unable to sustain infection in murine cells. More recently it has been demonstrated the use of humanized mice models (Van Duyne et al., 2009).

Studies in non-human primates (NHP; i.e.: *Macaca rhesus*), when allowed, even if expensive gave some good results and have the advantage of sharing a high genetic background with humans. NHP are the natural host of a retrovirus of the same HIV family, SIV (Simiar Immunodeficiency Virus) which has a very low mutational rate compared to HIV. In some studies the SHIV, a hybrid virus composed of parts of the genome of HIV and SIV, has beer implied to create the infection model (Stapransan et al, 2010).

Although providing crucial information about viral immunobiology and vaccine design, it must be taken in account that important differences in the viral infection exist betweer humans and NHP. Data from NHP models should be critically evaluated for their predictive value in human trials (Shedlock et al., 2009).

3. Strategies and methods used in the development of anti-HIV vaccines

Like most vaccines, candidates for HIV vaccine contained weakened or killed forms of the virus or viral components which resembling original HIV and could be able to stimulate the immune system to develop an appropriate response. Taking in account all these considerations, in the past decades several aspects related to the vaccine composition, route of immunization and vaccine strategy have been tested in the effort to develop an effective HIV vaccine.

3.1 Vaccine composition
3.1.1 Immunogen production

Many techniques have been employed in order to produce relevant immunogenic HIV antigens, such as:

- chemical (eg. alcohols) or heat inactivated virus particles;
- viral proteins or peptides artificially synthesized (mimetopos) or produced by the insertion of relevant genes in biological vectors (recombinants);
- proteins expressed in the form of virus like particles (VLP), consisting of structurally preserved viral epitopes (i.e.: parts of the virus surface proteins), without the viral genetic material, thus preventing their replication.
- HIV genetic material to insert directly into cells that will express their products. Usually this material is inserted in the form of plasmids, which are molecules of extra-chromosomal circular DNA, with independent replication. The insertion of genetic material in the body can be made directly (eg. electroporation or gene guns using compressed gas) or through biological vectors.

Live attenuated virus vaccines have not been investigated in anti-HIV vaccines due to the risk of development of virulence, as evidenced in a model of NHP (Whatmore et al., 1995).

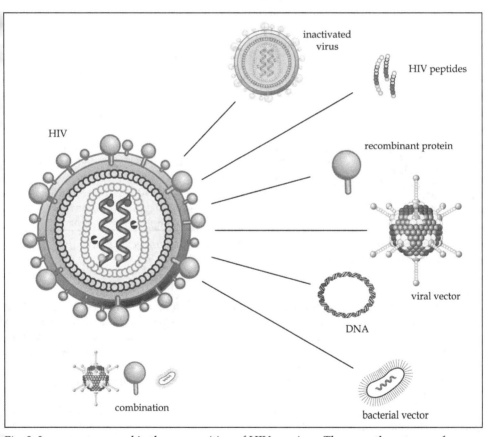

Fig. 3. Immunogens used in the composition of HIV vaccines. There are three types of immunogens: whole vital particle, peptides or recombinant proteins and genetic material of the virus, which may or may not be inserted within vectors. Sometimes the combination of different immunogens can be used (prime-boost strategy).

The advantages and disadvantages of some types of immunogens used in the development of HIV vaccines are summarized in Table 1.

PRODUCT	ADVANTAGE	DISADVANTAGE
Inactivated virus	- whole virus is included in the vaccine	-risk that the preparation contains active virus - difficult to produce in large scale -the response induced by chance is directed only to the type of virus
Peptide	-production relatively simple and inexpensive -safe	-un representative in terms of immunogenic epitopes
Recombinant proteins	-production relatively simple -safe	-low immunogenic
DNA	-production relatively simple and inexpensive	-there are gaps of knowledge about the integration of DNA in the human genome -low immunogenic
Vaccines based on biological vectors	-safe -it is possible to control the type and amount of HIV protein	- limited ability to incorporate HIV genes (in the case of viral vectors) - limited immunogenicity by the existence of prior immunity to the vector - production platforms more complex (viral vectors)

Table 1. Advantages and disadvantages of some types of immunogens used in the development of HIV vaccines

3.1.2 Adjuvants

A vaccine adjuvant is a component that potentiates the immune responses to an antigen and/or modulates it towards the desired immune responses (i.e.: with respect to immunoglobulin classes and induction of cytotoxic or helper T lymphocyte responses). In addition, certain adjuvants can be used to promote antibody responses at mucosal surfaces. Activation of innate immune system and in particular of dendritic cells (DCs) is a crucial mechanism by which adjuvants stimulate protective adaptive immunity against the vaccine antigen.

As immune response is typically initiated by activation of antigen presenting cells (APCs), notably dendritic cells (DCs). There has been significant interest in improving APC-stimulating adjuvants as a key step in constructing better vaccines

Adjuvants have several forms, ranging from mineral salts such as alum to oil-based emulsions. Moreover molecular adjuvants such as proteins, lipids, nucleic acids, carbohydrates, or chemical compounds have a known receptor in DCs (i.e.: Toll Like receptors - TLRs) and result in an improvement in the quantity or quality of the ensuing immune response (Kornbluth & Stone, 2006).

CLASS	EXAMPLE
CD40 agonists	CD40L or its derivates, Agonistic anti-CD40 antibodies, Heat shock protein (Hsp70)
NKT cell ligand	CD1d-binding NKT
TLRs agonists	poly(I:C), LPS, and imidazoquinolines act on TLR3, TLR4, and TLR7 (mDCs) imidazoquinolines and CpG ODP act on TLR7 and TLR9 (pDCs) flagellin act on TLR5 (Vassilieva et al., 2011)
NLRs agonists	MDP act on NOD2 and NALP3, extracellular ATP and pathogen RNA act on NALP3
Chemokines	MIP-1a, CCL19/EBI1-ligand and CCL21/SLC

Table 2. Molecular adjuvants for HIV vaccine strategy.

Many adjuvants have been developed in the past, but were never accepted for routine vaccination because of safety concerns (e.g. acute toxicity and the possibility of delayed side effects).

3.2 Route of administration

Vaccine delivery systems are the sum of pharmacologic technologies (including drug preparation, route of administration, site targeting, metabolism and toxicity) and have the principal aim to make the vaccine preparation faster and easier available to immune system. In its broadest sense, the concept of vaccine delivery systems can be expanded to include a diverse range of devices and physical delivery systems that are designed to improve the potency of vaccines or to allow immunization using novel, non-invasive routes (eg. gene-gun approach, devices designed to fire powdered vaccines into the skin through the use of helium gas and vaccine patches). Delivery systems may function to improve antigen access to lymph nodes in a number of ways:

a. increase antigens presenting cells (APCs), generally dendritic cells (DC), infiltration into the injection site;
b. promote the uptake of antigen in APCs through activating phagocytosis;
c. deliver antigen from the injection site to the local lymph node trough into the lymphatic system

Various routes of HIV vaccine administration have been used starting from the most common (eg. subcutaneous, intramuscular) to more specific such as mucosal with different outcomes. HIV transmission occurs through mucosal (specially of the genital tract) and many efforts have been done to better characterize the mucosal associated lymphoid tissue (MALT) and its involvement in early HIV infection, with the final purpose to use the mucosal route of immunization. For vaccine design, the choice of mucosal inductive site is critical in determining the distal effector site to which induced memory cells will home. In

HIV vaccine research, many mucosal sites were chosen to administer the immunogen: nasal mucosal (Vajdy & Singh, 2006), intratracheal/aerosol vaccination (Corbett et al., 2008), oral vaccination (Stahl-Hennig et al., 2007, N. Cuburu et al., 2007), rectal/colonic vaccination (Belyakov et al., 2006), intravaginal vaccination- (Pialoux et al., 2008).

3.3 Vaccination strategies
The vaccination strategy comprehends the combination of diverse types of vaccine (immunogen, adjuvant, route of immunization) with different schedules to increasing the vaccine potential immunogenic effect. In HIV vaccine several combinations of immunogens (inactivated virus, viral proteins, recombinant viral DNA), routes and schedules have been tested to augment the delivery of HIV antigens to the immune system.

For example, viral vectors are efficient to place HIV relevant epitopes within the target cells and, due to their composition, to stimulate the innate response, promoting an adjuvant effect, although it has been observed that the immunogenicity of these vectors could be affected by the competition between HIV and vector epitopes in the context of antigen presentation. For these reason it was developed the strategy to combined this type of vaccine with a vaccine based on HIV proteins or peptides in a such called prime-boost regimen.

Prime-boost strategy was first time used in 1992 in NHP studies (Hu et al., 1992). Briefly, it consists in the administration of one type of vaccine, such as a live-vector vaccine, followed by or together with a second type of vaccine, such as a recombinant subunit vaccine. The intent of this combination regimen is to induce different types of immune responses and enhance the overall immune response, a result that may not occur if only one type of vaccine were to be given for all doses (Ranasinghe et al., 2009).

3.4 Steps of vaccine development
The development of a vaccine is a process that requires several steps aiming to answer specific questions and to test concepts through experimental practice. Scientific knowledge generated from the execution of each stage or phase will give useful data for planning the next step.

The development of an effective vaccine against HIV infection, due to its unique aspects, will be an unprecedented challenge, and scientific rigor and discipline, statistical principles and bioethics should be required to achieve success.

The preliminary step is to generate more ideas. Established scientists in universities, research institutes and industry use the existing scientific knowledge and technology to develop ideas of how a vaccine might work.

From there, preclinical studies should be performed before human trials to assess whether a novel product has scientific merit to be a candidate vaccine. Such pre-clinical studies involve *in vitro* experiments and *in vivo* tests in available animal models to obtain information regarding the efficacy, toxicity and pharmacokinetics, using varying doses of the product being tested.

The transformation process of a candidate product in a vaccine logarithmic increases the cost and complexity of the research, as it moves from laboratory to clinical application. It is also important to emphasize that only a small percentage of the candidate products being studied in preclinical development is considered safe and promising enough to be evaluated in humans (clinical phase).

Once proven its potential as a vaccine candidate, the clinical phase of the study will start to evaluate safety, immunogenicity and efficacy of the product. Phases I-III are required for licensing the product. In the process of vaccine development, clinical trials may last for many years and the number of volunteers is increasing at every step. The goals set for each stage involves pharmacological and clinical issues, evaluated in a progressive manner throughout the process (www.ich.org - General Considerations for Clinical Trials).

The clinical trial itself begins in Phase I: the candidate vaccine is first evaluated in a small group of human volunteers in order to evaluate its safety, tolerability, pharmacokinetics and pharmacodynamics and identify possible side effects.

In Phase I trial it is also possible to evaluate efficacy markers (e.g.: the generation of antibodies and/or cytotoxic T response), allowing a preliminary assessment of the ability of the vaccine to generate an immune response. Once the safety of the candidate product has been checked, the research could proceed to the next step (Phase II).

The objective of Phase II is to test the candidate vaccine in a larger number of volunteers with two principal purposes: identify side effects related to the product use (within the perspective of future safety analysis, i.e.: toxicity) and collect preliminary indications of product potential effectiveness (efficacy).

Sometimes these aims are studied in different moments and the Phase II trials are divided into:

a.   Phase IIa: designed to determine the optimal dose of vaccine (dose-response studies).

b.   Phase IIb: designed to study the vaccine efficacy.

The Phase III trials are the last stage before possible licensing of the vaccine for marketing. They are randomized controlled trials, often multi-centric, involving large numbers of patients. The primary objective of this step is to evaluate the effectiveness of the product. Achieving a high level of effectiveness at this stage, however, does not necessarily guarantee that the product is effective in the general population, which will be evaluated in phase IV.

Phase IV trials, also called post-evaluation of efficacy, are pharmacovigilance studies performed after licensing the product and that aim to measure the effect of the product in a population. The importance of this phase is to assess the real impact of a vaccine in the epidemic.

The conduct of clinical trials involving prophylactic and therapeutic vaccines for HIV remains a challenge. In terms of design and implementing Phase I and early Phase II are relatively easy to do, although studies involving analysis of effectiveness show a higher degree of complexity. For prophylactic vaccines, the statistical requirements to demonstrate a real prevention of infection require a very large number of patients and they are sometimes prohibitive. Clinical trials for HIV vaccines require the appropriate preclinical studies and the development of better laboratory markers of efficacy.

The role of society is essential for the success of all the program to develop HIV vaccines and the establishment of a genuine dialogue with the community facilitates clinical research with HIV vaccines.

4. Current outlook

Obtaining an HIV vaccine has been one of the biggest challenges of this century. To date numerous clinical trials have been conducted to test candidate products as prophylactic vaccine.

Most initial approaches have focused on the gp120 HIV envelope protein. At least thirteen different gp120 candidates have been evaluated in Phase I trials in the USA predominantly through the AIDS Vaccine Evaluation Group, showing to be safe and immunogenic in diverse populations. They have induced neutralizing antibody, but rarely induced CD8+ cytotoxic T lymphocytes (CTL). Moreover it was very difficult to induce and maintain the high anti-gp120 antibody titers necessary to have any hope of neutralizing an HIV exposure. The availability of several recombinant vectors (adenovirus, canarypox) carrying HIV gens (gag, pol, nef or env) has provided interesting results characterized principally by a poly-functional CTL responses.

Currently, about 20 clinical trials are underway, most protocols for Phase I.

PROTOCOL	SPONSOR	PRODUCT	N	TRIAL SITE	fase
HVTN 082	NIAID, HVTN	VRC-HIVDNA016-00-VP; VRC-HIVADV014-00-VP		USA	I
PedVacc001 & PedVacc002	Medical Research Council	MVA.HIVA	48	Kenya	I
HVTN 078	NIAID, EuroVacc, HVTN	NYVAC-B; VRC-HIVADV038-00-VP	80	Switerzland	I/II
HVTN 505	NIAID, HVTN	VRC-HIVDNA016-00-VP; VRC-HIVADV014-00-VP	1,350	US	II
B001	IAVI, University of Rochester Medical Center	Prime: VRC-HIVDNA016-00-VP Adenovirus serotype 35 vector. Ad35-GRIN/ENV consists of two vectors: Ad35-GRIN vector with *gag*, reverse transcriptase, integrase, and *nef*Ad35-ENV vector with gp140 *env*	42	USA	I
HIVIS 05	Swedish Institute for Infectious disease Control	MVA-CMDR	24	Sweden	I
P001	IAVI, Indian Council of Medical Research, Tuberculosis Research Centre, Chennai; National AIDS Research Institute, Pune	Prime: ADVAX (DNA vaccine containing env, gag, pol, nef and tat) Boost: TBC-M4 (MVA vector with env, gag, RT, rev, tat and nef)	32	India	I
Tiantianvaccinia HIV Vaccine	Chinese Center for Disease Control and Prevention, National Vaccine and SerumInstitute, Peking Union Medical College	HIV-1 CN54 gag, pol and env genes with DNA and rTV vectors	80	China	I
Ad5HVR48.ENVA.01	NIAID, Brigham and Women's Hospital	Recombinant Adenovirus HIV-1 Vaccine, Ad5HVR48.ENVA.01	48	USA	I
HVTN205	GeoVax, HVTN	Prime: DNA vaccine containing gag, pol, env, rat,rev, vpu Boost: MVA vaccine containing gag, pol, env	225	USA, Peru	II
HVTN 073	HVTN, SAAVI, Brigham and Women's Hospital CRS, Fenway Community Health, Clinical Research Boston,	Prime: SAAVI DNA-C2 Boost: SAAVI MVA-C; DNA plasmid vaccine with *gag, RT, tat, nef, env*	48	USA, South Africa	I

PROTOCOL	SPONSOR	PRODUCT	N	TRIAL SITE	fase
	Crossroads, Chris Hani BaragwanathHospita				
VRC 015 (08-1-0171)	NIAID, VRC, NIH Clinical Center	Multiclade Recombinant HIV-1 Adenoviral Vector Vaccine, VRCHIVADV014-00-VP	40	USA	I
Ad26.ENVA.01	NIAID, IPCAVD, Brigham and Women's Hospital, Beth Israel Deaconess Medical Center, Crucell	Recombinant adenovirus serotype 26 (rAd26) vaccine	48	USA	I
NCHECR-AE1	NCHECR, University of New South Wales, Thai Red Cross AIDS Research Centre	A candidate prophylactic DNA prime-rFPV boost HIV vaccination strategy (rFPV-HIV-AE;pHIS-HIV-AE)	8	Thailand	I/II
VRC 012	NIAID, VRC	HIV-1 adenovirus vector vaccine VRC-HIVADV027-00VP: dose escalation and prime-boost with an HIV-1 adenovirus vector vaccine, VRC-HIVADV038-00-VP	35	USA	I
HVTN 077	NIAID, HVTN, Alabama Vaccine, San Francisco Vaccine and Prevention, Hope Clinic of the Emory Vaccine Center, NY Blood Ctr./Union Square, NY Blood Ctr./Bronx, University of Rochester HVTN	Recombinant Adenoviral Subtype 35 (rAd35) and Subtype 5 (rAd5) HIV-1 Vaccines When Given as a Heterologous Prime-Boost Regimen or as Boosts to a Recombinant DNA Vaccine in Healthy, Ad5-Naïve and Ad5-Exposed (VRC-HIVDNA044-00-VP;VRC-HIVADV027-00-VP;VRC-HIVADV038-00-VP)	192	USA	I
HPTN 027	HVTN, International Maternal Pediatric Adolescent AIDS Clinical Trials Group,Makerere University, Johns Hopkins University, Mulago Hospital, Sanofi-Pasteur	Canarypox viral vector with *env* and *gag-pol*	50	Uganda	I
HVRF-380-131004	Moscow Institute of Immunology, FederalMedical and Biological Agency, Russian Federation Ministry of Education and Science	VICHREPOL with polyoxidonium adjuvant	15	Russia	I
RV 138; B011	Walter Reed Army Institute of Research, US Military HIV	Sanofi Pasteur Live Recombinant ALVAC-HIV (vCP205, HIV-1 Env/Gag/Pol) subcutaneously, intradermally, or intramuscularly	36	USA	I
EnvDNA	St. Jude's Children's Research Hospital	Recombinant HIV-1 multi-envelope DNA plasmid vaccine with *env*	6	USA	I
RV 156A	NIAID, HVTN, VRC, MHRP, Makerere U.	VRC-HIVADV014-00-VP alone or as a boost to VRCHIVDNA009-00-VP	30	Uganda	I

Table 3. Ongoing clinical trials (www.avac.org/ht/a/GetDocumentAction/i/3436).

The results of Phase II and Phase III major prophylactic trials are summarized above.

4.1 VAX 004 trial (Phase III, USA 1998-2002)

The phase III VAX 004 trial enrolled 5,403 USA participants between 1998 and 1999. Volunteers received 7 injections of either vaccine or placebo (ratio, 2:1) over 30 months. The study vaccine contained 2 rgp120 HIV-1 envelope antigens (300 mg each of two recombinant proteins rgp120/HIV-1 MN and GNE8) (AIDSVAX B/B; VaxGen) that had been derived from 2 different subtype B strains and that were adsorbed onto 600 mg of alum. GNE8 gp120 was cloned directly from peripheral-blood mononuclear cells and had the CCR5 phenotype; the GNE8 gp120 DNA sequence was deposited in GenBank.

The vaccine did not prevent HIV-1 acquisition and there was no overall protective effect (Flynn et al., 2005).

4.2 STEP trial (Phase II, USA, 2004-2007)

On December 13, 2004, the HIV Vaccine Trials Network (HVTN) began recruiting for the STEP study, a 3,000-participant phase II clinical trial of a novel HIV vaccine, at sites in North America, South America, the Caribbean and Australia.

The trial was co-funded by the National Institute of Allergy and Infectious Diseases (NIAID/NIH, USA), and the pharmaceutical company Merck & Co. Merck developed the experimental vaccine called V520 which contains a adenoviral vector rAd5 carrying three subtype B HIV genes (gag/pol/nef). The vaccine was administered in prime-boost regimen at 0, 1 and 6 months. The follow up of vaccinated subjects showed the lack of efficacy of this vaccine, as well as an increment in HIV-1 infection in individuals with prior immunity to adenovirus. Adenovirus vectors and many other viral vectors currently used in HIV vaccines, will induce a rapid memory immune response against the vector. This results in an impediment to the development of a T cell response against the inserted antigen.

For this reason the phase II trial was closed in September 2007 and other vaccine protocols in progress including the same vector vaccine such as the HVTN503 (Phambili) were cancelled or modificated (Barouch & Korber, 2010).

While the final results of STEP have been disappointing, this study has raised its contribution to redefine the priorities in HIV vaccines research field, demonstrating the need to focus on basic research, preclinical and clinical studies.

4.3 RV144 trial (Phase III, Thailand, 2003-2009)

The phase III HIV vaccine RV144 involved more than 16,000 young Thailandese adults at variable risk for infection between October 2003 and September 2009. Ever six months, volunteers received a prime-boost vaccination including six injections of a vaccine called ALVAC-HIV (vCP1521, Sanofi Pasteur) with the last two of the six injections being a combination of that vaccine and another one called AIDSVAX B/E (gp120, Genentech).

ALVACHIV consists of a viral vector containing genetically engineered versions of three HIV genes (env, gag and pro).The ALVAC vector is an inert form of canarypox, a bird virus which cannot cause disease or replicate in humans. AIDSVAX B/E is composed of genetically engineered gp120. The RV 144 protocol was sponsored by the Surgeon General of the United States Army and conducted by the Thailand Ministry of Public Health with support from the United States Army Medical Research and Materiel Command and the NIAD/NIH.

The rate of HIV infection among volunteers who received the experimental vaccine being tested in the trial was 31% lower than the rate of HIV infection among volunteers who received placebo (Rerks-Ngarm et al., 2009).
Although showing only a modest benefit, this work has renewed optimism in this field of research. However, criticisms related primarily to the study design and statistical method employed to analyse data generated debate about the results (Cohen, 2009; Letvin, 2009).

4.4 Dendritic cell based immunotreatment

In addition to trials aimed at obtaining prophylactic HIV vaccine, has been also developed protocols for therapeutic vaccination using dendritic cells (DC) for the treatment of individuals already infected with HIV.

DCs are potent antigen presenting cells that act as controllers and regulators of the immune system and are the only cells capable of fully activate naive CD4 lymphocytes and thus initiate a specific response (Banchereau & Steinman, 1998). In the context of an HIV vaccine

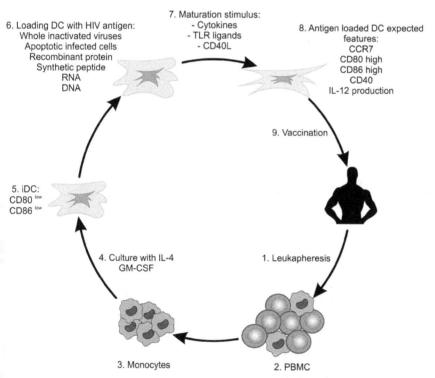

Fig. 4. Treatment of HIV infected patients with monocyte-derived DCs. Peripheral blood mononuclear cells (PBMC) are obtained by leukapheresis and monocytes are separated and cultured in the presence of IL-4 and GM-CSF to obtain immature DCs (iDCs). iDCs are loaded with the antigen of interest and are activated by different stimuli for maturation. Mature DCs (MDCs), potentially able to migrate and to present antigens, are reinoculate into the patient.

AUTHORS	n	TYPE OF ANTIGEN	IMMUNOGENICITY ASSESSMENT
Kundu et al., 1998	6	Recombinant HIV-1 MN gp160 or HLA-A2-restricted synthetic peptides of envelope, Gag, and Pol	Envelope-specific CTL- and lymphocyte-proliferative responses, IFN-gamma and IL-2 production, peptide-specific lymphocyte-proliferative responses
Lu W et al., 2004	18	Chemically inactivated autologous HIV-1	Serum neutralizingantibodytiters, HIV-1-specific interferon-γ (IFN-γ) expressing CD4+ T and CD8+ cells, HIV-1-specific IL-2- expressing CD4+ T cells, HIV-1 gag–specific CD8+ T cells, HIV-1 gag–specific CD8+ T cells expressing perforin
Garcia F et al.,2005	12	Heat-inactivated autologous human immunodeficiency virus type 1 (HIV-1)	Lymphoproliferation, Th1 cell levels, cytotoxic T lymphocyte [CTL] levels, serum neutralizingantibodytiters and changes in lymphoid tissue
Ide F et al., 2006	4	HIV-1-derived cytotoxic T lymphocytes (CTL) peptides	IFN-g production in CD8 lymphocytes
Connolly NC et al., 2008	18	Gag, Env, and Pol peptides	Gamma interferon (IFN-γ)-producing cells (PBMC)
Ghandhi RT et al., 2009	29	Viral vector (canarypox) expressing HIV-1 envandgag and a synthetic polypeptide encompassing epitopes from nefandpol	Gamma interferon (IFN-γ)-producing cells (PBMC), lymphocyte-proliferative responses
Garcia F et al, 2011	24	Heat-inactivated autologous human immunodeficiency virus type 1 (HIV-1)	Lymphoproliferation, serum neutralizing antibody titers, ELISPOT

Table 4. Parameters used in the post-vaccine immune response assessment
HLA= **Human Leukocyte Antigen.** IL-2= **Interleukin-2** . PBMCs=Peripheral Blood Mononuclear Cells.

becomes desirable to induce a specific and effective activation of the immune system against the viral chronic infection.

Protocols of immunotherapy with DCs began in the late 1990 and since then a growing number of studies evaluating this strategy. Because it is an individualized protocol, the number of individuals in the tests is always limited, never exceeding a few tens of individuals.

It is a strategy that involves the collection of mononuclear cells from HIV-infected individual, separation of monocytes and stimulation of these cells with cytokines to differentiate into immature dendritic cells. Dendritic cells are then sensitized (pulsed or loaded) with the antigen of interest, activated and reinoculated into the individuals (Figure 4). The objective of this strategy is to stimulate the immune response by enhancing antigen presentation mediated by dendritic cells.

An overview of the works conducted so far (Table 4) shows although that the products are always safe and the results are quite heterogeneous (Kundu et al., 1998; García et al., 2005, 2011; Ide at al., 2006; Connolly et al., 2008, Lu et al., 2004, Ghandhi, 2009)

Considering the difficulty to obtain an HIV prophylactic vaccine, the immunotherapy offers a unique opportunity to study the mechanisms of immune response against the virus and contribute to the definition of correlates of protection in HIV infection. Knowledge generated from studies of DC-based immunotherapy may contribute also to the development of prophylactic vaccines.

5. Conclusions

Despite numerous difficulties and great scientific challenges that must be overcome to obtain an HIV vaccine, the extraordinary advance in biomedical research and the remarkable progress achieved show clear reasons for optimism.

Knowledge has been accumulated on the biology and diversity of HIV; new methods have been used for the production of immunologically relevant antigens; the study of immune response in exposed not-infected individuals and in elite controllers has generated important information regarding the type of effective immune response against HIV. Furthermore, immunotherapy protocols in infected individuals provide a unique opportunity to studying immune mechanisms against the virus.

Lessons from the failure of the previous protocols can effectively guide the design and refinement of the next generation of candidate vaccines. In this scenario, the perspective is that knowledge of the various interdisciplinary areas of science can provide an environment leading to overcome these scientific challenges.

6. References

Banchereau, J., Steinman, R.M. (1998). Dendritic cells and the control of immunity. *Nature* , Vol 392, No. 6673, (Mar 1998), pp. 245-252, ISSN 0028-0836.

Barouch, D.H., Korber B. (2010). HIV-1 vaccine development after STEP. Annu Rev Med, Vol. 61, (Feb 2010), pp.153-167, ISSN 0066-4219.

Belyakov, I.M., Kuznetsov, V.A., Kelsall, B., Klinman, D., Moniuszko, M., Lemon, M., Markham, P.D., Pal, R., Clements, J.D., Lewis, M.G., Strober, W., Franchini, G. and Berzofsky J.A. (2006). Impact of vaccine-induced mucosal high-avidity CD8+ CTLs in delay of AIDS viral dissemination from mucosa. Blood, Vol. 107, pp. 3258–3264, ISSN 1528-0020.

Brenchley, J.M., Schacker, T.W., Ruff, L.E., Price, D.A., Taylor, J.H., Beilman G.J., Nguyen P.L., Khoruts, A., Larson M., Haase, A.T., Douek, D.C. (2004). CD4+ T cell depletion during all stages of HIV disease occurs predominantly in the gastrointestinal tract. *J Exp Med*, Vol. 200, No. 6, (Sep 2004), pp. 749-759, ISSN 0022-1007.

Cadogan, M., Dalgleish, A.G. (2008). HIV immunopathogenesis and strategies for intervention. *Lancet Infect Dis*, Vol. 8, No. 11, pp:675-684. ISSN 1473-3099.

Carr, A. (2000). HIV protease inhibitor-related lipodystrophy syndrome. *Clin Infect Dis*, Vol 30, Suppl 2, pp.S135-42, ISSN 1537-6591

Cohen, J. (2009). HIV/AIDS research. Beyond Thailand: making sense of a qualified AIDS vaccine "success". *Science*, Vol. 326, No. 5953, pp. 652-653, ISSN 1095-9203.

Connolly, N.C., Whiteside, T.L., Wilson, C., Kondragunta, V., Rinaldo, C.R., Riddler, S.A. (2008). Therapeutic immunization with human immunodeficiency virus type 1 (HIV-1) peptide-loaded dendritic cells is safe and induces immunogenicity in HIV-1-infected individuals. *Clin. Vac. Immunol.* Vol. 15, No 2, pp. 284-92, ISSN 1556-679X.

Corbett M., Bogers, W.M., Heeney, J.L., Gerber, S., Genin, C., Didierlaurent, A., Oostermeijer, H., Dubbes, R., Braskamp, G., Lerondel, S., Gomez, C.E., Esteban, M., Wagner, R., Kondova, I., Mooij, P., Balla-Jhagjhoorsingh, S., Beenhakker, N., Koopman, G., van der Burg, S., Kraehenbuhl, J.P. and Le Pape, A. (2008). Aerosol immunization with NYVAC and MVA vectored vaccines is safe, simple, and immunogenic. *Proc Natl Acad Sci USA*, Vol. 105, pp. 2046–2051, ISSN 1091-6490.

Cuburu, N., Kweon. M.N., Song, J.H., Hervouet, C., Luci, C., Sun, J.B., Hofman, P., Holmgren, J., Anjuere, F. and Czerkinsky, C. (2007). Sublingual immunization induces broad-based systemic and mucosal immune responses in mice. *Vaccine* Vol. 25, pp. 8598–8610, ISSN 0264-410X.

Dolin, R. (1995). Human studies in the development of human immunodeficiency virus vaccines. *J Infect Dis*. Vol. 172, No. 5, pp.1175-1183,ISSN 1537-6613.

Dunham, R., Pagliardini, P., Gordon, S., Sumpter, B., Engram, J., Moanna, A., Paiardini, M., Mandl, J.N., Lawson, B., Garg, S., McClure, H.M., Xu, Y.X., Ibegbu, C., Easley, K., Katz, N., Pandrea, I., Apetrei, C., Sodora, D.L., Staprans, S.I., Feinberg, M.B., Silvestri, G. (2006). The AIDS resistence of naturally SIVinfected sooty mangabeys is independent of cellular immunity to the virus. *Blood*, Vol. 108, No 1, pp. 209-217, ISSN 1528-0020.

Egger, M., Hirschel, B., Francioli, P., Sudre, P., Wirz, M., Flepp, M., Rickenbach, M., Malinverni, R., Vernazza, P., Battegay, M.(1997). Impact of new antiretroviral combination therapies in HIV infected patients in Switzerland: prospective multicentre study. Swiss HIV Cohort Study. *BMJ*, Vol. 315, pp. 1194-1199, ISSN 09598138.

Fischl, M.A., Richman, D.D., Grieco, M.H., Gottlieb, M.S., Volberding, P.A., Laskin, O.L., Leedom, J.M., Groopman, J.E., Mildvan, D. Schooley, R.T et al. (1987). The efficacy of azidothymidine (AZT) in the treatment of patients with AIDS and AIDS-related complex. A double-blind, placebo-controlled trial. *N Engl J Med*, Vol.317, pp. 185-191, ISSN 1533-4406.

Flynn, N.M., Forthal, D.N., Harro, C.D., Judson, F.N., Mayer, K..H., Para ,M.F.; rgp120 HIV Vaccine Study Group. (2005). Placebo-ControlledPhase 3 Trial of a RecombinantGlycoprotein 120 Vaccine to Prevent HIV-1 Infection. J Infect Dis, Vol. 91, pp. 654–65, ISSN ISSN 1537-6613.

García, F., Lejeune, M., Climent, N., Gil, C., Alcamí, J., Morente, V., Alós, L., Ruiz, A., Setoain, J., Fumero, E., Castro, P., López, A., Cruceta, A., Piera, C., Florence, E., Pereira, A., Libois, A., González, N., Guilá, M., Caballero, M., Lomeña, F., Joseph, J., Miró, J.M., Pumarola, T., Plana, M., Gatell, J.M., Gallart, T. (2005). Therapeutic Immunization with dendritic cells loaded with heat-inactivated autologous HIV-1 in patients with chronic HIV-1 Infection. *J. Infect. Dis.* Vol. 191, pp. 1680-1685, ISSN 1537-6613.

García, F., Climent, N., Assoumou, L., Gil, C., González, N., Alcamí, J., León, A., Romeu,. J., Dalmau J., Martínez-Picado, J., Lifson, J., Autran, B., Costagliola, D., Clotet, B., Gatell, J.M., Plana, M., Gallart, T. DCV2/MANON07- AIDS Vaccine Research Objective Study Group. (2011). A therapeutic dendritic cell-based vaccine for HIV-1 infection. J Infect Dis, Vol 203, No. 4, pp. 473-478, ISSN 1537-6613.

Gaschen, B., Taylor, J., Yusim, K., Foley, B., Gao, F., Lang, D., Novitsky, V., Haynes, B., Hahn, B.H., Bhattacharya, T., Korber, B. (2002) Diversity considerations in HIV-1 vaccine selection. *Science*, Vol. 296, No 5577, pp. 2354–2360, ISSN 1095-9203.

Gandhi RT, O'Neill D, Bosch RJ, Chan ES, Bucy RP, Shopis J, Baglyos L, Adams E, Fox L, Purdue L, Marshak A, Flynn T, Masih R, Schock B, Mildvan D, Schlesinger SJ, Marovich MA, Bhardwaj N, Jacobson JM; AIDS Clinical Trials Group A5130 team. (2009). A randomized therapeutic vaccine trial of canarypox-HIV-pulsed dendritic cells vs. canarypox-HIV alone in HIV-1-infected patients on antiretroviral therapy. Vaccine, Vol 27, No. 43, pp. 6088-6094, ISSN 0264-410X.

Hawkins, T. (2010). Understanding and managing the adverse effects of antiretroviral therapy. *Antiviral Res*, Vol 85, No 1, pp. 201-209, ISSN 0166-3542.

Heyward, W.L., MacQueen, K.M., Goldenthal, K.L. (1998). HIV vaccine development and evaluation: realistic expectations. AIDS Res&Hum Retroviruses, Vol. 14, Suppl 3:S205-10, ISSN 1931-8405.

Hladik, F., Desbien, A., Lang, J., Wang, L., Ding, Y., Holte, S., Wilson, A., Xu, Y., Moerbe, M., Schmechel, S., McElrath, M.J. (2003). Most highly exposed seronegative men lack HIV-1-specific, IFN-gamma-secreting T cells. *J Immunol*, Vol. 171, No 5, pp. 2671-83, ISSN 1550-6606.

Hu, S.L., Abrams, K., Barber, G.N., Moran, P., Zarling, J.M., Langlois, A.J., Kuller, L., Morton, W.R., Benveniste, R.E. (1992). Protection of macaques against SIV infection by subunit vaccines of SIV envelope glycoprotein gp160. *Science,* Vol. 255, No. 5043, pp. 456-459, ISSN 1095-9203.

Ide, F., Nakamura, T., Tomizawa, M., Kawana-Tachikawa, A., Odawara, T., Hosoya, N. and Iwamoto, A. (2006). Peptide-loaded dendritic-cell vaccination followed by treatment interruption for chronic HIV-1 infection: a phase 1 trial. *J. Med. Virol,* Vol. 78, No. 6, pp. 711-718, ISSN 1096-9071.

Kornbluth, R.S., Stone, G.W. (2006). Immunostimulatory combinations: designing the next generation of vaccine adjuvants. J Leukoc Biol, Vol. 80, No. 5, pp.1084-1102, ISSN 0741-5400.

Kozlowski, P.A., Neutra, M.R. (2003). The role of mucosal immunity in prevention of HIV transmission. Curr Mol Med, Vol. 3, No 3, pp. 217-228, ISSN 1566-5240.

Kundu, S.K., Engleman, E., Benike, C., Shapero, M.H., Dupuis, M., van Schooten, W.C., Eibl, M., Merigan, T.C. (1998). A pilot clinical trial of HIV antigen-pulsed allogeneic and autologous dendritic cell therapy in HIVinfected patients. AIDS Res. Hum. Retrovir. Vol. 14, pp. 551–560, ISSN 1931-8405.

Lederman, M.M., Alter, G., Daskalakis, D.C., Rodriguez, B., Sieg, S.F., Hardy, G., Cho, M., Anthony, D., Harding, C., Weinberg, A., Silverman, R.H., Douek, D.C., Margolis, L., Goldstein, D.B., Carrington, M., Goedert, J.J. (2010). Determinants of protection among HIV-exposed seronegative persons: an overview. J Infect Dis, Vol. 202, Suppl 3:S333-8, ISSN 1537-6613.

Letvin, N.L. (2009). Virology. Moving forward in HIV vaccine development. Science, Vol. 26, No 5957, pp. 1196-8, ISSN 1095-9203.

Lu, W., Arraes, L.C., Ferreira, W.T., Andrieu, J.M. (2004). Therapeutic dendritic-cell vaccine for chronic HIV-1 infection. Nat. Med, Vol, 10, pp. 1359–65, ISSN 1078-8956.

Mattapallil, J.J., Douek, D.C., Hill, B., Nishimura, Y., Martin ,M., Roederer, M. (2005). Massive infection and loss of memory CD4+ Tcells in multiple tissues during acute SIV infection. Nature, Vol. 434, pp. 1093–1097, ISSN 0028-0836.

Menéndez-Arias L. (2010). Molecular basis of human immunodeficiency virus drug resistance: an update. Antiviral Res. Vol. 85, No. 1, pp. 210-231, ISSN 0166-3542.

Parren, P.W., Marx, P.A., Hessell, A.J., Luckay, A., Harouse, J., Cheng-Mayer, C., Moore, J.P. and Burton, D.R. (2001). Antibody protects macaques against vaginal challenge with a pathogenic R5 simian/human immunodeficiency virus at serum levels giving complete neutralization in vitro. J Virol, Vol. 75, No. 17, pp. 8340-8347, ISSN 1098-5514.

Pialoux, G., Hocini, H., Perusat, S., Silberman, B., Salmon-Ceron, D., Slama, L., Journot, V., Mathieu, E., Gaillard, C., Petitprez, K., Launay, O. and Chene, G. (2008). Phase I study of a candidate vaccine based on recombinant HIV-1 gp160 (MN/LAI) administered by the mucosal route to HIV-seronegative volunteers: The ANRS VAC14 study. Vaccine, Vol. 26, pp. 2657–2666, ISSN 0264-410X.

Poropatich, K., Sullivan, D.J.Jr. (2011). Human immunodeficiency virus type 1 long-term non-progressors: the viral, genetic and immunological basis for disease non-progression. J Gen Virol, Vol. 92 Pt 2, pp. 247-68, ISSN 1465-2099.

Ranasinghe, C., Ramshaw, I.A. (2009). Genetic heterologous prime–boost vaccination strategies for improved systemic and mucosal immunity. Expert Rev Vaccines , Vol. 8, pp. 1171–1181, ISSN 1476-0584.

Rerks-Ngarm, S., Pitisuttithum, P., Nitayaphan, S., Kaewkungwal, J., Chiu, J., Paris, R., Premsri, N., Namwat, C., de Souza, M., Adams, E., Benenson, M., Gurunathan, S., Tartaglia, J., McNeil, J.G., Francis, D.P., Stablein, D., Birx, D.L., Chunsuttiwat, S., Khamboonruang, C., Thongcharoen, P., Robb, M.L., Michael, N.L., Kunasol, P., Kim, J.H. and MOPH-TAVEG Investigators. (2009). Vaccination with ALVAC and

AIDSVAX to prevent HIV-1 infection in Thailand. , Vol. 361, No. 23, pp. 2209-2220, ISSN 1533-4406.

Rowland-Jones, S.L., Dong, T., Fowke, K.R., Kimani, J., Krausa, P., Newell, H., Blanchard, T., Ariyoshi, K., Oyugi, J., Ngugi, E., Bwayo, J., MacDonald, K.S., McMichael, A.J. and Plummer, F.A. (1998). Cytotoxic T cell responses to multiple conserved HIV epitopes in HIV-resistant prostitutes in Nairobi. *J Clin Invest*, Vol. 102, No. 9, pp. 1758-1765, ISSN 1558-8238.

Shedlock, D.J., Silvestri, G., Weiner, D.B. (2009). Monkeying around with HIV vaccines: using rhesus macaques to define 'gatekeepers' for clinical trials. *Nat Rev Immunol*, Vol. 9, No. 10, pp. 717-728, ISSN 1474-1733.

Stahl-Hennig, C., Kuate, S., Franz M., Suh, Y.S., Stoiber, H., Sauermann, U., Tenner-Racz, K., Norley, S., Park, K.S., Sung, Y.C., Steinman, R., Racz, P., and Uberla, K. (2007) Atraumatic oral spray immunization with replication-deficient viral vector vaccines. *J Virol*, Vol. 81, pp.13180–13190, ISSN 1098-5514.

Stapransa, S.I., Feinberga, M.B., Shiverb, J.W. and Casimiro, D.R. (2010). Role of nonhuman primates in the evaluation of candidate AIDS vaccines: an industry perspective. Current Opinion in HIV and AIDS, Vol. 5, No. 5, pp. 377–385, ISSN 1746-6318.

Sumpter, B., Dunham, R., Gordon, S., Engram, J., Hennessy, M., Kinter, A., Paiardini, M., Cervasi, B., Klatt, N., McClure, H., Milush, J.M., Staprans, S., Sodora, D.L. and Silvestri, G. (2007). Correlates of preserved CD4(+) T cell homeostasis during natural, non-pathogenic simian immunodeficiency virus infection of sooty mangabeys: implications for AIDS pathogenesis. *J. Immunol*, Vol. 178, No. 3, pp. 1680-1691, ISSN 1550-6606.

Vajdy, M. and Singh M. (2006). Intranasal delivery of vaccines against HIV. *Expert OpinDrug Deliv*, Vol. 3, pp. 247–259, ISSN 1742-5247.

Van Duyne, R., Pedati, C., Guendel, I., Carpio, L., Kehn-Hall, K., Saifuddin, M., Kashanchi, F. (2009). The utilization of humanized mouse models for the study of human retroviral infections. *Retrovirology*, Vol. 6, pp. 76, ISSN 1742-4690.

Vassilieva, E.V., Wang, B.Z., Vzorov, A.N., Wang, L., Wang, Y.C., Bozja, J., Xu, R., Compans, R.W. (2011). Enhanced Mucosal Immune Responses to HIV Virus-Like Particles Containing a Membrane-Anchored Adjuvant. *MBio*, Vol. 2, No. 1, ISSN 2150-7511.

Walker, B.D. (2007). Elite control of HIV Infection: implications for vaccines and treatment. *Top HIV Med*, Vol. 15, No. 4, pp. 134-136, ISSN 1542-8826.

Wawer, M.J., Sewankambo, N.K., Serwadda, D., Quinn, T.C., Paxton, L.A., Kiwanuka, N., Wabwire-Mangen, F., Li , C., Lutalo, T., Nalugoda, F., Gaydos, C.A., Moulton, L.H., Meehan, M.O., Ahmed, S., Gray, R.H. (1999). Control of sexually transmitted diseases for AIDS prevention in Uganda: a randomized community trial. Rakai Project Study Group. *Lancet*, Vol 353, pp. 525-535, ISSN 0140-6736.

Whatmore, A.M., Cook, N., Hall, G.A., Sharpe, S., Rud, E.W., Cranage, M.P. (1995). Repair and evolution of nef in vivo modulates simian immunodeficiency virus virulence. *J. Virol*, Vol. 69, pp.5117–5123, ISSN 1098-5514.

Towards Universal Acess: Scaling up priority HIV/AIDS Interventions in the health sector. WHO, UNAIDS, UNICEF, 2007. www.who.int/entity/hiv/mediacentre/universal_access_progress_report_en.pdf

www.ich.org - General Considerations for Clinical Trials

www.hivresourcetracking.org/treatments/vaccines

www.avac.org/ht/a/GetDocumentAction/i/3436

9

Towards a Functional Cure for HIV Infection: The Potential Contribution of Therapeutic Vaccination

Maja A. Sommerfelt
Bionor Pharma ASA
Norway

1. Introduction

Human immunodeficiency virus (HIV-1) currently infects 33.3 million people globally. In 2009, 1.8 million people died from acquired immunodeficiency syndrome (AIDS) marking a decline in AIDS deaths by 19% since 1999, the estimated peak of the pandemic. This is largely due to the introduction of combination antiretroviral therapy (ART) in 1996 and its expanding access in recent years. However, despite continued efforts to improve ART availability worldwide, only 5 of the estimated 15 million people living with HIV-1 in low- and middle-income countries have access (UNAIDS, 2010). Furthermore, the number of new infections continues to outpace the number of people being put on ART each day. ART is costly, and places a formidable financial burden on healthcare services. This in turn compromises efforts for universal access.

Combination ART has made a significant impact on HIV-1 morbidity and mortality (Vittinghoff et al., 1999, Palella et al., 2006) and represents the 'gold standard' for HIV-1 treatment. Despite early optimism that combination ART could potentially eradicate infection (Perelson et al., 1996, Ho, 1997), it has since become clear that virus invariably returns if ART is stopped. As a result, ART remains a daily lifelong treatment requiring a high level of compliance to avoid the development of (multi) drug resistance.

Where ART is available, the diagnosis 'AIDS' becomes less frequent, and HIV-1 infection may no longer be considered a irrevocable terminal disease but rather a chronic manageable infection. However, recent studies have observed that ART does not restore life expectancy completely (Neuhaus et al., 2010a; The Antiretroviral Therapy Cohort, 2008). Furthermore, as those living with HIV-1 do become older, age-related toxicities emerge (Powderly, 2007, 2010) as well as other ART co-morbidities such as increased risk of cardiovascular disease, metabolic disorders, neurocognitive abnormalities, liver and renal disease, bone disorders, malignancy and frailty (Deeks & Phillips, 2009).

Untreated HIV-1 infection is characterised by a substantial depletion of CD4+ T-cells in the mucosa as well as a gradual progressive decline of CD4+ T-cells in peripheral blood. When CD4+ T-cell levels in peripheral blood fall below 200 cells/mm³, immune competence is reduced leading to susceptibility to opportunistic infections and conditions that characterise AIDS as well as significant increases in viral load (Levy, 2007). It is primarily the level of CD4+ T-cells in peripheral blood that determines the requirement for ART (Panel on Antiretroviral Guidelines for Adults and Adolescents, 2011).

In recent years it has become apparent that disease progression in HIV-1 infection is not simply due to a loss of CD4+ T-cells as a result of chronic cytopathic viral infection. Instead, HIV-1 infection is accompanied by a progressive generalised immune activation (Neuhaus et al., 2010b; Kuller et al., 2008). Indeed, expression of the activation marker CD38 particularly on CD8+ T-cells has been found to be more predictive of disease progression than viral load (Giorgi et al., 1993; Hazenberg et al., 2003). Although immune activation may be reduced on effective ART, it is not completely absent but remains higher than in uninfected individuals. This may in part explain the loss and/or lack of optimal gain in CD4+ T-cell counts despite effective viral suppression below the level of detection (Hunt et al., 2003). It is intriguing that a similar immune activation is also observed in rhesus macaques infected with simian immunodeficiency virus (SIVsmm or SIVagm) but not in the natural host for these viruses, the sooty mangabey and African green monkey respectively, despite high viral loads (Silvestri et al., 2003). Furthermore, HIV-2 in contrast to HIV-1, is associated with slower disease progression and lower levels of immune activation (Sousa et al., 2002).

The underlying causes of the generalised immune activation associated with HIV-1 infection are presently not fully understood, but are probably associated with multiple mechanisms. These may include reactivation of latent viruses during HIV-1 infection, such as cytomegalovirus (CMV) or Epstein-Barr virus (EBV). The most widely considered mechanism is based on the significant depletion of CD4+ T-cells in the mucosa leading to a disruption of the gut lining and translocation of microbial flora to the systemic immune system (Brenchley et al., 2006). HIV-1 is known to incorporate host human leukocyte antigens (HLA) into its envelope during budding, that may play a role in immune activation. Furthermore, the conserved C5 region of gp120 may also be involved in immune activation (Cadogan & Dalgleish, 2008) by virtue of similarity with the peptide binding domains of HLA molecules. This region of gp120 has been shown to bind peptide and promote activation of antigen-specific T-cell clones (Sheikh et al., 2000).

A small percent (<5%) of individuals have been found to control HIV-1 infection for long periods in the absence of ART. Virus levels, although very low – are never eliminated in these individuals (Hunt et al., 2011). These elite and viraemic controllers (that have a low viral load) have been shown to have narrow cell-mediated immune responses preferentially targeting Gag, and lower immune activation (Rosenberg et al., 1997; Zuniga et al., 2006; Walker, 2007; Saez-Cirion et al., 2007; Binley et al., 1997; Kiepiela et al., 2007). The fact that some individuals can control HIV-1 viraemia suggests that long-term immunological control of HIV-1 infection is possible. This therefore provides credence to the concept of therapeutic vaccination as a means to confer relevant immune stimulation that can ultimately lead to a sustained virological response, emulating a long-term nonprogressor status where the risk of virus transmission is reduced. As a result, more focus will need to be directed to understanding the mechanism(s) behind the control of HIV-1 in elite and viraemic controllers (Autran et al., 2011).

Long-term control of HIV-1 infection in the absence of ART forms the basis for the term 'functional cure' where virus and immune activation levels become equivalent to that found in elite controllers or natural virus suppressors (Jeffries, 2010). In contrast, a 'sterilising cure' relates to HIV-1 eradication, that is, the permanent removal of the HIV-1 by the complete elimination of viral reservoirs. The eradication concept has been inspired by 'The Berlin Patient' who received a bone marrow transplant from a donor that had the CCR5 Δ32 mutation rendering the cells resistant to virus strains using this co-receptor for infection (Hütter et al., 2009). The Berlin patient has remained virus-free for four years to date (Allers et al., 2011).

Therapeutic vaccines have the advantage of being able to penetrate sanctuary sites less well accessed by ART such as lymphoid tissue (Pantaleo et al., 1991; Fox et al., 1991) and the central nervous system (Alexaki et al., 2008), that represent regions for viral persistence. This relates to therapeutic interventions targeting both the virus itself as well as HIV-associated immune activation. This chapter will discuss the potential contribution of therapeutic vaccination to achieve a functional cure for HIV-1 infection.

2. HIV-1 persistence in reservoirs

The failure of ART to eradicate HIV-1 infection lies in the observation that HIV-1 remains quiescent in latent reservoirs. Latently infected resting CD4+ cells (either naive or long lived memory cells) carry transcriptionally silent HIV-1 and represent the predominant reservoir of HIV-1 infection. Other cells may also act as reservoirs (Reviewed in Alexaki et al., 2008) such as macrophages, dendritic cells and astrocytes (where HIV-1 infection occurs via a CD4-independent mechanism). It is these latent reservoirs that represent the major challenge to eradication of HIV-1 infection. More than 80% of individuals on suppressive ART have persistent viraemia below the level of detection (Maldarelli et al., 2007). This low level viraemia is not reduced further despite ART intensification (Dinoso et al., 2009) supporting the concept that HIV-1 rebounds on ART cessation from the rapid reactivation of virus from latently infected cells rather than from continuous ongoing low level replication (Joos et al., 2008). Long lived memory cells comprise approximately 1 cell per million with an extremely low decay rate explaining why 73 years is required to eliminate HIV-1 from infected individuals (Finzi et al., 1999, Siliciano, 2010).

It is clear that to achieve a functional cure, therapeutic vaccination will need to induce not only effective antigen-specific immune responses but also combat the generalised immune activation induced by HIV-1.

3. The concept of a functional cure

The ultimate aim of a functional cure for HIV-1 infection is to induce long-term remission by depleting virus reservoirs to such an extent that a 'controller' status is achieved. In this way virus is maintained at low levels for long periods of time in the absence of ART, equivalent to that observed in known HIV-1 controllers (Lambotte et al., 2005) natural virus suppressors (Sajadi et al., 2007) and elite controllers (Deeks & Walker, 2007). This concept can be compared to achieving a sustained virological response for hepatitis C virus (HCV) infection following interferon/ribavirin treatment. If a sustained virological response is observed for HCV (undetectable virus for at least 6 months), the patient is considered cured. The potential for curing HCV infection is theoretically greater than for HIV-1 since HCV, a separate genus *Hepacivirus* within the virus family Flaviviridae, replicates solely in the cytoplasm of infected cells. As such, on cell division, the virus may remain in only one of the daughter cells. In contrast, HIV-1 is a retrovirus that integrates into the host genome and as such, on cell division will be automatically present in both daughter cells.

A sustained virological response for HIV-1 could be envisaged as either:

a. Indefinite virus control below the limits of detection (<50 copies HIV-1 RNA/ml) (equivalent to a sterilising cure/eradication).

b. Long-term low level virus replication, as for a natural virus suppressor or long-term non progressor, with concomitant low levels of immune activation (equivalent to a functional cure).

Approaches towards eradication include attempts to purge reservoirs by selective activation of latently infected cells (such as memory cells) in the presence of ART such that released virus may not infect and replicate in neighbouring cells (Richman et al., 2009). Agents include histone deacetylase inhibitors, cytokines, such as IL-2 and IL-7, as well as bryostatin, the protein kinase C activator (Kovochich et al., 2011). However, such interventions may also be associated with side effects, resistance and high cost.

Maintaining HIV-1-infected cells in a continuously latent (transcriptionally silent) state, akin to true latency characteristic of herpesviruses, represents the opposite extreme that has received less attention. HIV-1 is produced from activated CD4+ T-cells. At present it is not clear how HIV-1 can be maintained transcriptionally silent whilst still allowing for the CD4+ T-cell activation required to mount an immune response.

3.1 Functional cure and treatment interruption

In order to demonstrate a sustained virological response (functional cure) for patients that are well controlled on ART, treatment will ultimately need to be stopped in order to show that virus levels remain controlled (low/undetectable).

Treatment interruption has been intensely investigated in the past as a means to overcome the limitations of lifelong ART which include side effects, drug resistance and high cost. Today, treatment interruption *per se*, is viewed with scepticism due to safety concerns arising from the SMART study, the largest treatment interruption study to date (El-Sadr et al., 2006). In the SMART study and numerous previous smaller studies, ART was interrupted without any additional immunological support. Treatment interruption in the SMART study was CD4-guided, where ART was discontinued when CD4 levels rose above 350 cells/mm^3 and resumed if CD4 counts fell below 250 cells/mm^3. However, the study was prematurely halted since patients in the treatment conservation group (treatment interruption) experienced greater side effects and adverse events than those in the continuous ART arm. The SMART study therefore concluded that treatment interruption was not safe and that ART should remain a continuous life-long treatment. These safety concerns have affected the design of all treatment interruption trials including those for therapeutic vaccines. Interestingly, a more recent large study of the Swiss Cohort, has suggested that treatment interruption of up to six months can be safely tolerated particularly if patients are well monitored (Kauffman et al., 2011).

Earlier clinical studies have shown that upon cessation of ART, and in the absence of therapeutic immunisation, CD4+ T-cell counts and virus load rebound to preART levels (i.e. the preART set point) (Oxenius et al., 2002a; Wit et al., 2005; Oxenius et al., 2002b; Mata et al., 2005). However, not all patients have available preART viral load information and therefore efforts have been made to identify alternate markers that may predict where the viral load may settle on treatment interruption in the absence of any other intervention. This is necessary in order to determine whether an intervention has lowered the viral load set point in a subject. Proviral DNA levels at baseline have been shown to correlate with the preART viral load, (Yerly et al., 2005), however, this approach will require further validation before it can be taken in to routine use. Until alternative markers are available, preART RNA values will remain the best predictor of the viral load set point that may be obtained on treatment interruption in the absence of therapeutic immunisation. Consequently, the effect of different therapeutic interventions on the viral load will therefore be compared to the preART values.

CD4+ T-cell counts represent the major parameter that determines the need for ART initiation. For this reason, earlier efforts within therapeutic vaccination aimed to improve CD4+ T-cell counts in order to slow disease progression. However, in light of the SILCAAT and ESPRIT studies that focused on improving CD4+ T-cell counts using IL-2 (which provides nonspecific immune stimulation unlike a therapeutic vaccine that is antigen-specific), the conclusion was that improving CD4 counts *per se* was not associated with clinical benefit (INSIGHT-ESPRIT and SILCAAT Study groups, 2009). Consequently, reducing viral load now represents the unequivocal major endpoint for any therapeutic vaccine or intervention aimed at effecting a functional cure or ultimately eradication.

The current scepticism regarding treatment interruption means that inclusion criteria for patients in such studies will take in to consideration both preART and nadir (lowest ever) CD4+ T-cell counts since this has been shown to be a critical parameter in determining the outcome of treatment interruption (Willberg & Nixon, 2007). In subjects with low CD4+ T-cells nadir (200-250 cells/mm^3), CD4+ T-cell levels fall rapidly on treatment interruption requiring earlier re-initiation of ART (Toulson et al., 2005). Patients selected may therefore be relatively newly infected and have robust preART CD4+ T-cell levels and less well established viral reservoirs.

3.1.1 Functional cure scenario 1: Long lasting remission on ART interruption

One approach towards a functional cure could involve therapeutic vaccination in combination with ART followed by treatment interruption with the aim of providing long lasting sustained virological suppression. The advantage of immunising individuals in the presence of ART is that patients have usually regained CD4+ T-cell counts, including naive CD4+ T-cells that can be stimulated to target HIV-1. Furthermore, virus replication is controlled allowing for immunisation in the absence of circulating virus. The immunisation itself will provide some immune activation as CD4+ T-cells harbouring virus become activated leading to a virus burst which would nevertheless be contained by ART. It would therefore be important to allow for vaccine-induced immune activation to subside before stopping ART. Antigen-specific therapeutic vaccines inducing cell-mediated immune responses against gene products from multiply spliced RNA such as Tat may function in the presence of ART and remove infected cells. This is because these early gene products are not targeted by current antiretroviral therapy. Furthermore, Tat expression is not dependent on the activation state of the infected cell and is therefore also synthesized in quiescent T-cells in the absence of virus replication (Wu & Marsh, 2001). In contrast, for therapeutic vaccines targeting products requiring the expression of structural genes such as Gag and Env, ART would need to be stopped in order for the immune system to identify HIV-1 infected cells expressing these antigens.

Therapeutic vaccination using antigen-specific immune stimulation could be combined with other interventions to provide a long-lasting reduction of HIV-1-associated generalised immune activation and consequently reduce the level of viral rebound even further. The aim would be that when patients are removed from ART, CD4+ T-cell counts would remain sustained and a virus set point would be established at a level compatible with a long-term non-progressor, or elite controller for a significant period of time (Figure 1). The therapeutic vaccine may also attenuate the height of the initial peak rebound so that it does not necessarily overshoot the preART value. This scenario may be most beneficial for newly infected subjects that have robust CD4 T-cell counts.

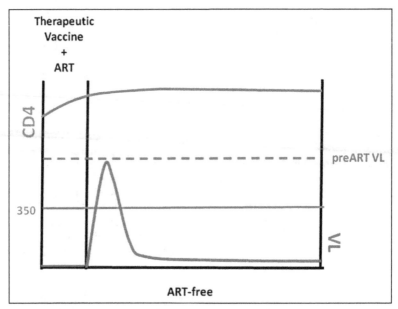

Stippled line at 350 indicates CD4 count below which ART should be initiated. Thick solid line: CD4 count. Thin line: viral load (VL). Dashed line: PreART viral load

Fig. 1. Scenario 1: Therapeutic vaccination in combination with ART leading to sustained virological response (long-lasting remission). Viral rebound may not necessarily overshoot the preART viral load. CD4+ T-cell levels would remain above the level of 350 cells/mm³ that necessitates a return to ART according to current guidelines

3.1.2 Functional cure scenario 2: Remission following intermittent ART

It is possible that on treatment interruption as in scenario 1, viral load levels may stabilize at a lower set point, but not sufficiently low to be compatible with an HIV controller. This may be the case for individuals that started ART later on in disease course, where the number of viral reservoirs is greater, and the CD4+ T-cell nadir lower. To address this, therapeutic vaccination may be used to allow ART to become safely intermittent and where the viral set point may be sequentially reduced following multiple cycles of ART and booster immunisations with the therapeutic vaccine (Figure 2). In such a scenario, due to the safety concerns, the duration of the ART-free period should not exceed the 6 month time period shown to be safe in the Swiss cohort study (Kauffman et al., 2011). This approach of intermittent ART in combination with therapeutic immunisation and booster immunisations has not been investigated to date and may be viewed with scepticism due to the safety concerns arising from the SMART study. However, the underlying basis for the SMART study, i.e. a need to combat ART side effects, drug resistance and high cost remain relevant issues that need to be resolved.

Similarly to scenario 1, therapeutic vaccination may also attenuate the size of the initial peak of rebound during the first treatment interruption allowing the set point to establish below the preART level. Following subsequent booster immunisations on ART in this scenario, as the viral load set point is lowered, CD4+ T-cell decline would also become less marked and would ultimately stabilise above the level necessitating ART (350 cells/mm³).

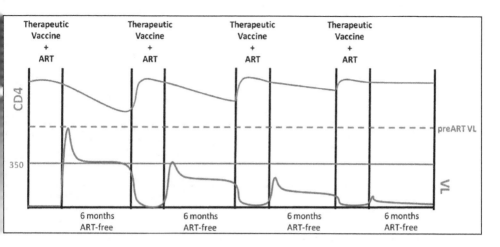

Stippled line at 350 indicates CD4 count below which ART should be initiated. Thick solid line: CD4 count. Thin line: viral load (VL). Dashed line: PreART viral load

Fig. 2. Scenario 2: Functional cure over time: intermittent ART supported by therapeutic vaccination, where viral rebound achieves a lower set point for each successive treatment interruption with a concomitant slower CD4+ T-cell decline over time

Any therapeutic vaccination approach involving treatment interruption involves concerns that viral reservoirs would become repopulated. It is interesting to note that viral reservoirs are also repopulated in elite controller patients since they never manage to eliminate their virus despite maintaining a viral set point below the level of detection (Hunt et al., 2011).

3.1.3 Functional cure scenario 3: On continuous ART
Although potentially applicable to all patient categories, this third scenario for achieving a functional cure on continuous ART may be particularly suited for subjects where treatment interruption is not considered a viable option due to poor CD4+ T-cell reconstitution on ART, low CD4+ T-cell nadir or a very high preART viral load set point. This approach could involve combining continuous ART with therapeutic vaccination and reservoir purging agents (Figure 3).

In this scenario, subjects would be maintained on continuous ART. Therapeutic vaccination would be carried out in the presence of ART as in scenarios 1 and 2 with the aim of generating more effective responses to HIV-1. However, instead of removing patients from ART as in scenarios 1 and 2, reservoir purging agents would be used to reverse latency and allow for the expression of viral genes. Viral replication and spread would be hindered due to the presence of ART. Expression of viral genes would render infected cells 'visible' to the immune system allowing for their removal as a consequence of the improved immune responses resulting from therapeutic immunisation. However, to show ultimately that viral reservoirs have been reduced significantly or even fully depleted, subjects will need to be removed from ART.

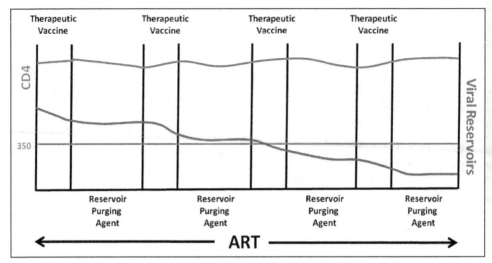

Stippled line at 350 indicates CD4 count below which ART should be initiated. Thick solid line: CD4 count. Thin line: viral reservoirs

Fig. 3. Scenario 3: Subjects remain on continuous ART. Therapeutic vaccination takes place in the presence of ART and the immune responses generated can remove infected cells that release virus following the use of reservoir purging agents. This procedure may need to be repeated to gradually remove virus reservoirs over time

3.2 Functional cure and treatment naive patients
Therapeutic vaccination of individuals that are treatment naive would be an attractive proposition in regions where ART availability is incomplete and where the financial burden to sustain life long treatment is greatest. In this case, subjects would be immunised in the presence of circulating virus to improve and direct immune responses to important epitopes such that viral load is decreased, CD4+ T-cell numbers have the potential to increase and the initiation of treatment delayed. However, therapeutic vaccination itself may result in a transient immune activation that could result in the seeding of further reservoirs with functional and 'fit' (replication competent) virus.

Treatment naive individuals currently represent a study population where the effects of therapeutic vaccination on viral load and CD4+ T-cell counts can be readily observed. However, clinical trials involving treatment naive subjects will likely involve enrolment of patients that are early in disease course and where ART is not yet indicated. Such patients would likely have robust CD4+ T-cell counts and viral loads below 100 000 copies/ml. It is likely that viral reservoirs in these patients would be less well established. The more robust the CD4+ T-cell count, the more likely that the patient may provide an immunological response to the therapeutic vaccine.

4. Approaches to therapeutic vaccination in clinical development

A number of different approaches to HIV-1 therapeutic vaccination are currently in clinical development, although not necessarily at this point in time directly aiming to achieve a functional cure (Tables 1-3). The majority of products aim to induce T-cell immunity whereas a minority aim to induce antibody responses to specific viral antigens. The viral antigens used as therapeutic vaccine candidates include peptides, polypeptides, fusion proteins, recombinant proteins, DNA, RNA either alone or with viral vectors such as poxviruses or adenoviruses, as well as inactivated autologous virus. These antigens can be injected directly or via *ex vivo* bombardment of autologous dendritic cells that are re-infused into the patient. The overall objective of therapeutic vaccine candidates is to reduce viral load, although some also aim to concurrently sustain CD4+ T-cell counts upon ART interruption.

The potency of *ex vivo* stimulation of dendritic cells with inactivated autologous virus was first appreciated following the original studies by Lu et al., (2004) and Garcia et al., (2005) where subjects experienced a significant although transient reduction of viral load. Such approaches require access to autologous virus prior to ART initiation either for purification and inactivation or use as the basis for amplification of viral genes. This approach requires access to advanced technology and may require intermittent boosting to maintain the effect. Therapeutic vaccines are also being developed that aim to target dendritic cells *in situ*. This usually involves intradermal administration. Since intradermal injection requires trained personnel, alternative approaches are being developed to target dendritic cells such as topical patches/plasters.

Company	Product	Clinical phase	Technology
Argos Therapeutics	AGS-004	II n=34 NCT00672191	Autologous DCs co-electroporated with amplified *in vitro* transcribed RNA encoding CD40L and autologous HIV-1 antigens derived from the patient's own plasma taken immediately prior to the initiation of ART.
Baylor University/ ANRS	DC Vaccine	I n=19 NCT00796770	DALIA study: *Ex vivo* administration of Lipopeptides to Nef, Gag and Env to DCs followed by reinfusion to patient
Bionor Pharma	Vacc-4x	IIb n=137 NCT00659789	Peptides to conserved domains of HIV p24 injected intradermally with GM-CSF.
Genetic Immunity	LC002	II n=16 NCT00918840	Clade B DNA in nanoparticles and delivered to DCs in a patch (Dermavir).
NIAID/ Profectus Biosciences	MRK Ad5 HIV-1 gag	II n=120 NCT00080106	Replication defective adenovirus vector carrying HIV-1 gag.

Table 1. Therapeutic vaccine candidates immunising subjects on ART with a treatment interruption phase in the study. DC:dendritic cell, TI: treatment interruption. NCT provides the clinical trial identifier for trials listed on www.clinicaltrials.gov

Viral vectors derived from adenoviruses or poxviruses have also been extensively used to deliver DNA-based vaccines most often in a prime boost strategy. For such approaches it will likely be necessary to determine the serological status of vaccine recipients to the viruses that have been used as a basis for these vectors since prior immunity may negatively affect vaccine efficacy. Similarly, maintenance of vaccine effect may require boosting using a heterologous virus vector, to avoid inhibitory effects of prior vaccine-induced immunity to the original vector.

Although the induction of neutralising antibodies remains the major goal for an effective preventative vaccine, therapeutic vaccines aim to induce antibody responses to other viral antigens such as the HIV-1 Tat protein. Earlier studies have shown that loss of antibody responses to Tat correlated with disease progression (van Baalen et al., 1997; Rezza et al., 2005). Such a vaccine may also address pathogenic effects of Tat released from infected cells (Ensoli et al., 1993).

Company	Product	Clinical phase	Technology
Imperial College	GTU-MultiHIV-B (FIT06)	I n=30 NCT01130376	DNA plasmid. Intradermal injections in combination with GM-CSF and IL-2 as well as a growth hormone.
Univ. Oxford Med Research Council.	MVA.HIVco nsv	I n=20 NCT01024842	MVA vector encoding a DNA that carries conserved domains in Gag, Vif, Pol, Env.
University Pennsylvania / Drexel University	PENNVAX B,GENEVA X IL-12-4532, pIL15EAM	I n=38 NCT00775424	PENNVAX-B is a DNA vaccine encodes synthetic HIV-1 envelope protein, Gag and Pol. GENEVAX and pIL15 are DNA adjuvants (IL-12 and IL-15)
Massachusetts General Hospital	DNA	I n=21 NCT00833781	Dendritic cells transfected with vectors encoding consensus (clade B) HIV Gag and Nef mRNA.
NIAID	HIV Antigens & IL-12	I n=60 NCT01266616	Plasmid DNA with IL-12 to enhance the response.

Table 2. Therapeutic vaccine candidates in clinical development where therapeutic vaccination occurs in the presence of continuous ART. DC: dendritic cell. NCT provides the clinical trial identifier for trials listed on www.clinicaltrials.gov

5. The challenges facing therapeutic vaccination

No preventative vaccine has yet been developed for HIV-1 infection. This is despite intense efforts since the virus was first isolated in 1983 (Barre-Sinoussi et al., 1983). The challenges faced by preventative and therapeutic vaccines are similar in that HIV-1 shows extensive genetic variation and a propensity for immune escape. Furthermore, human populations are also varied and this is characterised by a variety of human leukocyte antigens (HLA). HLA function to present HIV-1 epitopes at the surface of infected cells to allow for recognition and removal by cytotoxic T-lymphocytes. The association of certain HLA with virus control (e.g. HLA-B57) and disease progression (e.g. B35) has recently been highlighted

(International HIV Controllers Study Study, 2010). However these HLA alleles are not present in a large proportion of individuals. It has been suggested that patients in clinical studies should be HLA tested to help explain and understand the results (Li et al., 2011). One salient difference between the preventative and therapeutic vaccines lies in their objectives. At present it is considered remote that a vaccine can be developed that will yield sterilising immunity and complete protection from HIV-1 infection. For this reason, the objective of a preventative vaccine is now to prevent infection as far as is possible, and should infection occur the immune system will be sufficiently primed to ensure that the disease course is milder (Johnston & Fauci, 2007). This was the aim of the STEP trial, which used an adenovirus vector. However, unexpectedly, prior exposure to adenovirus infection resulted in greater susceptibility to HIV-1 infection in study participants (Buchbinder et al., 2008).

Company	Product	Clinical phase	Technology
Genetic Immunity	LC002	II n=36 NCT00711230	Clade B DNA incorporated into nanoparticles and delivered to DCs in a patch (Dermavir).
SEEK (previously PepTcell)	HIV-v	I n=55 NCT01071031	Mixture of polypeptide T-cell epitope sequences to conserved domains of HIV (internal proteins). Single subcutaneous injection
Statens seruminstitutt, DK, EU clinical trials partnership	AFO-18	I n=20 NCT01141205	Peptides representing 3 CD4 and 17 CD8 minimal HIV epitopes. Adjuvant CAF01.
Thymon	TUTI-16	I/II n=24 NCT00848211	Tat Lipopeptide. Subcutaneous injection, acts as own adjuvant.
FIT Biotech	FIT06 (GTU-MultiHIV-B)	II n=60	DNA plasmid using GTU® Technology patented by FIT Biotech (Gene Transport Unit). Gag, Rev, Nef, Tat. Clade B.
Hospital Clinic of Barcelona	DCV2	I/II n=60 NCT00402142	Autologous dendritic cell pulsed *ex vivo* with patient's own virus.
Istituto Superiore di Sanita	ISS T003	II n= 160 NCT01029548	Inactivated Tat protein injected intradermally (i.d.) to induce antibodies to Tat. This study is an observational cohort.

Table 3. Therapeutic vaccine candidates in clinical development immunising subjects that are treatment naive.

6. Conclusion

The complexity of HIV-1 infection represents a challenge to achieving a functional cure or ultimately eradication of infection. A number of scenarios have been suggested in this chapter where therapeutic vaccination is combined with ART and also potentially with virus purging agents. At present it is unlikely that any one scenario will suit all purposes, indeed, the choice of approach will likely depend upon the availability of ART, how far advanced the infection is on diagnosis and when during the disease course ART was initiated since these considerations will influence the size of viral reservoir.

It is unlikely that there will ever be a single product that will either prevent HIV-1 infection completely or eradicate HIV-1 infection. Therefore, combinations may be more appropriate. Harnessing the immune system is a rational approach to combine with ART bearing in mind that the immune system may penetrate regions of the body not reached by current therapy. Combination ART has been more successful than monotherapy. Similarly combining ART with therapeutic vaccination and/or virus purging agents will likely be more effective than any of these interventions on their own. The recent Thai study provides is an example where two preventative vaccine candidates that had not shown effect earlier, provided an improved response leading to a marginally significant effect when combined (Reks-Ngarm et al., 2009).

Ultimately a therapeutic vaccine will need to confer effective immune responses in all individuals regardless whether they possess HLA compatible with virus control or not. It is therefore important that therapeutic vaccine candidates take into consideration genetic variation in both human and viral populations in order to be able to elicit the most effective responses leading to control of infection. Strictly, the term 'functional cure' can be considered misleading since virus is not completely removed from the body, but rather the patient experiences remission from symptoms. The term 'functional control' would therefore be more appropriate.

Eradication approaches will require much research and development, where both novel and known compounds will be tested in new ways to determine a potential effect on eradication without incurring too many side effects. It may therefore take significant time before such products are available on the market. In contrast, a functional cure may be achievable in the shorter term and represent a more realistic goal since virus reduction has been shown for a number of therapeutic vaccine candidates. Approaches that aim to successfully combat HIV-1 infection will need to address both the virus (virus-specific approaches including ART and therapeutic vaccines) as well as the generalized immune activation that drives the infection. It is likely that to achieve a functional cure, a combination of different interventions may ultimately be required.

7. Acknowledgments

This work has been partly supported by a grant from the Research Council of Norway GLOBVAC programme. Many thanks to Birger Sørensen, Ingebjørg Baksaas, Vidar Wendel-Hansen and Giuseppe Pantaleo for reading and commenting the manuscript.

8. References

Alexaki, A.; Liu, Y. & Wigdahl B. (2008). Cellular reservoirs of HIV-1 and their role in viral persistence. *Curr. HIV Res.* 6:388-400.

Allers, K.; Hütter, G.; Hofmann, J.; Loddenkemper, C.; Rieger, K.; Thiel, E.; Schneider, T. (2009). Evidence for the cure of HIV infection by CCR5Δ32/Δ32 stem cell transplantation. *Blood* 117:2791-99.

Autran, B.; Descours, B.; Avettand-Fenoel, V. & Rouzioux, C. (2011). Elite controllers as a model of functional cure. *Curr. Opin. HIV and AIDS* 6:181-187.

Barré-Sinoussi, F., Chermann, J.C., Rey, F., Nugeyre, M.T., Chamaret, S., Gruest, J., Dauguet, C., Axler-Blin, C., Vézinet-Brun, F., Rouziousx, C., Rosenbaum, W., Montagnier, L. (1983). Isolation of a T-lymphotropic retrovirus from a patient at risk for acquired immunodeficiency syndrome AIDS. *Science* 220:868-71.

Binley, J.M.; Klasse, P.J., Cao, Y.; Jones, I.; Markowitz, M.; Ho, D.D. & Moore, J.P.(1997). Differential regulation of the antibody responses to Gag and Env proteins of human immunodeficiency virus type 1. *J. Virol.* 71:2799-2809

Brenchley, J.M. Price, D.A.; Schacker, T.W.; Asher, T.E.; Silvestri, G.; Rao, S.; Kazzaz, Z.; Bornstein, E.; Lambotte, O.; Altmann, D.; Blazar, B.R.; Rodriguez, B.; Teixeira-Johnson, L.; Landay, A.; Martin, J.N.; Hecht, F.M.; Picker, L.J.; Lederman, M.M.; Deeks, S.G. & Douek, D.C. (2006). Microbial translocation is a cause of systemic immune activation in chronic HIV infection. *Nat. Med.* 12:1365-71

Buchbinder, S.P.; Mehrotra, D.V.; Duerr, A.; Fitzgerald, D.A.; Mogg, R.; Li, D. Gilbert, P.B.; Lama, J.R.; Marmor, M.; del Rio, C.; McElrath, J.; Casimiro, D.R.; Gottesdiener, K.M.; Chodakewitz, J.A.; Corey, L. & Robertson, M.N. The Step Study Protocol Team (2008). *Lancet* 372:1881–93

Cadogan, M. & Dalgleish, A.G. (2008). Pathogenesis of HIV: non-specific immune hyperactivity and its implications for vaccines. *Clinical Medicine* 8:267-71.

Deeks, S.G. & Phillips, A.N. (2009). HIV infection, antiretroviral treatment, ageing and non-AIDS-related morbidity. *BMJ* 338:a3172.

Deeks, S.G. & Walker, B.D. (2007). Human immunodeficiency virus controllers: mechanisms of durable virus control in the absence of therapy. *Immunity* 27:406-416.

Dinoso, J.B.; Kim, S.Y.; Wiegand, A.M.; Palmer, S.E.; Gange, S.J.; Cranmer, L.; O'Shea, A.; Callender, M.; Spivak, A., Brennan, T.; Kearney, M.F.; Proschan, M.A.; Mican, J.M.; Rehm, C.A.; Coffin, J.M.; Mellors, J.W.; Siliciano, R.F. & Maldarelli, F. (2009). Treatment intensification does not reduce residual HIV-1 viraemia in patients in highly active antiretroviral therapy. *Proc. Nat. Acad. Sci. USA* 106:9403-08.

El-Sadr, W.M., Lundgren, J.D.; Neaton, J.D.; Gordin, F.; Abrams, D.; Arduino, R.C.; Babiker, A.; Burman, W.; Clumeck, N.; Cohen, C.J., Cohn, D.; Cooper, D.; Darbyshire, J.; Emery, S.; Fätkenheuer, G.; Gazzard, B.; Grund, B.; Hoy, J.; Klingman, K.; Losso, M.; Markowitz, N.; Neuhaus, J.; Phillips, A.; Rappoport, C. & the SMART Study Group. CD4+ count-guided interruption of antiretroviral treatment. *N. Engl. J. Med.* 2006; 355:2283-96

Ensoli, B.; Buonaguro, L.; Barillari, G.; Fiorelli, V.; Gendelman, R.; Morgan, R.A.; Wingfield, P. & Gallo, R.C. (1993) Release, uptake, and effects of extracellular human immunodeficiency virus type 1 Tat protein on cell growth and viral transactivation. *J. Virol* 67:277–87.

Finzi, D.; Blankson, J.; Siliciano, J.D.; Margolick, J.B.; Chadwick, K.; Pierson, T.; Smith, K.; Lisziewicz, J.; Lori, F.; Flexner, C.; Quinn, T.C.; Chaisson, R.E.; Rosenberg, E.; Walker, B.; Gange, S.; Gallant, J. & Siliciano, R.F. (1999). Latent infection of CD4+ T cells provides a mechanism for lifelong persistence of HIV-1, even in patients on effective combination therapy. *Nat. Med.* 5:512–517.

Fox, C.H.; Tenner-Racz, K.; Firpo, A.; Pizzo, P.A. & Fauci, A.S. (1991) Lymphoid germinal centers are reservoirs of human immunodeficiency virus type 1 RNA. *J. Infect. Dis.* 164:1051–57.

Garcia, F.; García, F.; Lejeune, M.; Climent, N.; Gil, C.; Alcamí, J.; Morente, V.; Alós, L.; Ruiz, A.; Setoain, J.; Fumero, E.; Castro, P.; López, A.; Cruceta, A.; Piera, C.; Florence, E.; Pereira, A.; Libois, A.; González, N.; Guilá, M.; Caballero, M.; Lomeña, F.; Joseph, J.; Miró, J.M.; Pumarola, T.; Plana, M.; Gatell, J.M. & Gallart, T. (2005). Therapeutic immunization with dendritic cells loaded with heat-inactivated autologous HIV-1 in patients with chronic HIV-1 infection. *J. Infect. Dis.* 191:1680-5

Giorgi, J.V.; Liu, Z.; Hultin, L.E.; Cumberland, W.G.; Hennessey, K. & Detels, R. (1993). Elevated levels of CD38+CD8+ T cells in HIV infection add to the prognostic value of low CD4+ T-cell levels: Results of 6 years follow-up. The Los Angeles Center, Multicenter AIDS Cohort Study. *J. Acquir. Immune Def. Syndr.* 6:904-12.

Hazenberg, M.D.; Otto, S.A.; van Benthem, B.H.; Roos, M.T.; Coutinho, R.A.; Lange, J.M.; Hamann, D.; Prins, M. & Miedema, F. (2003). Persistent immune activation in HIV-1 infection is associated with progression to AIDS. *AIDS* 17:1881-8.

Ho, D.D. (1997). How far can you knock down HIV? An interview with David D. Ho, MD. Interview by Mark Mascolini. *J. Int. Assoc. Physicians AIDS Care.* 3:40-4.

Hunt, P.W.; Martin, J.N.; Sinclair, E.; Bredt, B.; Hagos, E.; Lampiris, H. & Deeks, S.G. (2003). T cell activation is associated with lower CD4+ T-cell gains in human immunodeficiency virus-infected patients with sustained viral suppression during antiretroviral therapy. *J. Infect. Dis.* 187:1534-43.

Hunt, PW.; Hatano, H.; Sinclair, E.; Lee, T-H.; Busch, MP.; Martib, JN.; McCune, JM. & Deeks, SG. (2011). HIV-specific CD4+ T cells may contribute to viral persistence in HIV controllers. *Clin. Infec. Dis.* 52:681-7.

Hütter, G.; Nowak, D.; Mossner, M.; Ganepola, S.; Musig, A.; Allers, K.; Schneider, T.; Hofmann, J.; Kucherer, C.; Blau, O.; Blau, IW.; Hofmann, WK. & Thiel, E. (2009). Long-Term Control of HIV by CCR5 Delta32/Delta32 Stem-Cell Transplantation. *N. Engl. J. Med.* 360:692-8.

INSIGHT-ESPRIT and SILCCAT study Groups. (2009). Interleukin-2 therapy in patients with HIV infection. *N. Engl. J. Med.* 361:1548-59.

International HIV Controllers Study. (2010). The major genetic determinants of HIV-1 control affect HLA class I peptide presentation. *Science* 330:1551-7

Jeffries, RJ. (2010). Workshop report: Towards a cure: HIV reservoirs and strategies to control them. *Journal of the International AIDS Society* 13(Suppl. 3):I1. (http://www.jiasociety.org/content/13/S3/I1)[Accessed 11th July 2011]

Johnston, M. & Fauci, A. (2007). An HIV Vaccine – Evolving concepts. *N. Engl. J. Med.* 356:2073-81

Joos, B.; Fischer, M.; Kuster, H.; Pillai, S.K.; Wong, J.K.; Böni, J.; Hirscheld, B.; Webera, R.; Trkolaa, A.; Günthard, H.F.; & The Swiss HIV Cohort Study (2008). HIV rebounds from latently infected cells, rather than from continuing low-level replication. *Proc. Natl. Acad. Sci. USA* 105:16725-30.

Kaufmann, GR.; Elzi, L.; Weber, R.; Furrer, H.; Giulieri, S.; Vernazza, P.; Bernasconi, E.; Hirschel, B. & Battegay, M.; the Swiss HIV Cohort Study (2011). Interruptions of cART limits CD4 T-cell recovery and increases the risk of opportunistic complications and death. *AIDS* 25:441-451.

Kiepiela, P.; Ngumbela, K.; Thobakgale, C.; Ramduth, D.; Honeyborne, I.; Moodley, E.; Reddy, S.; de Pierres, C.; Mncube, Z.; Mkhwanazi, N.; Bishop, K.; van der Stok, M.; Nair, K.; Khan, N.; Crawford, H.; Payne, R.; Leslie, A.; Prado, J.; Prendergast, A.; Frater, J.; McCarthy, N.; Brander, C.; Learn, G.H.; Nickle, D.; Rousseau, C.; Coovadia, H.; Mullins, J.I.; Heckerman, D.; Walker, B.D.; Goulder, P. (2007). CD8+ T-cell responses to different HIV proteins have discordant associations with viral load. *Nat. Med.* 13:46-53.

Kovochich, M.; Marsden, M.D. & Zack, J. (2011). Activation of latent HIV using drug-loaded nanoparticles. *PLoS ONE* 6 (4):e18270.

Kuller, L.H.; Tracy, R.; Belloso, W.; De Wit, S.; Drummond, F.; Lane, H.C.; Ledergerber, B.; Lundgren, J.; Neuhaus, J.; Nixon, D.; Paton, N.I. & Neaton, J.D. INSIGHT SMART Study Group (2008) Inflammatory and Coagulation Biomarkers and Mortality in Patients with HIV Infection. *Plos Med.* Oct 21;5(10):e203.

Lambotte, O.; Boufassa, F.; Madec, Y.; Nguyen, A.; Goujard, C.; Meyer, L.; Rouzioux, C.; Venet, A. & Delfraissy, J.F. SEROCO-HEMOCO Study Group (2005). HIV controllers: a homogeneous group of HIV-1 infected patients with spontaneous control of viral replication. *Clin. Infect. Dis.* 41:1053-1056.

Levy J. (2007). Overall features of HIV pathogenesis: prognosis for long-term survival. In: *HIV and the Pathogenesis of AIDS* 3rd Edition pp317-357. ASM Press. ISBN-13 978-1-55581-393-2.

Li, J.Z.; Brumme, Z.L.. Brumme,, C.J.; Wang, H.; Spritzler, J.; Robertson, M.N.; Lederman, M.M.; Carrington, M.;Walker, B.D.; Schooley,R.T.; & Kuritzkes, D.R. for the AIDS Clinical Trials Group A5197 Study Team (2011). Factors associated with viral Rebound in HIV-1-infected individuals enrolled in a therapeutic HIV-1 gag vaccine trial. *J. Infect. Dis.* 203:976–83

Lu, W.; Arraes, L.C.; Ferreira, W.T. & Andrieu, J. M. (2004). Therapeutic dendritic cell vaccine for chronic HIV-1 infection. *Nat. Med.* 10:1359-65

Maldarelli, F.; Palmer, S.; King, M.S.; Wiegand, A.; Polis, M.A.; Mican, J.; Kovacs, J.A.; Davey, R.T.; Rock-Kress, D.; Dewar, R.; Liu, S.; Metcalf, J.A.; Rehm, C.; Brun, S.C.; Hanna, G.J.; Kempf, D.J.; Coffin, J.M. & Mellors, J.W. (2007). ART suppresses plasma HIV-1 RNA to a stable set point predicted by pretherapy viremia. *PLOS Pathog.* 13:e46

Mata, R.C.; Viciana, P.; de Alarcon, A.; Lopez-Cortes, L.F.; Gomez-Vera, J.; Trastoy, M. & Cisneros, J.M. (2005). Discontinuation of antiretroviral therapy in patients with chronic HIV infection: Clinical, virologic, and immunologic consequences. *AIDS Patient Care STDS* 19:550–562.

Neuhaus, J.; Angus, B.; Kowalska, J.D.; La Rosa, A.; Sampson, J.; Wentworth, D. & Mocroft, A. INSIGHT SMART and ESPRIT study groups. (2010a). Risk of all-cause mortality associated with nonfatal AIDS and serious non-AIDS events among adults infected with HIV. *AIDS* 24: 697-706.

Neuhaus, J.; Jacobs, D.R. Jr.; Baker, J.V.; Calmy, A.; Duprez, D.; La Rosa, A.; Kuller, L.H.; Pett, S.L.; Ristola, M.; Ross, M.J.; Shlipak, M.G.; Tracy, R. & Neaton, J.D. (2010b)

Markers of inflammation, coagulation and renal function are elevated in adults with HIV infection. *J. Infect. Dis.* 201:1788-1795.

Oxenius, A.; Price, D.A.; Dawson, S.J.; Günthard, H.F.; Fischer, M.; Perrin, L.; Ramirez, E.; Fagard, C.; Hirschel, B.; Scullard, G.; Weber, J.N.; McLean, A.R. & Phillips RE; Swiss HIV cohort study (2002a). Residual HIV-specific CD4 and CD8 T cell frequencies after prolonged antiretroviral therapy reflect pretreatment plasma virus load. *AIDS* 16:2317-22.

Oxenius, A.; Price, D.A.; Günthard, H.F.; Dawson, S.J.; Fagard, C.; Perrin, L.; Fischer, M.; Weber, R.; Plana, M.; García, F.; Hirschel, B.; McLean, A. & Phillips, R.E. (2002b). Stimulation of HIV-specific cellular immunity by structured treatment interruption fails to enhance viral control in chronic HIV infection. *Proc. Natl. Acad. Sci. USA* 99:13747-13752.

Palella, FJ, Jr., Baker, R.K.; Moorman, A.C.; Chmiel, J.S.; Wood, K.C.; Brooks, J.T. & Holmberg, S.D. HIV Outpatient Study Investigators (2006). Mortality in the Highly Active Antiretroviral Therapy Era. Changing Causes of Death and Disease in the HIV Outpatient Study. *J. Acquir. Immune Def. Syndr.* 43:27-34

Panel on Antiretroviral Guidelines for Adults and Adolescents. Guidelines for the use of antiretroviral agents in HIV-1-infected adults and adolescents. Department of Health and Human Services. January 10, 2011; 1–166. Available at http://www.aidsinfo.nih.gov/ContentFiles/AdultandAdolescentGL.pdf [Accessed 7th May 2011]

Pantaleo, G.; Graziosi, C. & Butini, L. (1991). Lymphoid organs function as major reservoirs for human immunodeficiency virus. *Proc. Natl. Acad. Sci. USA* 88:9838–42.

Perelson, AS.; Neumann, AU.; Markowitz, M.; Leonard, J.M. & Ho, D.D. (1996). HIV-1 dynamic in vivo: Infected cell lifespan, and viral generation time. *Science* 271:1582-86.

Powderly, W. (2007). The three ages of antiretroviral therapy – its evolution and the emergence of long-term safety concerns. *European Infectious Disease* 1:19-25.

Powderly, W. (2010). Growing old with HIV-dealing with co-morbidities. *Journal of the International AIDS Society* 13(Suppl 4):025.

Rerks-Ngarm, S.; Pitisuttithum, P.; Nitayaphan, S.; Kaewkungwal, J.; Chiu, J.; Paris, R.; Premsri, N.; Namwat, C.; de Souza, M.; Adams, E.; Benenson, M.; Gurunathan, S.; Tartaglia, J.; McNeil, J.G.; Francis, D.P.; Stablein, D.; Birx, D.L.; Chunsuttiwat, S.; Khamboonruang, C.; Thongcharoen, P.; Robb, M.L.; Michael, N.L., Kunasol, P. & Kim, J.H. MOPH-TAVEG Investigators (2009). Vaccination with ALVAC and AIDSVAX to Prevent HIV-1 Infection in Thailand. *N. Engl. J. Med.* 361:2209-20.

Rezza, G.; Fiorelli, V.; Dorrucci, M.; Ciccozzi, M.; Tripiciano, A.; Scoglio, A.; Collacchi, B.; Ruiz-Alvarez, M.; Giannetto, C.; Caputo, A.; Tomasoni, L.; Castelli, F.; Sciandra, M.; Sinicco, A.; Ensoli, F.; Buttò, S. & Ensoli, B. (2005). The presence of anti-Tat antibodies is predictive of long-term nonprogression to AIDS or severe immunodeficiency: findings in a cohort of HIV-1 seroconverters. *J. Infect. Dis.* 191:1321-4.

Richman, DD.; Margolis, DM.; Delaney, M.; Greene, WC.; Hazuda, D. & Pomerantz RJ. (2009). The challenge of finding a cure for HIV infection. *Science* 323:1304-1307.

Rosenberg, E.S.; Billingsley, J.M.; Caliendo, A.M.; Boswell, S.L.; Sax, P.E.; Kalams, S.A. & Walker, B.D.(1997). Vigorous HIV-1-specific CD4+ T cell responses associated with control of viremia. *Science* 278:1447 -50.

Sáez-Cirión, A.; Lacabaratz, C.; Lambotte, O.; Versmisse, P.; Urrutia, A.; Boufassa, F.; Barré-Sinoussi, F.; Delfraissy, J.F.; Sinet, M.; Pancino, G. & Venet, A. Agence Nationale de Recherches sur le Sida EP36 HIV Controllers Study Group (2007). HIV controllers exhibit potent CD8 T cell capacity to suppress HIV infection *ex vivo* and peculiar cytotoxic T lymphocyte activation phenotype. *Proc. Natl. Acad. Sci. USA* 104:6776-81.

Sajadi, M.M.; Heredia, A.; Le, N.; Constantine, N.T. & Redfield, R.R. (2007). Natural virus suppressors: Control of viral replication in the absence of therapy. *AIDS* 19:517-9.

Schooley, R.T.; Spritzler, J.; Wang, H.; Lederman, M.M.; Havlir, D.; Kuritzkes, D.R.; Pollard, R.; Battaglia, C.; Robertson, M.; Mehrotra, D.; Casimiro, D.; Cox, K. & Schock, B.; AIDS Clinical Trials Group 5197 Study Team (2010). AIDS clinical trials group 5197: A placebo-controlled trial of immunization of HIV-1 infected persons with replication deficient adenovirus type 5 vaccine expressing HIV-1 core protein. *J. Inf. Dis.* 202:705-16.

Sheikh, J.; Souberbielle B.; Westby, M.; Austen, B. & Dalgleish, A.G. (2000). HIV gp120 plus specific peptides are recognized in a similar way to specific HLA plus peptide by HLA restricted antigen specific cell lines. *Viral Immunol.* 13:9-17.

Siliciano, RF. (2010). Prospects of curing HIV infection. *Top. HIV Med.* 18:104-8.

Silvestri G.; Sodora D.L.; Koup, R.A.; Silvestri, G.; Sodora, D.L.; Koup, R.A.; Paiardini, M.; O'Neil, S.P.; McClure, H.M.; Staprans, S.I. & Feinberg, M.B. (2003). Nonpathogenic SIV infection of sooty managebeys is characterised by limited bystander immunopathology despite chronic high level viremia. *Immunity* 18:441-52.

Sousa, A.E.; Carneiro, J.; Meier-Schellersheim, M.; Grossman, Z. & Victorino, R.M. (2002). CD4 T-cell depletion is linked directly to immune activation in the pathogenesis of HIV-1 and HIV-2 but only indirectly to viral load. *J. Immunol.* 169:3400-6.

The Antiretroviral Therapy Cohort Collaboration (2008). Life expectancy of individuals on combination antiretroviral therapy in high-income countries: a collaborative analysis of 14 cohort studies. *Lancet* 372:293-9

Toulson, A.R.; Harrigan, R.; Heath, K.; Yip, B.; Brumme, Z.L.; Harris, M.; Hogg, R.S. & Montaner, J.S. (2005). Treatment interruption of highly active antiretroviral therapy in patients with nadir CD4 cell counts >200 Cells/mm[3]. *J. Infect. Dis.* 192:1787–93.

UNAIDS Report on the Global AIDS Epidemic (2010). ISBN 978-92-9173-871-7. Available at http://www.unaids.org [Accessed 11th July 2011]

van Baalen, C.A.; Pontesilli, O.; Huisman, R.C.; Geretti, A.M.; Klein, M.R.; de Wolf, F.; Miedema, F.; Gruters, R.A.; & Osterhaus, A.D. (1997). Human immunodeficiency virus type 1 Rev- and Tat-specific cytotoxic T lymphocyte frequencies inversely correlate with rapid progression to AIDS. *J. Gen. Virol.* 78:1913–18.

Vittinghoff, E.; Scheer, S., O'Malley, P.; Colfax, G.; Holmberg, S.D. & Buchbinder, S.P. (1999). Combination antiretroviral therapy and recent declines in AIDS incidence and mortality. *J. Infect. Dis.* 179:717-20.

Walker B. (2007). Elite control of HIV infection: Implications for vaccines and treatments. *Top. HIV Med.* 15:134-6.

Willberg, C.B. & Nixon, D.F. (2007). Treatment interruption in chronic HIV-1 infection: does it deliver? *Curr. Opin. HIV AIDS* 2:26-30.

Wit, F.W.; Blanckenberg, D.H.; Brinkman, K.; Prins, J.M.; van der Ende, M.E.; Schneider, M.M.; Mulder, J.W.; de Wolf, F. & Lange, J.M. ATHENA Study Group.(2005). Safety of long-term interruption of successful anti-retroviral therapy: the ATHENA cohort study. *AIDS* 19:345-48.

Wong, J.K.; Hezareh, M.; Günthard, H.F.; Havlir, D.V.; Ignacio, C.C.; Spina, C.A. & Richman, D.D. (1997). Recovery of replication competent HIV despite prolonged suppression of plasma viraemia. *Science* 278:1291-5.

Wu, Y. & Marsh, J.W. (2001). Selective transcription and modulation of resting T cell activity by preintegrated HIV DNA. *Science* 293:1503-6.

Yerly, S.; Günthard, H.F.; Fagard, C.; Joos, B.; Perneger, T.V.; Hirschel, B.; & Perrin, L. Swiss HIV Cohort Study. (2004). Proviral HIV-DNA predicts viral rebound and viral setpoint after structured treatment interruptions *AIDS.* 24;18:1951-3.

Zuñiga, R.; Lucchetti, A.; Galvan, P.; Sanchez, S.; Sanchez, C.; Hernandez, A.; Sanchez, H.; Frahm, N.; Linde, C.H.; Hewitt, H.S.; Hildebrand, W.; Altfeld, M.; Allen, T.M.; Walker, B.D.; Korber, B.T.; Leitner, T.; Sanchez, J. & Brander, C. (2006). Relative dominance of Gag p24-specific cytotoxic T-lymphocytes is associated with human immunodeficiency virus control. *J. Virol.* 80:3122-5.

Part 4

Beyond Conventional

10

Substance Abuse Treatment Utilizing Medication Assisted Treatment as HIV Prevention

Thomas F Kresina, Robert Lubran and Laura W. Cheever

Centre for Substance Abuse Treatment, Substance Abuse and Mental Health Services Administration and HIV/AIDS Bureau, Health Resources and Services Administration USA

1. Introduction

International guidelines have been developed for the use of medications in the treatment of substance use disorders (WHO, 2008; WHO, 2009). Medications used in the detoxification from drug abuse and dependence provide symptomatic relief of drug and alcohol withdrawal. For long term treatment or medical maintenance treatment, medications eliminate the physiological effects of drug use by blocking drug-receptor binding in the brain and are an important part of the recovery process. The use of medication assistant treatment (MAT) is part of a comprehensive treatment plan for drug and alcohol dependence that addresses the medical, social, and psychological needs of the patient (SAMHSA, 2005; SAMHSA, 2009). An effective long term treatment paradigm for the successful treatment of alcohol or opioid dependence is the concomitant use of medications that block the effects of drug use in concert with behavior change counseling and psychotherapy. Medications which have demonstrated effectiveness in the long term treatment of opioid dependence are methadone, buprenorphine (subutex®, suboxone®), and naltrexone (Revia®, Depade®) or extended release injectable naltrexone (vivitrol®). Pharmacotherapies used in the treatment of alcohol dependence include acamprosate (Campral®), disulfiram (antabuse®, antabus®) and naltrexone (Revia®, Depade®) or extended release injectable naltrexone (vivitrol®).

Time in treatment is a reliable indicator for successful treatment of drug dependence. Patients remain in treatment for longer periods of time when they perceive that their health care environment is supportive and non-stigmatizing, have a good patient-provider relationship, and feel that their needs are identified and met. Access to community-based substance abuse treatment that includes MAT is fundamental to achieving broad service coverage. Given that substance abuse treatment is Human Immunodeficiency Virus (HIV) prevention and the frequent co-morbidity of substance abuse and HIV infection, the provision of prevention, care and treatment for both need to be addressed in a coordinated manner for ideal patient outcomes. There are several models to achieve excellent patient outcomes for both HIV infection and the treatment of substance abuse (Proeschold-Bell et al 2010; Weiss et al, 2011). The highest level of coordinated care model has MAT and HIV services fully integrated with both the same medical record and health providers for both services. Alternatively, MAT and HIV services can be separately managed but co-located to allow convenient utilization of both MAT and HIV services in another form of "one stop shopping". A third approach is coordinated care and treatment where MAT and HIV services are provided at distinct locations, and case managers, peer facilitators, or others promote coordination of referrals. This third model can pose significant barriers to substance users who are heavily stigmatized and medically disenfranchised and who have multiple competing medical, psychological and social needs that limit access to care. MAT programs that offer comprehensive services and care options can best contribute to improving the health of these individuals thereby reducing HIV infection in the community.

2. Drug and alcohol use and their linkage to HIV infection

Exposure to the HIV can result in a patent viral infection. HIV infection can occur via two transmission routes: direct injection of the virus through the use of injection equipment infected with HIV and through sexual contact with an infected individual. There is a direct linkage between these disparate behaviours and drug and alcohol use.

For people who inject drugs, there is a risk of HIV infection when the injection equipment is reused and not sterilized after use or when there is direct sharing of the injection equipment with individuals who may be infected with HIV. Drug users who are under the influence of drugs may engage in risk behaviours for HIV that they would not while sober. In addition, for drug users who develop dependence, withdrawal induced drug cravings may result in the exchange of sex for money or drugs or other behaviours that increase risk of HIV acquisition. Similarly, alcohol consumption increases sexual risk-taking including high risk behaviors (Figure 1). That includes sexual acts without the use of condoms and an increased number of sexual partners. Concurrent sexual partnerships are a significant risk factor for the transmission of HIV (Epstein & Morris, 2011). Alcohol can also be an important contributor in the progression of HIV infection to acquired immune deficiency syndrome (AIDS) (Hahn & Samet , 2010). Alcohol consumption is an important consideration in the medical management of patients with HIV infection, particularly those co-infected with the hepatitis C virus (HCV) (Edlin et al 2001). Studies have also shown that alcohol consumption can modify drug metabolism in the liver, and thereby potentially influence the effectiveness of HIV antiretroviral therapy. Alcohol-induced cirrhosis can result in changes in drug metabolism in the liver through compromised liver function. Research has shown that alcohol consumption greater than 50 g/day (4–5 drinks) is a risk factor for disease progression for patients with HIV/HCV co-infection.

All substance abuse, whether the use of opioids, stimulants, or excessive alcohol, can negatively influence the course of HIV disease progression when the use results in low antiretroviral adherence or facilitates missed medical appointments. Substance abuse has been associated with less access to antiretroviral medications, lower medication adherence, and increased mortality among HIV infected patients.

2.1 Alcohol abuse, medication assisted treatment and HIV infection

Alcohol abuse and dependence are global problems of major medical importance with high societal impact (WHO, 2010). In determining the global burden of disease, the World Health Organization (WHO) has noted that a leading cause of disability is alcohol and drug use disorders. Alcohol consumption is estimated to cause 4% of the total of Disability-Adjusted

Life Years and 3.2% of deaths, globally. The WHO estimates that about 2 billion individuals worldwide consume alcoholic beverages.

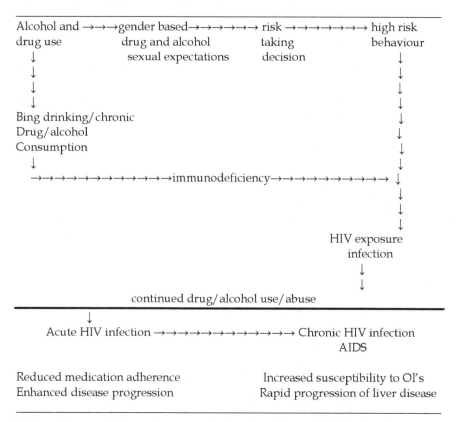

Fig. 1. Interactions and linkages between drug and alcohol use and abuse in the course of HIV infection and AIDS.

Alcoholic beverage consumption can be described based on quantity. Abstainers or light/occasional drinkers comprise roughly 40% of a general population while moderate drinkers comprise about 35% of the general population. Both groups comprise approximately 55–75% of a general medical practice. At-risk drinkers, those with hazardous drinking patterns or quantities, and alcohol abusers, those with harmful drinking (meeting the required clinical criteria) comprise approximately 20% of the population and 20–35% of a general medical practice. At-risk drinkers are males who drink more than two drinks a day or greater than four drinks per occasion. For females and individuals over the age of 65, at-risk drinkers are those who drink greater than one drink per day or greater than three drinks per occasion. These individuals consume alcohol at levels that place them at-risk for alcohol-related social and/or medical problems (Dufour, 1999). These at-risk individuals are best managed through the use of brief interventions that can be provided by primary care physicians, health care providers or specialists, upon training. Usually these brief interventions are outpatient interventions that include some form of counseling.

Approximately 76.3 million individuals have a diagnosable alcohol use disorder. Alcohol and drug use disorders are defined clinically as alcohol/drug abuse or dependence (WHO, 2004). Diagnostic and Statistical Manual of Mental Disorders-4th edition (DSM-IV) definitions of abuse and dependence are maladaptive patterns of alcohol or drug use that result in clinically significant impairment or distress as well as significant behavior modifications. Individuals with alcohol dependence comprise approximately 5% of the population and around 5-10% of a general medical practice. Alcohol abusers and alcohol-dependent individuals exhibit a varying degree of social and/or medical dysfunction. These individuals require intensive treatment, including structured counseling and/or pharmacotherapy (Fiellin et al., 2000). Severely involved dependent patients have been traditionally thought of requiring treatment in a specialty setting. However, studies (Fiellin et al., 2000a) have shown that primary care physicians may also have an important role in providing treatment to these individuals.

Pharmacotherapy for alcohol dependence is an important adjunct to behavioral therapies to reduce the risk of relapse to drinking after an initial period of abstinence (SAMHSA, 2009). Pharmacotherapy for alcohol consumption is also important for patients with co-occurring conditions such as patients with HIV and/or HCV infection(s) where alcohol consumption can augment disease progression. For these patients alcohol dependence treatment has been reported with either acamprosate, naltrexone, vivitrol or disulfiram (Collins et al, 2006). Acamprosate and naltrexone have different mechanisms of action and modify different behavioral aspects of alcohol dependence. Acamprosate is a long acting compound that prolongs periods of abstinence by normalizing glutamateric neurotransmission. Glutamateric neurotransmission in the brain is dysregulated during chronic alcohol consumption and withdrawal. Naltrexone is a fast acting opioid receptor antagonist that reduces heavy drinking through a decrease of the reward effects of ethanol. An evidence-based risk –benefits assessment can be used to inform health care providers on medication choice (Mason, 2003). However, the safety and efficacy of treatment using both medications for alcohol dependence has been shown in double blind studies (Kiefer & Wiedemann, 2004). Disulfiram, another pharmacotherpy option, blocks the oxidation of alcohol at the acetaldehyde stage of its metabolism. The increase in the levels of acetaldehyde resulting in a series of unpleasant symptoms (e.g., flushing, headache, and vomiting). Although disulfiram is widely used, particulalry is the setting of opioid dependence, superior data of studies support the use of naltrexone and acamprosate as pharmacologic treatments of alcoholism (Kiefer et al 2005). For resource limited settings, a series of factors acting synergistically may be creating the "perfect storm" promoting alcohol availability, alcohol consumption, and reducing alcohol control policies, thereby increasing the need for public health efforts (Table 1) to reduce alcohol consumption the beyond the use of medication-assisted treatment for alcohol abuse and dependence (Caetano & Laranjeira, 2006).

Use of alcohol may impact the care and course of HIV infection for an individual patient (Baum et al, 2010; Hahn & Samet, 2010). Optimal management of HIV infected patients with alcohol problems requires recognition of the impact of alcohol on a number of issues: patient's linkage to medical care; adherence to anti-retroviral treatment, impact on co-morbid conditions (such as HCV infection), liver function, and the stage of HIV disease. Due to its many ramifications, the clinical approach to the HIV infected patient with alcohol problems takes on a high priority, yet it is similar in many ways to the standard optimal approach to any medical patient (Bogart et al., 2000). It requires the effective screening for

Public Health Educational Efforts to Prevent HIV Transmssion in the Context of Aclohol Consumption :

- Public education to inform youth and adults of the harms associated with at-risk alcohol consumption
- Education of women of the gender related issues regarding alcohol use and abuse
- Public education on changing societal norms for heavy drinking, and awareness of HIV related risk, including condom use
- Beverage industry collaboration to promote responsible drinking.

Integration of targeted alcohol information, education and interventions in HIV/AIDS prevention programs for persons at high risk for HIV/AIDS:

- Women of child-bearing age
- HIV-positive persons and their partners
- Anti-retroviral treatment patients
- Sex trade workers and truckers
- Injection drug users
- MSM

Brief Interventions. Screening, brief advice & motivational interventions for at-risk drinkers

- By HIV healthcare workers
- By HIV peer outreach workers
- By VCT and anti-retroviral professionals

Detoxification

- Community-based detoxification for acute stabilization prior to outpatient or residential treatment
- Hospital detoxificaion - as medically required

Specialty treatment for alcohol abusers and dependent persons

- Inpatient or residential treatment
- Therapeutic Community Model
- Outpatient treatment and Aftercare- Community drop-in centers for alcohol-free activities and outreach, peer support
- Supportive Residential- Half-way or similar residential support post-discharge
- Treatment approaches- Motivational Interviewing, Cognitive Behavioral, and 12-step based treatmen, Relapse Prevention, and Peer Support
- Medications (Naltrexone, Acamprosate, Disulfiram, Vivitrol)

Peer Recovery Community Support

Table 1. Approaches to Alcohol Use and Abuse in HIV/AIDS

the prevalent condition of alcohol abuse, assessment of the severity of the alcohol problem, and skills to intervene effectively to reduce the harm associated with alcohol use/abuse. New strategies to target alcohol use/ abuse in HIV populations need to be implemented in the context of existing recommended HIV clinical approaches. Addressing alcohol problems in HIV-infected persons has the potential to improve the overall management of HIV disease in a substantial proportion of the population

2.2 Illicit opioid abuse, medication assisted treatment and HIV infection
Based on the 2010 World Drug Report (UNODC, 2010) from the United Nations Office on
Drugs and Crime (UNODC), it is estimated that between 175- 250 million people from
almost every country, or 5 percent of the global population age 15-64, have used illicit drugs
at least once in the last 12 months. Cannabis is by far the most widely used drug, followed
by stimulants, such as amphetamines and ecstasy, then cocaine use and then opioids. While
most individuals occasionally use or have casually tried illicit drugs, UNODC estimates that
there are between 18-38 million problem drug users. These individuals consume most of the
drugs and likely fulfill the criteria for a diagnosis of drug abuse or dependence.
These medical co-occurring conditions are specifically prevalent in injection drug users
(IDU). Estimates for IDU's are available for at least 130 countries with approximately 78% of
the 13.2 million IDU's living in developing or transitional countries (Aceijas et al 2004).
Forty-one countries have reported a high prevalence (>5%) of HIV infection in this high-risk
population. Globally, IDU's now account for at least 10% of all new HIV infections which
are estimated at 5 million per year (IHRDP, 2006). In chronic HIV infection, AIDS has been
reported as the leading cause of death in IDUs (Chin, 2007). Epidemiological data of HIV
infection show that generalized HIV epidemics can result from diffusion transmission of
HIV from high risk groups, such as IDUs. Thus, it is important for countries and regions to
undertake surveillance studies to identify current alcohol and drug use patterns and
develop best practices for the treatment of individuals who use and abuse alcohol and illicit
drugs.
Drug dependence is a chronic, relapsing neurophysiological disease resulting from the
prolonged effects of drug(s) on the brain. The neurochemical abnormalities resulting from
chronic use are the underlying cause of many of the observed physical and behavioral
aspects of abuse and dependence. The brain abnormalities associated with addiction are
wide ranging, complex, and long lasting (Chana et al 2006; Goodkin et al 1998; Langford et
al 2003). They can involve abnormal brain signaling pathways, psychological conditioning
or stress and social factors that result in cravings leading to a predisposition to relapse even
months or years after drug(s) use cessation. Thus, substance abuse/dependence can be
most effectively addressed in a multifaceted medical-based paradigm that comprises a
comprehensive program of interventions that are delivered through the course of long term
treatment. Such comprehensive treatment programs include behavioral, social rehabilitative
components, as well as biological (pharmacological) components Table 2. Behavioral
therapy interventions have been extensively researched and are critical components of the
treatment of all drug addictions. Social rehabilitative components are also important and
may prove suited to certain treatment environments.
In the United States, opioid abuse/dependence can be treated in two differing medical
paradigms. In the highly regulated and structured environment, methadone is dispensed
daily at Opioid Treatment Programs (OTPs). These OTPs are increasingly providing "wrap-
around" services to address important patient needs, enhance time in treatment, and
promote recovery. Alternatively, buprenorphine can be prescribed in a primary care health
care setting similar to other illnesses to reduce the stigma/discrimination of drug
dependence. Both medical paradigms need to address the reduced quality of life, physical
and mental functioning, compared to the general population that is associated with drug
abuse/dependence (Millson et al. 2006). In addition, multiple comorbidities are associated
with substance abuse and dependence that also contribute to the lower quality of life

Drug Use, Abuse and Dependence

(1)PREVENTION OF DRUG INITIATION
Individual targeted interventions through the life span
Family targeted interventions
Community interventions

(2)IDENTIFICATION OF SUBSTANE USE CONDITIONS
Screening for drug use
Case finding
Assessment & Diagnosis

(3)INITIATION AND ENGAGEMENT IN DRUG TREATMENT
Brief intervention
Promoting Engagement, case management/ care navagators
Detoxification/ Withdrawal Management
Assessment of social, co-morbid medical conditions and co-occurring
disorders

(4) LONG TERM TREATMENT OF SUBSTANCE USE ILLNESS
Psychosocial
Pharmacotherapy
Treatment of co-morbid medical conditions and co-occurring disorders
Promotion of treatment engagement & social stability through legal, social, educational,
financial support

(5) PRIMARY CARE AND POST TREATMENT MANAGEMENT OF PATIENT
Recovery
Relapse prevention
Rehabilitation
Medical Home

Table 2. Elements of the Continuum of Care in the Treatment of Opioid Abuse/Dependence

experienced and documented by opioid dependent individuals. Life priorities of opioid users have been reported as concern about HIV and treatment of infection with HIV, housing, money, and protection from violence (Mizuno et al, 2003).

Substance abuse is a complex medical disorder composed of multiple physiologic, social and behavioral problems often interrelated with psychological illness. Health care providers need to screen substance misusing patients for psychological illness (Schuckit, 2006). Although it can be difficult to ascertain whether substance abuse, psychological illness, or infectious comorbidities should be addressed first, an initial focus on the medical treatment of drug abuse is often necessary to create sufficient patient stability from which other treatments can begin. Stability is further increased with both mental health services and substance abuse treatment, subsequently enhancing the medical outcomes of treatment for comorbidities.

In the United States, multiple pharmacological treatments, including both agonists and antagonists have been developed and approved by the Food and Drug Administration for specific drug dependence. Currently, medications and evidence-based treatment paridigms utilizing these pharmacotherapies are available for the treatment of nicotine, alcohol, and opioid substance use disorders. Although none are available for stimulants, such as cocaine and methamphetamine, many potential medications are now being developed for these drugs of abuse and are expected to be available over the next few years. An effective treatment strategy for drug abuse and dependence is to match a comprehensive treatment plan to the individual's particular substance abuse problems and needs. Desired treatment outcomes should: a) reduce dependence on drugs of abuse, b) reduce morbidity and mortality of and associated with drugs of abuse, and c) maximize the patients' abilities to access services and achieve social integration.

2.2.1 Medication assited treatment utilizing methadone

In most countries that utilize MAT for the treatment of opioid dependence, methadone is the pharmacotherapy of choice. Methadone is usually the least expensive medication and when used in evidence-based treatment paridigms is cost effective and can result in abstenence from illicit drug use over time and the achievement of recovery (Connock et al 2007; Skinner et al 2011). Methadone is a synthetic μ-opioid receptor agonist with pharmacological properties qualitatively similar to morphine and was originally used to treat the painful symptoms of withdrawal from heroin and other opioids (Gowing et al 2006; Payte & Zweben , 1998). Administered daily as an oral dose for the treatment of opioid dependence, an individual therapeutic dosage is determined to maintain an asymptomatic state and stabilize a patient, without episodes of opioid overmedication or withdrawal. The therapeutic dosage for a patient is a function of many factors including: absorption, metabolism, drug-drug interactions, physiology, diet and the use of alternative medications. Minimum retention time in treatment varies for residential and outpatient methadone treatment programs. The National Institutes of Health consensus panel on opioid-addiction treatment (NIH, 1997) concluded that individuals treated for fewer than three months with methadone do not show substantial medical gain. As time in treatment progresses, study outcomes have reported partial reductions of illicit opioid use progressing to abstinence. Relapse to opioid use is common when methadone is discontinued without further support or behavioral treatment. In the United States, OTPs or methadone maintenance treatment programs, MMTP, under the certification of the Substance Abuse and Mental Health Services Administration (SAMHSA), dispense methadone and can provide a comprehensive therapeutic milieu comprised of primary medical care, psychosocial counseling, vocational rehabilitation, HIV testing and counseling, hepatitis C education and testing and other vital medical and social services. Methadone treatment is effective as both primary and secondary HIV prevention (Kerr et al 2004) and cost-effective to society (Barnett et al 2001; Doran et al 2003). In addition to improving health outcomes, methadone treatment also substantially improves the quality of life of patients over the course of methadone treatment (Giacomuzzi et al 2005).

Barriers to retention in methadone treatment include the severity of drug, medical and social problems at initiation of treatment, as well as patient readiness for treatment and motivation. Integrating multiple components of the drug treatment program is fundamental to successful treatment outcomes. Treatment programs that offer a broader array of "wrap-around" services and a greater frequency of services have reported improved retention in treatment and treatment outcomes (Fiellin et al 2003). Programs responsive to the severity of drug abuse during initial stages of drug treatment have been shown to produce positive treatment outcomes based on greater retention time in treatment and patient satisfaction with treatment services. Maximum retention time in methadone treatment is associated with comprehensive treatment, provision of frequent health service, as well as appropriate methadone dosing (Litwin et al 2001).

2.2.2 Medication assited treatment utilizing buprenorphine
In the United States and globally, primary care physicians can expand the accessibility of substance abuse treatment while mitigating the stigma associated with drug use and treatment through an outpatient treatment setting in primary care and the use of buprenorphine. However, in the United States, buprenorphine-only OTPs have been recently developed where buprenorphine is provided to opioid dependent patents under the highly regulated rules and regulations that apply to methadone. Buprenorphine, a partial mu-receptor opiate agonist (Ling & Smith 2002), differs significantly from full agonists. Most significantly, buprenorphine has a plateau of its agonist properties at higher doses. This results in an improved safety profile compared with a full agonist. Specifically, buprenorphine has a favorable 'ceiling effect' on respiratory depression precluding overdose potential (Walsh et al 1994). However, the abuse of other substances that may enhance respiratory depression (e.g., benzodiazepines) remains a contraindication with buprenorphine as with methadone. Improved safety and thrice weekly flexible dosing promotes patient acceptance. In addition, buprenorphine has two features that decrease street diversion. Buprenorphine can precipitate opiate withdrawal when buprenorphine is taken by an opiate dependent patient (Schuh et al. 1996) and buprenorphine can be marketed both alone (Subutex®) and in combination with naloxone (Suboxone®). In the latter formulation, if it is crushed and injected, acute opiate withdrawal symptoms will ocuur which are a potent disincentive for prescription opioid abuse (Yokell et al. 2011).

2.2.3 Medication assited treatment utilizing naltrexone
Naltrexone is a non-narcotic long-acting, opioid antagonist that blocks the euphoric effects of opioids binding the mu opioid receptor. Unlike methadone, there is no negative reinforcement (opioid withdrawal) upon discontinuation. Due to naltrexone's opioid antagonism, patients must abstain from opioids for a minimum of seven days prior to starting treatment to avoid the precipitation of opioid withdrawal. The effectiveness of naltrexone treatment depends upon patient motivation and social support system (Greenstein et al 1983). Thus, in cultures where there is strong family or social support for the patient in care, oral naltrexone has been shown to be effective in the prevention of relapse to heroin use (Krupitsky et al 2010). Because of a lack of positive reinforcing effects with naltrexone and low motivation on the part of many patients, as well as, poor clinician acceptability, it is not widely prescribed for the treatment of opioid dependence in the United States.

Vivitrol is an injectable extended-release formulation of naltrexone that has recently been approved for the treatment of opioid abuse and dependence. Vivitrol addresses the concern of medication adherence as a monthly injectable formulation and has been shown to be more effective than oral naltrexone (Krupitskya & Blokhina, 2010). This was also shown in a recent Phase 3 clinical trial that confirmed vivitrol's safety and efficacy in the prevention of relapse to heroin use in a cohort of injection drug users. A higher retention in care and higher rates of opioid-free urine screens were observed along with a significant reduction in opioid craving compared to placebo. Currently, studies are underway to determine the most efficacious service model(s) for the use of vivitrol in the treatment of relapse prevention to heroin use.

3. Medication assisted treatment: Stages of treatment and recovery

The stages or phase of MAT are shown in Table 3. The patient travels through these three stages of treatment, sometimes linearly and sometimes with oscillations between phases. The ultimate goal upon entering MAT is a good clinical outcome which includes the

---

- Induction
  - Medication is chosen based on clinical and patient circumstances
  - MAT initiation where initial dosing of medication is observed and dosing titration is performed by a clinician
  - Dosing and dose titration is based on expression and control of withdrawal symptoms and is a critical period in terms of risk of opioid overdose in treatment
  - procedures for patient observation during and after dose titration are incorporated into the clinic setting
  - Induction can last 7-10 days with the goal of obtaining a therapeutic dose of opioid medication
- Stabilization
  - stabilization phase occurs when the patient no longer exhibits drug seeking behavior or craving
  - The correct dosage of medication is critical (overdosing versus underdosing) as well as successful participation of the patient in behavioral therapies and rehabilitation services
  - MAT provider determines stabilization based on patient symptoms, not on opioid free urine samples
  - Individual patient health (e.g. pregnancy, liver disease, etc.), other medical treatments including HAART and TB treatments, and other drug use or alcohol consumption affects stabilization
- Maintenance
  - Maintenance pharmacotherapy occurs when the patient is responding optimally to medication treatment and routine dose adjustments are not needed.
  - Patients at this stage have stopped using illicit opioid and resumed productive lifestyles away from the local drug culture.
  - It is also at this stage that patients should have minimal or normal medical needs and can move away from intensive drug treatment settings and receive their medications in a primary care/community setting.
  - Typically take home medication of controlled medications is allowed for patients
  - If maintenance phase cannot be reached, other drug dependence treatment approaches should be explored to complement MAT

Table 3. Stages or Phases of MAT

recovery from opioid abuse and dependence and social reintegration back into society. The individual in recovery is a functioning member of the community and contributes to the social fiber and health of the community. Thus, a foundation of MAT is the obtainment of Recovery from opioid abuse and dependence (Davidson & White , 2007).

The recovery process is the individual way in which a person actively manages their substance use disorder with efforts to reclaim full functional and meaningful lives in the community. Recovery is personal process of growth and change which embraces hope, autonomy and the elements that result in establishing a satisfying and productive life. MAT is a recovery oriented system of care when integrated with other medical, social and rehabilitative services in support of the individual's and family's long term efforts to reclaim full and meaningful lives in the community. Important in recovery is the provision of comprehensive services in the context of MAT but also a supportive, enabling environment that fosters individual responsibility over one's health and empowerment to change to a healthy lifestyle (Sowers, 2005).

MAT, as a recovery orientated system of care, has four phases as shown in Table 4, along with a set of recovery oriented goals, strategies, and services (White & Mojer-Torres, 2010). An important consideration in phase four, long term sustained recovery, is the personal decision to continue with medical maintenance of pharmacotherapy or to taper the medication. In either case, the home or living environment is critical to the prevention of relapse to opioid use. To prevent relapse of opioid use the individual in recovery needs a drug free environment. While significant gains have been made through national prevention programs such as "Drug Free Communities", it remains a Herculean task to keep a community entirely free of illicit drug use. Thus, for long term recovery the home or living environment is where recovery is nucleated (Ashcraft et al, 2008). Local peer recovery programs as well as recovery oriented systems of care that link to or provide individualized, quality long term supportive care are critical (Jason & Ferrari, 2010). These settings provide a network of people to support abstinence as well as a low risk environment to support recovery. Receiving abstinence support, guidance and information from a recovery home, that is committed to long term sobriety, reduces the risk of relapse to illicit opioid use. These homes need to be considered as a fundamental component in the development and maintenance of the public health of communities.

4. Service models for medication assisted treatment

Health service programs deliver MAT in a regulatory environment where both the federal government and state/local government provide a regulatory framework for the access to and delivery of medications that are controlled by international convention (Kresina et al, 2009). In the United States, state and local regulation can enhance the federal regulations but they can not negate the federal regulations. The MAT federal regulations can be found in the Code of Federal Regulations (CFR, 2002) and establish procedures to determine if a health practitioner is qualified to dispense methadone in the treatment of opioid abuse and dependence in opioid treatment programs, as well as, the quantity of methadone that can be provided for unsupervised use by patients. Thus, the federal regulations address the balance needed in the use of controlled medications for treatment versus the restrictions to limit diversion of the controlled medication (Yokell et al 2011).

The MAT federal regulations do not regulate the health service models that can be use to maximize access to MAT as well as time in treatment. These are two important

- *Recovery initiation and stabilization*
  - o Major goal- eliminate use of illicit opioid use for at least twenty-four hours as well as other drug of abuse
    - ▪ Educate the patient about the risk and benefits of pharmacotherapy
    - ▪ Provide a choice of alternate/supplemental therapeutic approaches
    - ▪ Identify patient's treatment needs and engage early
    - ▪ Minimize sedative and side effects of medication
    - ▪ Asses safety and adequacy of each dose after administration
    - ▪ Discourage self medication of withdrawal symptoms
    - ▪ Assess and initially address medical, social, legal, family and other problems
    - ▪ Develop initial coping and craving strategies
- *Early recovery and rehabilitation*
  - o Major goal- empower individuals to cope with life problems, medical needs co-occurring disorders vocational and educational needs, family problems, legal issues and develop long term goals for education, employment and family reconciliation
    - ▪ Insure medication dose promotes daily comfort
    - ▪ Link patient to family and peer-recovery support
    - ▪ Develop recovery plan
    - ▪ Assess and initially address personal strengths and needs
- *Recovery Maintenance*
  - o Major goal- patient assumes primary responsibility for their life
    - ▪ Patient receives needed integrated services
    - ▪ Patient is active in community recovery support programs
    - ▪ Patient receives take home medication from an OTP
    - ▪ Decision on medical maintenance or tapering of pharmacotherapy
- *Long-term Sustained Recovery*
  - o Major goal- continued primary responsibility for life
    - ▪ Taper from pharmacotherapy- quarterly or biannual check-up from substance abuse treatment program
    - ▪ Continuing pharmacotherapy- continued regular check-up with substance abuse treatment provider
    - ▪ Continued engagement with peer-based recovery support program
    - ▪ Patient becomes a recovery support for other patients

Table 4. Phases and Goals of MAT Recovery Oriented Systems of Care

characteristics to maximize as one designs model MAT programs to ensure good clinical and public health outcomes. Barrier free access to MAT is important for obtaining maximal public health impact and reaching all opioid abusing individuals seeking treatment. Research studies have shown that the more time in MAT the better the treatment outcome. Thus, MAT programs providing comprehensive services as part of the continuum of care (see Table 2) in an enabling environment result in quality and effective substance abuse treatment services that promote individual well-being and improved community health.

4.1 Integrated models of medication assisted treatment

Health service models for MAT that provide comprehensive services interface substance abuse treatment services with primary medical care and social/rehabilitation services. That interface can be comprehensive through the integration of substance abuse treatment services, primary medical care, infectious disease prevention, care and treatment and social/rehabilitation services. An integrated care and treatment model, where MAT services are provided within primary care using a single medical record, minimizes the sigma and discrimination associated with drug treatment services while improving overall health outcomes in a cost-effective manner (Collins et al 2010).

For OTPs dispensing methadone, primary medical care and social/rehabilitation services are integrated on-site in the structured environment where methadone is dispensed (Freidman et al 1999; Kresina et al 2008). Based on patient needs, various types of health services can be integrated into OTP MAT services including primary care, mental health, and infectious diseases. Specific limiting factors for the integration of services have been shown to be the organizational structure of the OTP and cost.

Buprenorphine, a less regulated opioid agonist medication, is approved in the United States for office based opioid treatment. An office based setting provides enhanced treatment access to MAT using buprenorphine in a less stigmatized environment enabling integrated medical care of infectious diseases and co-morbid conditions (Gunderson & Fiellin , 2008). Multiple models have been piloted for the integration of MAT using buprenorphine within HIV primary care (Sullivan et al 2006). These include an on-site combination of addiction treatment/HIV specialist treatment; a HIV primary care physician prescribing buprenorphine; a non-physician health care provider integrating medical care and substance abuse treatment services using buprenorphine; and a community outreach model where buprenorphine is provided along with medical services in a mobile van. These pilot projects have uncovered barriers to integrating MAT using buprenorphine within HIV primary care that are both financial and regulatory. Regulatory challenges include licensing and training restrictions imposed by the Drug Addiction Treatment Act of 2000 and confidentiality regulations for alcohol and drug treatment records (Schackman et al 2006). A recent study has shown that in a primary care setting that used buprenorphine, prescription opioid dependent patients showed better clinical outcomes compared to patients who were dependent on heroin (Moore et al, 2007).

Naltrexone is a non-narcotic and therefore non-controlled medication for the treatment of opioid abuse as well as alcohol abuse. Naltrexone integrated with mental health services, particularly psychosocial treatment has been shown to be an effective maintenance treatment for reducing heroin use after detoxification (Minozzi et al. 2006). In addition, using clonidine and naltrexone together has been shown to be successfully integrated into a primary care setting (O'Connor et al. 1997). In this study retention in care and successful detoxification from opioid abuse was observed with MAT using either naltrexone or buprenorphine. In other care settings, treatment of alcohol use disorders using naltrexone has been successfully integrated into the treatment of patients who have tuberculosis (Greenfield et al. 2010). Current efforts are determining the optimum conditions to integrate vivitrol (extended release naltrexone) into HIV primary care programs. Additionally, how to integrate vivitrol into an OTP setting and in primary medical care as a relapse prevention intervention for patients following their completion of maintenance treatment with either methadone or buprenorphine, is currently moving forward.

4.2 Coordinated care models of medication assisted treament

Health service models for MAT that provide comprehensive services can connect substance abuse treatment services with primary medical care and social/rehabilitation services in a non-integrated but coordinated fashion. Here, MAT services coordinate with primary medical care and social/rehabilitation services to promote good patient outcomes and enhance community health. MAT, health services and social/rehabilitation services can be separately managed with a different network of health care providers but co-located to allow convenient utilization of primary care, MAT and other services. An additional coordinated approach provides primary care, MAT and other services at distinct locations through a differing network of health care providers. As shown in a recent study where twice as many patients retained in MAT when the MAT services were provided at single location compared to referral of MAT to a distant location (Lucas et al 2010), providing needed health services at distinct locations is less than optimal. However, coordinated programs can be effective when case managers, peer facilitators, care navigators or others promote or support service utilization at the various locations. For example, a referral system intervention was modeled with linkages to treatment services for substance use, mental health and social services for HIV+ patients receiving HIV primary care (Zaller et al. 2007). Patients receiving the intervention were referred to MAT either at an OTP or in an office based setting that prescribed buprenorphine. An alternative model provided highly stable OTP patients with 28 days of methadone doses and required monthly check-ins. Successful patients were noted to have increased family and social activities and failed patients were provided stepped treatment intensification (King et al. 2006). Community -wide health service delivery programs also provide an alternative to integration through enhanced access to networked drug treatment and co-morbidity health services (Neufeld et al 2010).

Unique to buprenorphine is the model that a substance abuse treatment specialist provides the initial treatment (induction) with buprenorphine until the patient is stabilized. Then the patient is transferred/referred to a primary care physician who can then provide maintenance buprenorphine treatment and medical primary care. This so called 'wheel and spoke model' allows for substance abuse treatment specialists to manage the more difficult portion of buprenorphine treatment (early treatment -or induction phase) while the primary care medical program manages the long term maintenance phase of buprenorphine treatment (BBI, 2008). This model is important in the United States since the Drug Addiction Treatment Act of 2000 limits the number of patients a qualified buprenorphine treatment provider can manage in their practice (DATA, 2000). This model has been adapted to HIV+ patients where the buprenorphine induction is performed by the substance abuse treatment specialist and then the patient is transferred/ referred to the HIV primary care physician (Basu et al. 2006).

Coordinated MAT for patients seeking relapse prevention interventions after detoxification from opioid use can be provided by naltrexone or the recently approved vivitrol. As noted earlier, naltrexone it is not widely prescribed for the treatment of opioid dependence in the United States, but is provided as an office based treatment for opioid dependence after detoxification. In addition, studies have shown that the extended release formulations are effective in reducing opioid use and retaining patients in care after detoxification (Comer et al 2006; Kunoe et al. 2010). Fishman et al 2010 has shown good clinical outcomes (retention in care and reduced opioid use) for adolescents receiving vivitrol over a four month period. This study is important because of the limted use of controlled pharmacotherapies in adolescent populations as part of national regulatory frameworks.

5. Preventing HIV infection by integration of medication assisted treatment into HIV prevention services

Important HIV prevention interventions for people who inject drugs are the provision of clean needles and syringe through syringe service programs and associated HIV testing and counseling programs. These HIV prevention interventions, when integrated into MAT programs, maximize the enrollment in treatment programs for opioid and alcohol abuse, and thereby maximize HIV prevention efforts (Kidorf et al 2009; Lloyd et all 2005). Maximizing HIV prevention efforts targeting peple who use drugs and those dependent on opioids and alcohol are critcial to prevent HIV infection in these most-at –risk populations. Integrating drug abuse treatment and early HIV prevention interventions, particulaly HIV testing and counseling, are important as components of the newly emerging Seek,Test, Treat and Retain" strategy (Crawford & Vlahov, 2010; Taege, 2011). This is an engagement and retention strategy that outreach workers can employ with injection drug users to reduce their risk for HIV infection. By utilizing outreach workers to seek out most-at-risk people who inject drugs, establish their HIV status through HIV testing, followed by sexual risk reduction councelling, HIV risk behaviors can be addressed with subsequent emphasis on treatment for their substance use disorder.

Unfortuately, there is not signifcant integration of HIV testing and counseling in OTPs. In the US, while approaximely 90% of opioid treatment programs provide some form of federally mandated HIV/AIDS education, only 74% of opiod treatment progams offered HIV testing (Kresina et al 2005). These services appear underutilized in that approximately one-in-three persons receiveving subtance abuse treatment also received HIV testing and counselling (Pollack & D'Aunno, 2010). Globally, although subtantial efforts are being made to increase the availability of HIV testing, most-at-risk populations remain underserved with regard to HIV prevention service utilization. It is estimated that only 10% of persons at-risk for HIV infection receive HIV testing. Thus, strategies such as opt-out testing, home-based testing, dor-to-door testing as well as providing dedicated HIV testings counselors at point-of-service locations are being utilized to enhance the uptake of HIV testing for people who use alcohol and inject drugs. Studies have shown that most-at-risk populations prefer point-of-service HIV testing, however, this intervention requires additional measures to support HIV positive individuals entering into HIV care and treatment (Keller et al 2011).

6. Preventing HIV transmission by integration of medication assisted treatment into HIV care and treatment

A significant factor in not reducing the global HIV epidemic is the lack of entrance into HIV care and treatment by most-at-risk populations. These populations, which include illicit drug users and alcohol abusers, encounter numerous barriers in accessing HIV care and treatment. In addition, once in treatment these individuals often suffer stigma and discrimination as they receive their needed medical care. The result is an increase in the prevalence of medical and psychiatric co-morbidities as well as social issues and high risk behaviors, in addition to worse clinical outcomes with a higher mortality rate compared to the non-drug and non-alcohol using populations infected with HIV (Altice et al 2010).

The increased mortally rate noted in people who inject drugs is related to their late presentation for HIV care. Patients who present late for care and treatment of HIV/AIDS are at a higher risk of significant clinical complications and are thus more difficult to clinically manage. Late presentation for treatment of HIV/AIDS is a common scenario leading to death (Moreno et al 2010). A recent study has documented a highly lethal neurological syndrome found in HIV-infected drug abusers (Newsome et al 2011). Although rare, the newly described syndrome is highly lethal with a mean survival time of 21 days after diagnosis. The authors suggest that access and initiation of antiretroviral therapy may provide a better outcome for these patients. In addition, substance abuse treatment, particularly MAT, which has been shown to enhance the health status, reduce mortality and quality of life of injection drug users, would be an important adjunct to anti-retroviral treatment for these patients. Thus, as noted earlier integrating both MAT with anti-retroviral treatment in a HIV primary care setting is a paradigm to optimize health outcomes and the health status of HIV-infected injection drug users.

How MAT is integrated in HIV primary care programs depends on the country's regulatory framework. In the United States, all medications accept methadone, can be prescribes to patients in a HIV primary care or outpatient HIV clinical care setting. The federal regulations in the United States require methadone to be dispenses in OTPs. However, in this setting studies have shown that HIV care and anti-retroviral treatment can be effectively prescribed either as directly observed therapy or as routine care. Other countries, such as Australia, have less stringent federal regulations for prescribing controlled medications and all medications comprising MAT can be provided in a primary care setting. In either case, the important aspect of providing integrated MAT and HIV primary care is the single location/clinic. In that case, the patient can receive all the needed services to support their recovery from drug/alcohol dependence as well as care and treatment for HIV infection.

7. Essential health interventions for the prevention of HIV infection in people who inject opioids

The WHO, UNODC and UNAIDS has approved and advocates for a package of essential interventions for the prevention, treatment and care of HIV for people who inject drugs (WHO, 2009a). These evidence based intervention, shown in Table 6, need three important characteristics in their implementation to maximize effectiveness. These interventions need to be part of a public health policy that is human rights based, gender responsive, and community owned.

As noted earlier, no single intervention alone will prevent or reverse to growing national HIV epidemics due to injection drug use and abuse. However, the greatest impact will be obtained when the interventions are provided through an integrated services platform in a comprehensive fashion. And in order to reach all of those seeking HIV prevention, care and treatment services, health service platforms need to provide an enabling environment that establishes confidentiality. In addition, they also need to develop patient –provider trusting relationships. Both community outreach and peer –to-peer services can promote full service utilization. The national Ministries of Health need to embrace and support these health services and interventions through a supportive legal and policy framework validating their place in the public health area and in society as they improve community health.

Prevention, Care and Treatment for People Who Inject Drugs
1. Needle and Syringe Programmes (NSP)/Syringe Service Programs (SSP)
2. Drug dependence treatment including Medication Assisted Treatment (MAT) and Opioid Substitution Treatment (OST)
3. HIV Testing and Counselling
4. Antiretroviral Therapy (ART)
5. Prevention and Treatment of Sexually Transmitted Infection (STI)
6. Condom distribution programs for People Who Inject Drugs and their sex partners
7. Targeted information, education and communication (IEC) for People Who Inject Drugs and their sex partners
8. Vaccination, diagnosis and treatment of viral hepatitis infection
9. Prevention, diagnosis and treatment of tuberculosis

Table 5. Listing of Internationally Accepted Essential Interventions for HIV

8. Conclusion

Substance abuse treatment is HIV prevention. The use of medication assisted treatment as a component of a comprehensive treatment plan for those individuals who abuse opioids and/or alcohol is an effective, evidence-based treatment paradigm that results in good medical outcomes including a reduction in HIV transmission as well as a reduction of incident infections in opioid and alcohol abusing populations.

9. References

Aceijas, C., Stimson, G.V., Hickman, M., & Rhodes, T. (2004) Global overview of injecting drug use and HIV infection among injection drug users. *Acquir Immun Defic Syndr* vol 18 no 17 pp 2295-2303.

Altice, FL., Kamarulzaman, A., Soriano, V., Schechter, M., & Friedland, GH. (2010) Treatment of medical, psychiatric and substance use comorbidities in people infected with HIV who use drugs. *The Lancet* vol 376 no 9738 pp367-387.

Ashcraft, L., Anthony, W.A,&, Martin C. (2008) Home is where recovery begins. *Behav Health* vol 28 no 5 pp 13-15.

Barnett, P.G., Zaric, G.S.& Brandeau, M..L.(2001) The cost-effectiveness of buprenorphine maintenance therapy for opiate addiction in the United States. *Addiction.* vol 96 no 9 pp1267-78.

Basu, S., Smith-Rohrberg, D., Bruce, R.D.& Altice, F.L. (2006) Models for integrating buprenorphine therapy into the primary HIV care setting. Clin Infect Dis vol 42 no 5 pp 716-721

Baum, MK., Rafie, C., Lai, S., Sales, S., Page, JB., & Campa, A. (2010) Alcohol use accelerates HIV disease progression. *AIDS Res Hum Retroviruses* vol 26 no 5 pp 511-518.

BBI (2008) *Baltimore Buprenorphine Initiative Newsletter*. Baltimore Buprenorphine Initiative Updates. October 2008.Retreived from:
http://www.bsasinc.org/media/doc/Baltimore%20buprenorphine%20initiativene wsletteroctober200

Bogart, LM., Kelly, JA., Catz, SL., & Sosman. (2000) Impact of medical and nonmedical factors on physician decision making for HIV/AIDS antiretroviral treatment. *J Acquir Immune Defic Syndr* vol 23 no 5 pp 396-404.

Caetano, R. & Laranjeira, R. A. (2006) A 'perfect storm' in developing countries: economic growth and the alcohol industry. *Addict* vol 101 no 2 pp149-52.

CFR (2002) Part 8 Certification of Opioid Treatment Programs. *Code of Federal Regulations*. Title 42. Public Health. Chapter 1 Public Health Service, Department of Health and Human Services.. retrieved from:
http://www.access.gpo.gov/nara/cfr/waisidx_02/42cfr8_02.html

Chana, G., Everall, I.P., Crews, L., Langford, D., Adame, A., Grant, I., Cherner, M., Lazzaretto, D., Heaton, R., Ellis, R., Masliah, E. & HNRC Group (2006). Cognitive deficits and degeneration of interneurons in HIV+ methamphetamine users. *Neurology* vol 67 no 8 pp 1486-1489.

Chin, J. (2007). *The AIDS Pandemic: the collision of epidemiology with political correctness*. Oxford: Radcliffe Publishing. ISBN-13: 978-1846191183

Collins, C., Hewson, D.L., Munger, R. & Wade, T.(2010) Evolving models of behavioral health integration in primary care. *Milbank Memorial Fund Report*, New York available   at:
http://www.milbank.org/reports/10430EvolvingCare/EvolvingCare.pdf

Collins, G.B., McAllister, M.S. & Adury, K. (2006) Drug adjuncts for treating alcohol dependence. *Cleve Clin J Med*. vol 73 no 7 pp 641-644

Comer, S.D., Sullivan, M.A., Yu, E., Rothenberg, J.L., Kleber, H.D., Kampman, K., Dackis, C.& O'Brain, C.P.(2006) Injectable, sustained-release naltrexone for the treatment of opioid dependence. A randomized, placebo controlled trial. *Arch Gen Psychiatry*. vol 63 no 2 pp 210-218.

Connock, M., Juarez-Garcia, A., Jowett, S., Fre, E., Liu, Z., Taylor, R.J., Fry-Smith, A., Day, E., Lintzeris, N., Roberts, T., Burls, A. & Taylor , R.S.(2007) Methadone and buprenorphine for the management of opioid dependence: a systematic review and economic evaluation. *Health Technol Aassess* vol 11 no 9 pp 1-171.

Crawford, N.D. & Vlahov, D. (2010) Progress in HIV reduction and prevention among injection and noninjection drug users. *J Acquir Immune Defic Syndr* vol 55 suppl 2 ppS84-87.

DATA (2000). *Drug Addiction Treatment Act of 2000*. Public Law 106-310 106th Congress Retrieved from: http://www.naabt.org/documents/DATA2000LAWTEXT.pdf

Davidson, L.& White, W. (2007) The concept of recovery as an organizing principle for integrating mental health and addiction services. *J Behave Health Ser Res* vol 34 no 2 pp 109-120.

Doran, C.M., Shanahan, M., Mattick, R.., Ali, R., White, J.& Bell, J.(2003) Buprenorphine versus methadone maintenance: a cost-effectiveness analysis. *Drug Alcohol Depend*. vol 71no 3 pp295-302.

DSM-IV (1999), Substance Related Disorders. In *DSM-IV™ Diagnostic and Statistical Manual of Mental Disorders- 4th edition*. American Psychiatric Association Publishers, ISBN 0-89042-062-9, Washington, DC pp175-272.

Dufour, M. (1999). What is moderate drinking? Defining « drinks » and drinking levels. *Alcohol Res Health* vol 23 no 1 pp5-14.

Edlin, B.R., Seal, K.H., Lorvick, J., Kral, A.H., Ciccarone D.H. & Moore ,L.D. (2001) Is it justifiable to withhold treatment for hepatitis C from illicit-drug users?, *New England Journal of Medicine* vol 345 no 3 pp. 211–214.

Epstein, H., & Morris, M. (2011) Concurrent partnerships and HIV : An inconvenient truth. *J Int AIDS Soc* vol 14 no 1 pp13-23.

Fiellin, DA., Reid, MC., & O'Connor PG. (2000) New therapies for alcohol problems: application to primary care. *Am J Med* vol 108 no 3 pp227-237.

Fiellin, DA., Reid, MC., & O'Connor PG. (2000a). Screening for alcohol problems in primary care : a systematic review. *Arch Intern Med* vol 160 no 13 pp1977-1989.

Fiellin, D.A., Rosenheck, R.A. & Kosten, T.R..(2003) Coordination of medical care and opioid dependence treatment in primary care: A case report. *Substance Abuse* vol 24 no 1 pp 43-46.

Fishman, M.J., Winstanley, E.L., Curran, E., Garrett, S. & Subramanian, G. (2010) Treatment of opioid dependence in adolescents and young adults with extended release naltrexone: preliminary case-series and feasibility. *Addiction* vol 105 no 9 pp1669-1676.

Freidmann, P.D. Alexander, J.A., Jin, L. & D'Aunno, T.A. (1999) On-site primary care and mental health services in outpatient drug abuse treatment units. *J Behav Health Ser Res* vol 26 no 1 pp 80-94.

Giacomuzzi, S.M., Ertl, M., Kemmler, G., Riemer, Y. & Vigl, A. (2005) Sublingual buprenorphine and methadone maintenance treatment: a three year follow-up of quality of life assessment. *Scientific World* J vol 5 pp 452-68

Goodkin, K., Shapshak, P., Metsch, L.R., McCoy, C.B., Crandall, K.A., Kumar, M., Fujimura, R.K., McCoy, V., Zhang, B.T., Reyblat, S., Xin, K.Q. & Kumar, A.M. (1998). Cocaine abuse and HIV-1 infection: epidemiology and neuropathogenesis. *J Neuroimmunol.* vol 83 no 1-2 pp 88-101

Gowing, L., Ali, R. & White, J. (2006) Opioid antagonists under heavy sedation or anaesthesia for opioid withdrawal. *Cochrane Database Syst Rev* April 19, 2006, no 2 CD002022.

Greenfield, S.F., Shields, A., Connery, H.S., Livchits, V., Yanov, S.A., Lastimoso, C.S., Strelis, A.K., Mishustin, S.P., Fitzmaurice, G., Mathew, T.A., Shin, S. (2010) Integrated management of physician-delivered alcohol care for tuberculosis patients: Design and implementation. *Alcohol Clin Exp Res* vol 34 no 2 pp 317-330

Greenstein, R.A., Evan, B.D., McLellan, A.T. & O'Brien, C.P. (1983) Predictors of favorable outcome following naltrexone treatment. *Drug Alcohol Depend* vol 12 no 2 pp 173-180.

Gunderson, E.W. & Fiellin D.A..(2008) Office-based maintenance treatment of opioid dependence: how does it compare with traditional approaches? *CNS Drugs* vol 22 no 2 pp 99-111

Hahn, JA., & Samet, JH. (2010) Alcohol and HIV disease progression: weighing the evidence. *Curr HIV/AIDS Rep* vol 7 no 4 pp226-233.

IHRDP (International Harm Reduction Development Program). (2006). Harm reduction developments 2005: countries with injection-driven HIV epidemics. New York: Open Society Institute. Retrieved from: http://www.soros.org/initiatives/health/focus/ihrd/articles_publications/public ations/ihrdreport_20060417/ihrd_ar.pdf

Jason, L.A. & Ferrari J.R. (2010) Oxford House recovery homes: characteristics and effectiveness. *Psychol Serv* vol 7 no 2 pp 92-102.

Kerr, T., Wodak, A., Elliott, R., Montane,r JS.& Wood, E. (2004)Opioid substitution and HIV/AIDS treatment and prevention. *Lancet.* vol 364 no 9449 pp1918-9

Keller, S., Jones, J., & Erbelding, E. (2011) Choice of Rapid HIV testing and entrance into care in Baltimore City sexually transmitted infection clinics. *AIDS Patient Care* STD vol 24 no 4 pp237-243..

Kidorf, M., King, V.L., Neufeld, K., Peirce, J., Kolodner, K. & brooner, R.K. (2009) Improving substance abuse treatment enrollment in community syringe exchangers. *Addiction* vol 104 no 5 pp786-795.

Kiefer, F., Helwig, H., Tarnaske, T., Otte, C., Jahn, H. & Wiedermann, K (2005). Pharmacological relapse prevention of alcoholism: clinical predictors of outcome. *Eur Addict Res vol* 11 no 2 pp 83-91.

Kiefer, F. & Wiedemann, K. (2004) Combined therapy: what does acamprosate and naltrexone combination tell us? *Alcohol Alcohol* vol 39 no 6 pp 542-547.

King, V.L., Kidorf, M.S., Stoller, K.B., Schwartz, R., Kolodner, K.& Brooner, R.K.(2006) A 12 month controlled trial of medical methadone maintenance integrated into an adaptive treatment model. *J Sub Abuse Treat* vol 31 no4 pp 385-393.

Kresina, T.F., Bruce, R.D., Lubran, R. & Clark, H.W. (2008) Integration of viral hepatitis services into opioid treatment programs. *J Opiod Manag* vol 4 no 6 pp 369-381.

Kresina, T.F., Litwin, A., Marion, I., Lubran, R. & Clark, H.W. (2009) Federal government oversight and regulation of medication assisted treatment for the treatment of opioid dependence. *J Drug Policy Anal* vol 2 no 1 pp 1-23.

Kresina, T.F., Maxwell, C., Parrino, M.W. & Lubran, R. (2005). Testing and Counseling for Hepatitis B, Hepatitis C, and HIV Infections in Opioid Treatment Programs (OTP's). Summary results from two surveys. Abstract presented at the *2005 CDC HCV Prevention Conference.* Washington, DC

Krupitsky, E., Zvartau, E. & Woody, G. (2010). Use of naltrexone to treat opioid addiction in a country in which methadone and buprenorphine are not available. *Curr Psychiatry Rep* vol 12 no 5 pp 448-453.

Krupitskya, E.M. & Blokhina, E.A. (2010) Long-acting depot formulations of naltrexone for heroin dependence: a review. *Curr Opin Psychiatry* vol 23 pp 210–214

Kunoe, N., Lobmaier, P., Vederhus, J.K., Hjerkinn, B., Hegstad, S., Gosso,p M, Kristensen, O. & Waal, H. (2010) Retention in naltrexone implant treatment for opioid dependance. Drug Alcohol Depend vol 111 no 1-2 pp 166-169

Langford, D., Adame, A., Grigorian, A., Grant, I., McCutchan, J.A., Ellis, R.J., Marcotte, T.D. & Masliah, E. (2003). HIV Neurobehavioral Research Center Group. Patterns of selective neuronal damage in methamphetamine-user AIDS patients. *J Acquir Immun Defic Syndr.* vol 34: no 5 pp 467-474

Ling, W. &. Smith, D. (2002) Buprenorphine: blending practice and research. *J Sub Abuse Treat.* vol 23 no 2 pp 87-92

Litwin, A.H., Soloway, I.& Gourevitch, M.N. (2005) Integrating services for injection drug users infected with hepatitis C virus with methadone maintenance treatment: challenges and opportunities. *Clin Infect Dis* vol 40: Suppl 5 pp S339-3345

Lloyd, J.J., Ricketts, E.P., Strathdee, S.A., Cornelius, L.J., Bishai, D., Heuttner, S., Havens, J.R. & Latkin, C. (2005) Social contextual factors associated with entry into opiate agonist treatment among injection drug users. *Am J DrugAlcohol Abuse* vol 31 no 4 pp 555-570.

Lucas, G.M., Chaudhry, A., Hsu, J., Woodso, T., Lau, B., Olse, Y., Keruly, J.C., Fiellin, D.A., Finkelstein, R., Barditch-Crovo, P., Cook, K.& Moore, R.D. (2010) Clinic-based treatment of opioid –dependent HIV-infected patients versus referral to an opioid treatment program: a randomized trial. *Ann Intern Med* vol 152 no 11 pp 704-711

Mason BJ. (2003). Acamprosate and naltrexone treatment for alcohol dependence: an evidence based risk –benefits assessment. *Eur Neuropsychopharm* vol 13 no 6 pp 469-475.

Millson, P., Challacombe, L., Villeneuve, P.J, Strike, C.J., Fischer, B., Myers, T., Shore, R.& Hopkins, S. (2006). Determinants of health-related quality of life of opiate users at entry to low-threshold methadone programs. *Eur Addict Res* vol 12 no 2 pp 74-82.

Minozzi, S., Amato, L., Vecchi, S., Davoli, M., Kirchmayer, U. & Verster, A. (2006) Oral naltrexone maintenance treatment for opioid dependence. *Cochrane Database of Systematic Reviews* CD001333DOI:101002/14651858.CD001333.pub2

Moore, B.A., Fiellin, D.A., Barry, D.T., Sullivan, L.E., Chawarski, M.C.,O'Connor, P.G.& Shottenfeld, R.S. (2007) Primary care office-based buprenorphine treatment: comparison of heroin and prescription opioid dependent patients. *J Gen Intern Med* vol 22 no 4 pp 527-530

Moreno, S., Mocroft, A., & Monforte, A. (2010) Medical and social consequences of late presentation. *Antivir Ther* vol 12 Suppl 1 pp9-15.

Neufeld, K., Kidorf, M., King, V., Stoller, K., Clark, M., Peirce, J., & Brooner, R.K. (2010) Using enhanced and integrated services to improve response to standard methadone treatment : changing the clinical infrastructure of treatment networks. *J Subst Abuse Treat* vol 38 no 3 pp170-177.

Newsome, SD., Johnson, E., Pardo, C., McArthur, JC., & Nath, A. (2011) Fulminent encephalopathy with basal ganglia hyperintensities in HIV-infected drug users. *Neurology* vol 76 no 9 pp787-794.

NIH (National Institutes of Health). (1997) Effective Medical Treatment of Opiate Addiction. *NIH Consensus Statement.* Bethesda, MD: National Institutes of Health. no 15 pp:1-38.

O'Connor, P.G., Carroll, K.M., Shi J.M., Schottenfeld, R.S,. Kosten, T.R.& Rounsaville B.J. (1997). Three methods of opioid detoxification in a primary care setting. A randomized trial. *Ann Intern Med* vol 127 no 7 pp526-530

Payte, J.T & Zweben, J.E. (1998) Opioid maintenance therapies. In: *Principles of Addiction Medicine.* 2nd ed. Chevy Chase, MD: American Society of Addiction Medicine, Inc publisher pp 557-570

Pollack, H.A. & D'Aunno, T. (2010) HIV testing and counseling in the nation's outpatient subtance absue treatment system, 1995-205. *J Subst Abuse Treat* vol 38 no 4 pp307-316.

Proeschold-bell, R.J., Heine, A., Pence, B.W., McAdam, K & Quinlivan, E.B. (2010) A cross-site, comparitive effectivenss study of an integreated Hiv and subtance use treatment program. *AIDS Patient Care STDS* vol 24 no 10 pp 651-658.

SAMHSA (Substance Abuse and Mental Health Services Administation) (2005). Medication Assisted Treatment for Opioid Addiction in Opioid Treatment Programs. *A Treatment Improvement Protocol, TIP 43* Department of Health and Human Services Publication (SMA)-05-4048.

SAMHSA   (Substance Abuse and Mental Health Services Administation) (2009).Incorporating Alcohol Pharmacotherapies into Medical Practice. *A Treatment Improvement Protocol, TIP 43* Department of Health and Human Services Publication (SMA)-09-4380.

Schackman, B.R., Merrill, J.O., McCarty, D., Lev,i J.& Lubinsk,i C. (2006) Overcoming policy and financing barriers to integrated buprenorphine and HIV primary care. *Clin Infect Dis* vol 43 Suppl 4 pp S247-253

Schuckit, M.A. (2006) Comorbidity between substance use disorders and psychiatric conditions. *Addiction* vol 101: suppl 1 pp 76-88.

Schuh, K.J., Walsh, S.L., Bigelow, G.E., Preston, K.L. & Stitzer, M.L. (1996) Buprenorphine, morphine and naloxone effects during ascending morphine maintenance in humans. *J Pharm Exp Therap.* vol 278 no 2 pp 836-846.

Sinner, M.L., Haggarty, K.P., Fleming, C.B., Catalano, R.F. & Gainey, R.R. (2011) Opiate-addicted parents in methadone treatment: long term recovery, health and family relationship. *J Addict Dis* vol 30 no 1 pp 17-26.

Sowers W. (2005) Transforming systems of care: The American Association of Community Psychiatrists guidelines for recovery oriented services. *Community Mental Health J* vol 41 no 6 pp 757-774

Sullivan, L.E., Bruce, R.D., Haltiwanger, D., Lucas, G.M., Eldred, L., Finkelstein, R. & Fiellin, D.A..(2006) Initial strategies for integrating buprenorphine into HIV care settings in the United States. *Clin Infect Dis* vol 43 Suppl 4 pp S191-196

Taege,A. (2011) Seek and treat : HIV update 2011. *Cleve Clin J Med* vol 78 no 2 pp 95-100.

UNODC (2010). Executive Summary. *The World Drug report 2010.* United Nations Office on Drugs and Crime Publishers. ISBN 97-92-1-148256-0 Geneva. pp15-20.

Walsh, S.L., Preston, K.L., Stitzer, M.L., Cone, E.J. & Bigelow, G.E (1994). Clinical pharmacology of buprenorphine: ceiling effects at high doses. *Clin Pharm Therap.* vol 55 no 5 pp 569-580.

Weiss, L. Netherland, J., Egan, J.E., Flanigan, T.P., Finkelstein, R., Altice, F.L., & BHIVES Collaborative (2011). Integreationof buprenorphine/naloxone treatment into HIV clinical care: lessons from the BHIVES collaborative *J Acquir Immune Defic Syndr* vol 56 suppl 1 pp S68-75.

White W.L.& Mojer-Torres L (2010). *Recovery-oriented Methadone Maintenance.* Published by the Great Lakes Addiction Technology Transfer Center, the Philadelphia Department of Behavioral Health and Mental Retardation Services, and the NortheastAddiction Technology Transfer Center 2010. Retrieved from: http://www.ireta.org/resources/romm-exsum.pdf

WHO (World Health Organization) (2004). Alcohol consumption and beverage preferences. *Global Status Report on Alcohol 2004.* Department of Mental Health and Substance Abuse. World Health Organization Publishers. ISBN 92 4 156272 2 Geneva pp9-15.

WHO (World Health Organization) (2008). *Guidelines for the Psychosocially assisted pharmacological treatment of opioid dependence.* World Health Organization, WHO Press ISBN 978 92 4 154754 3 0 Geneva, Switzerland

WHO (World Health Organization) (2009). *Scaling up care for mental, neurological and substance use disorders.* mhGAP Mental Health Gap Action Programme. World Health Organization, WHO Press ISBN 978 92 4 159620 6 Geneva, Switzerland

WHO (World Health Organization) (2009a). *WHO,UNODC, UNAIDS Technical guide for countries to set targets for universal access to HIV prevention, treatment and care for injection drug users.* World Health Organization, WHO Press ISBN 978 92 4 159776 0 Geneva, Switzerland

WHO (World Health Organization) (2010). *Global strategy to reduce the harmfull use of alcohol.* WHO Press. ISBN 978 92 4 159993 1. Geneva, Switzerland

Yokell, M.A., Zaller, N.D., Green, T.C. & Rich, J.D. (2011) Buprenorphine and buprenorphine/naloxone diversion, misue and illicit use: An international review. *Curr Drug Abuse Rev* April 5 [Epub ahead of print]

Zaller, N., Gillani, F.S.& Rich, J.D.(2007) A model of integrated primary care for HIV-positve patients with underlying substance use and metal illness. *AIDS Care* vol 19 no 9 pp 1128-1133.

11

Micronutrient Synergy in the Control of HIV Infection and AIDS

Raxit J. Jariwalla, Aleksandra Niedzwiecki and Matthias Rath

Dr. Rath Research Institute, Santa Clara, CA

USA

1. Introduction

Acquired immune deficiency syndrome (AIDS) has become a global health pandemic and the most common cause of death among young adults aged 20-24 years (Patton et al., 2009). According to the UN/AIDS Global Report published in November 2010 (UNAIDS 2010), about 1.8 million persons died from AIDS-related causes in the year 2009 alone. At the end of that year, the epidemic had left behind totally 16.6 million orphans, defined as those under 18 who had lost one or both parents to AIDS. Since the beginning of the epidemic, nearly 30 million people have died from AIDS-related causes.

At the end of 2009, an estimated 30.8 million adults and 2.8 million children were living with HIV, the human immunodeficiency virus linked to AIDS; with women accounting for just over one-half of all adults living with HIV worldwide. During the same year, about 2.6 million persons became newly infected with HIV, including 370,000 children. Of all people living with HIV, about 68% reside in Sub-Saharan Africa (UNAIDS 2010).

Despite these gruesome statistics, there is no cure in sight. Current treatment is based on the use of antiretroviral (ARV) drugs targeted against HIV at various steps in viral replication (Sleaseman and Goodenow 2003). Although ARV drugs can reduce viral load in the bloodstream, they neither cure HIV infection nor restore the immune system to combat AIDS (Roederer 1998, Pakker et al., 1998). Virus is known to persist indefinitely in reservoirs of latently-infected cells and emergence of drug-resistant strains is common. Furthermore, the effectiveness of ARVs in having any clinical benefits at all depends upon a number of factors, particularly the CD4 count and the nutritional status of patients at the point at which ARV treatment is commenced (Hong et al., 2001, Paton et al., 2006). Additionally, drugs are higly toxic and are often associated with adverse side effects to various organs of the body, including the bone marrow and liver, (Fischl et al., 1987, Richman et al., 1987, Costello et al., 1988, Abrescia et al., 2008), cellular mitochondria (Carr et al., 2001), and with lipodystrophy and dyslipidemia (Carr et al., 1998).

Consequently, there is need for safe and effective, nontoxic therapy that can not only restore the immune system and keep virus multiplication/spread in check but also block AIDS progression without harming cells of the host. This review will focus on the relationship of nutrition to infection and immunity and evidence from experimental and clinical studies on the potential value of micronutrients and their combinations in controlling HIV infection and reducing symptoms associated with AIDS.

2. Nutritional deficiencies in HIV and AIDS

The relationship between nutrition, infection and immunity is well established since the early 1940's (Scrimshaw 2003, Webb and Villamor 2007). It is for instance well recognized that nutritional deficiency can lower immunity and predispose individuals to microbial infection. Conversely, nutritional supplementation can improve immune function and prevent/confer resistance to infection.

As the latent period between HIV infection and AIDS manifestation has been estimated at 8-10 years (Morgan et al 2002), nutritional cofactors, besides HIV, have been implicated in AIDS development (Beach et al., 1992, Baum et al., 1995, Jariwalla et al., 2008a, 2009). Furthermore, nutrient supplementation in asymptomatic HIV-infected individuals was shown to delay the onset of AIDS (Abrams et al., 1993, Tang et al., 1993), supporting involvement of nutritional status as a contributory factor in AIDS development.

It is universally known since the emergence of the AIDS epidemic in the early 1980's that nutritional deficiencies are prevalent in persons with HIV infection and AIDS (Gray 1984, Beach et al., 1992, Jariwalla 1995; see also Table 1). These deficits include: (i) specific micronutrient abnormalities such as reduced blood levels of the common ACE vitamins, minerals, trace elements including selenium, amino acids such as cysteine, and the tri-peptide glutathione, which displays a global systemic deficiency; (ii) macronutrient abnormalities such as protein calorie malnutrition, which has been linked to a wasting disease, characteristic of AIDS. Malnutrition has also been linked to the spread of AIDS and TB in developing countries and with reduced survival (Paton et al., 2006, Turchenko et al., 2008)

MICRONUTRIENT ABNORMALITIES	
Vitamins	Trace Elements
Vitamin A	Selenium
Vitamin B12	Zinc
Vitamin B6	
Vitamin C	Amino Acids
Vitamin E	Cysteine

Peptides
Glutathione

MACRONUTRIENT DEFECITS
Protein Calorie Malnutrition
Abnormal Lipids (Dyslipidemia)

Table 1. Commonly occurring nutritional deficiencies in HIV infection and AIDS

3. Impact of nutritional deficiencies

Micronutrient deficiencies in particular vitamin and mineral deficiencies can promote and strengthen microbial growth by weakening the immune system of the host, making it prone to acquiring new infections (Scrimshaw 2003, Webb and Villamor 2007; see Fig 1).

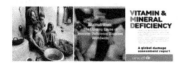
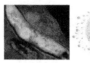

1) Weaken the host

- Make immune system less effective
- Increase susceptibility to infections and other diseases

2) Strengthen infectious agents

- Promote microbial growth
- Activate latent viruses
- Accelerate spread of infections

Fig. 1. Impact of micronutrient deficiencies on infectious diseases

4. Essential role of micronutrients in cell physiology and immunity

Micronutrients are essential for sustaining all cellular functions including metabolic reactions in the cytosol and biochemical functions within cellular organelles (Fig 2). Vitamins and minerals are needed in smaller amounts than proteins, fats and sugars but without them, cells cannot convert food into biological energy and build different body structures.

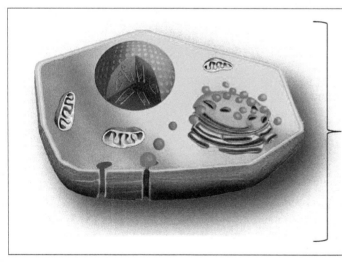

Vitamin C
Vitamin B1
Vitamin B2
Vitamin B3
Vitamin B5
Vitamin B6
Vitamin B12
Vitamin E
Vitamin D
Vitamin K
Vitamin A
Minerals
Trace Elements
Essential Amino Acids

Fig. 2. Micronutrients are essential for sustaining all cellular functions

Micronutrients are also critical for optimum functioning of the immune system including cell-mediated immunity, antibody production (humoral immunity) and optimum thymus function (Fig. 3).

The pathological basis of AIDS is a dysfunctional immune system clinically indicated by abnormally low levels of white blood cells. Micronutrients are essential for blood formation, including white blood cells. Of particular importance are: vitamin B-3, vitamin B-5, vitamin B-6, vitamin B-12, vitamin C, folic acid and iron. Any textbook of biology or biochemistry documents these scientific facts. Moreover, no less than nine Nobel Prizes in Medicine have been awarded to date on the discovery of the health benefits of vitamins, relevant to their role in cellular physiology and impact on the immune system (Nobel Prize Committee website, Nobelprize.org).

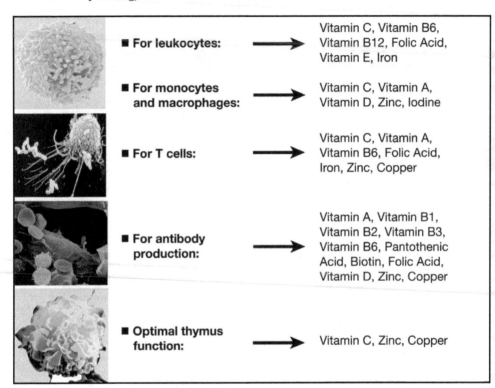

Fig. 3. Nutrients are critical for optimum immune defense of a host

5. Role of micronutrients in suppression of virus infection

Additionally, experimental studies have shown that specific micronutrients can suppress virus infection at various steps in the viral life cycle that include blocking (a) virus entry, (b) virus multiplication, (c) virus activation in latently infected cells and (d) virus spread (Fig 4).
Prevent viral entry into cells (Vitamin C, EGCG)
Stop viral multiplication (Vitamin C, N-Acetylcysteine)
Prevent activation of "silent" viruses (Vitamin C)
Limit spread of infections (Lysine, Vitamin C)
In the case of HIV, micronutrients have been shown to block virus expression at all stages of virus-host interactions, which include acute infection, chronic expression and activation from latently infected cells (Fig 5). The specific micronutrients demonstrated to affect different phases of virus infection are listed in Table 2. Most of them are reducing agents

with antioxidant properties. They include: vitamins C and E, amino acid thiols such as cysteine or its derivative N-acetyl cysteine (NAC), disulfides such as alpha-lipoic acid, tripeptides such as glutathione and its derivative glutathione monoester, polyphenols such as epigallo-catecheine gallate (EGCG from green tea) and the trace element selenium. Among them, ascorbic acid (vitamin C or ascorbate) is the most versatile, capable of blocking HIV replication in all phases of HIV infection namely, acute, chronic and latent infection (Harakeh et al., 1990; Harakeh and Jariwalla, 1991, 1995). Cysteine and glutathione monoester inhibit chronic HIV expression (Mihm et al., 1991; Kalebic et al., 1991) whereas NAC and selenium are effective in inhibiting HIV activation in latently-infected cells (Roederer et al., 1990, Harakeh and Jariwalla 1991; Sappey et al., 1994). It has been reported that alpha-lipoic acid can block acute infection (Bauer et al., 1991) and flavonoids including the polyphenol EGCG inhibit HIV at an early stage, blocking interaction of the virus with

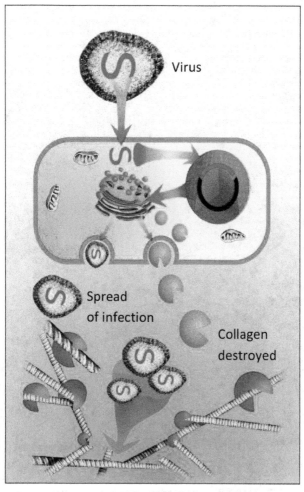

Fig. 4. Nutrients can directly suppress viral infections

host-cells receptor (Mahmood et al., 1993, Fassina et al., 2002). More recently, green tea extract enriched in such polyphenols (80% by weight) was shown to suppress HIV production in chronically and latently infected cells (Jariwalla et al., 2010).

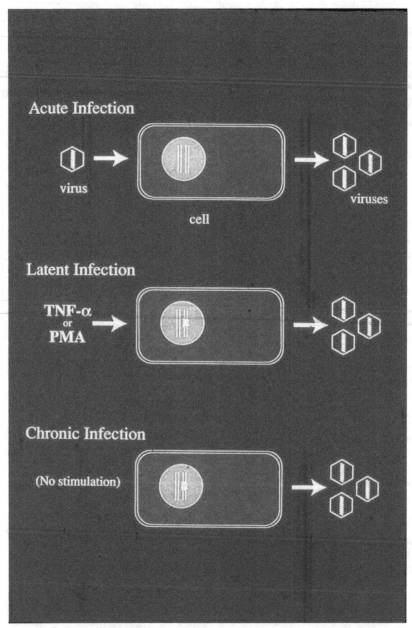

Fig. 5. Micronutrients can target different stages in HIV-host cell interaction

Nutrient	Inhibitory Effect Targeted at	Reference
Vitamin E	Latent infection	Suzuki *et al* 1993
Vitamin C	Acute, chronic and latent infection	Harakeh and Jariwalla (1991, 1995)
Cysteine, alpha-lipoic acid	Chronic and acute infection	Mihm *et al* 1991, Baur *et al* 1991
NAC, Selenium	Chronic and latent infection	Roederer *et al* 1990, Harakeh & Jariwalla 1991, Sappey *et al* 1994.
Glutathione monoester	Chronic infection	Kalebic *et al* 1991
Flavonoids, EGCG, green tea extract	Acute infection	Mahmood et al 1993, Fassina *et al* 2002, Jariwalla et al 2010
Nutrient mixture (NM)*	Synergistic HIV suppression in chronic and latent infection	Jariwalla *et al* 2010

Table 2. Action of micronutrients on phases of HIV infection
* containing (vitamin C, green tea extract, lysine, proline, arginine, NAC, selenium)

6. Our approach to controlling virus infection with nutrient synergy

Although specific, single nutrients have been shown to suppress HIV in previous studies, little attention has been directed at blocking virus expression with nutrient combinations. To investigate this, we have utilized the principle of nutrient synergy i.e. use of nutrients in combination at low to moderate (physiological) levels for prevention and control of disease (Rath and Niedzwiecki 1996, Rath et al., 2005, Jariwalla et al., 2008a, 2009). The principle underlying nutrient synergy is that nutrients work in the body in harmonious synergy, not isolation, and they allow for maximal benefits when used in combination at physiological doses. In nutrient synergy 1 + 1 is more than 2 (Fig 6). We have applied this principle to both experimental studies of HIV infection as well as the in vivo evaluation of a defined multi-micronutrient supplement in AIDS patients in a community wide setting.

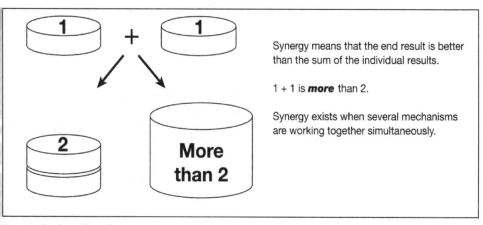

Synergy means that the end result is better than the sum of the individual results.

1 + 1 is **more** than 2.

Synergy exists when several mechanisms are working together simultaneously.

Fig. 6. The benefits of nutrient synergy

All nutrients work in our bodies in harmonious synergy, not in isolation.
Nutrient Synergy allows for achieving maximum health benefits and keeping cellular processes in balance using smaller quantities of nutrients. Use of single vitamins in very high-doses or a randomly selected nutrient combination is not recommended as an optimal approach to health.

7. Experimental studies in HIV infection

Studies conducted by us of micronutrient combinations in laboratory cultures of HIV infected cells have provided further support for nutritional efficacy in viral immunodeficiency disease (Jariwalla et al., 2010). In these studies, we compared the ability of micronutrient combinations to single nutrients in the suppression of HIV replication in both chronically and latently infected cells. H9-HTLV IIIB is a model, chronically-infected T lymphocytic cell line that constitutively produces HIV cytopathic virus in the cell culture supernatant (Popovic et al., 1984, Gallo et al., 1984, Harakeh et al., 1990, Harakeh and Jariwalla 1991). Exposure of these cells to low/moderate concentrations of single micronutrients such as ascorbic acid, green tea extract and the amino acids such lysine produced only small inhibitory effects on virus production. In contrast, exposure of cells to combinations of micronutrients conferred significantly greater HIV suppression compared to single nutrients, indicating a synergistic effect. A nutritional mixture (NM), consisting of vitamin C, green tea extract, amino acids (lysine, proline, arginine), NAC and selenium also gave enhanced suppression of HIV production in this cell line compared to single nutrients (Jariwalla et al., 2010; see also Table 2). A similar inhibitory effect on cytokine-stimulated virus expression was obtained in latently infected T cells, indicating that micronutrients cooperate to suppress virus expression in both chronically and latently-stimulated cells (Jariwalla et al., 2010; Table 2).

8. Clinical nutrition studies in AIDS patients

Based on the above scientific evidence of micronutrient effectiveness in laboratory cultures of virally-infected cells, we have incorporated the use of micronutrients in natural control of HIV infection. Our studies conducted in persons with AIDS symptoms have provided further support for micronutrient efficacy in viral immunodeficiency disease (Jariwalla et al., 2008a, 2009). This in vivo confirmation of micronutrient efficacy was demonstrated in AIDS patients in a community wide program conducted in South Africa between 2005 and 2008. In this community program, the Dr. Rath Foundation donated a micronutrient supplement to the South African National Civic Organization (SANCO) who distributed it among people affected by AIDS in various townships in South Africa.

The micronutrient supplement contained vitamins and trace elements (except iron) that are known to modulate the immune system (listed in Fig. 3) plus selenium, essential minerals and other important nutrients such as amino acids, green tea extract, bioflavonoids, N-acetyl cysteine, inositol and coenzyme Q10. This supplement was given to subjects to be taken 3 times a day with meals. The characteristics of participants, patient selection, informed consent, administration of questionnaire grading AIDS-defining symptoms and the evaluation methodology were reported previously (Jariwalla et al., 2008a, 2009).

The first township where a pilot nutritional program was evaluated was Khayelitsha, a township near Cape Town (Jariwalla et al., 2008a). In this pilot protocol, 56 AIDS patients completed all 3 examinations and their completed questionnaires were evaluated for changes in severity of symptoms seen after the first 3 visits (8-12) weeks from the beginning of micronutrient supplementation. Table 3 lists the AIDS-defining symptoms for Africa, other physical symptoms, pain symptoms and symptoms of well-being. Tables 4-6 show a summary of the impact on these symptoms from micronutrient supplementation. The results showed that within 10-12 weeks, the micronutrient supplement statistically significantly suppressed all AIDS-defining symptoms compared to baseline. The supplement also significantly suppressed other physical symptoms frequently seen in AIDS patients including state of well-being (Jariwalla et al., 2008a).

AIDS-Defining Symptoms	Symptoms of Well Being
Fever	Appetite
Diarrhoea	Energy
Cough	Enjoyment of life
Weight loss	Fear of future
TB	Concentration
Oppurtunistic infections	Anxiety
	Depression
Other Physical Symptoms	Insomnia
Swollen glands	Fatigue
Colds, flu	
Rashes	
Wounds, sores, ulcers	
Headache	
Bloating, gas	
Other physical symptoms	

Table 3. AIDS-Related Symptoms, Conditions and Diseases Monitored in Community Wide Micronutrient Program

The micronutrient supplement evaluated in Khayelitsha was also rolled out in KwaZulu Natal district (near Durban) where a very large group (522 patients) completed all 3 exams and questionnaires. Similar to Khayelitsha, the same trend in reduction of AIDS-defining symptoms, other physical AIDS-associated symptoms and pain symptoms was seen (Tables 4-6). The results were also confirmed in two other townships (Western Cape and Free State), for a total of 813 participants from all 4 townships (Tables 4-6).

Site	Total no of patients	% decrease in AIDS-defining symptoms from baseline after 3 visits *
Khayelitsha	50	33-61%
Kwazulu-Natal (KZN)	473	37-48%
Western Cape	153	51-78%
Free State	82	23-26%

Table 4. Impact of micronutrient supplementation on AIDS defining symptom in a community wide program
*8-12 weeks except Free State (= 40 weeks)

Site	Total no of patients	% decrease in other physical symptoms from baseline after 3 visits *
Khayelitsha	45	37-60%
Kwazulu-Natal (KZN)	522	17-54%
Western Cape	153	44-83%
Free State	78	17-47%

Table 5. Impact of micronutrient supplementation on other physical symptoms in AIDS patients in community wide program
* 8-12 weeks except Free State (= 40 weeks)

Site	Total no of patients	% decrease in pain symptoms from baseline after 3 visits *
Khayelitsha	44	38-49%
Kwazulu-Natal (KZN)	511	32-50%
Western Cape	149	43-64%
Free State	79	24-35%

Table 6. Impact of micronutrient supplementation on pain symptoms in AIDS patients in community wide program
* 8-12 weeks except Free State (= 40 weeks)

9. Conclusion

The results we have seen are not in isolation. Beneficial effects of micronutrients and their combinations have been seen in clinical studies conducted by other researchers as summarized in Table 7. These studies have evaluated nutrients in combination and reported beneficial effects on various outcomes including improvement in viral and immune parameters, antioxidant protection from cellular damage, slowing of disease progression, reduction of AIDS-related symptoms and improvement of birth outcomes in pregnant women. The impact of nutritional support and vitamin and micronutrient supplementation in the treatment of HIV and AIDS is a seriously under-investigated area. Repeated calls have been made for more studies in this area by international health agencies. Although micronutrients are not a cure for AIDS, in the absence of an effective cure or vaccine and in the face of the toxicity and limited efficacy of ARVs, they are a safe, effective and affordable way to halt progression towards and even reduce the symptoms of the AIDS disease and to improve the quality of life of AIDS patients.

The implications of micronutrient supplementation results for public health and control of infectious and immunodeficiency disease are enormous. If properly evaluated, micronutrients have the potential of being incorporated into strategies for fighting viral pandemics on a global scale. Implementation of the above positive findings could save millions of lives.

Micronutrient Supplement	Clinical change	Reference
Multivitamin Supplement	Delayed onset of AIDS in HIV positive asymptomatic persons	Abrams et al 1993, Tang et al 1993
N-acetylcysteine (NAC)	Increased survival compared to placebo	Herzenberg et al 1997
Vitamin C plus E	1) Reduced oxidative stress, viral load 2) Prevention of AZT-induced miochondrial damage	Allard et al 1998, de la Asuncion et al 1998
NAC plus vitamin C	Enhanced immune responses and reduced viral load in advanced AIDS	Muller et al 2000
Multivitamin Supplement	Reduced fetal death among HIV-infected Tanzanian women	Fawzi et al 1998, 2004
Multi-micronutrient Supplement	Increased survival among HIV-infected persons in Bangkok	Jiamton et al 2003
Micronutrient Supplement	Improved CD4 count	Kaiser et al 2006
Nutritional Supplements	Delayed AIDS progression in HIV-infected persons	Namulemia et al 2007
Alpha-lipoic acid	Enhanced blood glutathione and improved lymphocyte function	Jariwalla et al 2008b
Micronutrient Supplement (see text, page 8)	Reduced AIDS related and pain symptoms; improved state of well being	Jariwalla et al 2008a; 2009

Table 7. Clinical improvements seen upon micronutrient supplementation in HIV and AIDS patients, in peer-reviewed published studies.

10. Acknowledgement

We would like to thank Lisa Smith for help with formatting/presentation of the graphics and Anupriya Pandit for tabulating data and organizing references.

11. References

Abrams B, Duncan D & Hertz-Picciotto I. (1993). A prospective study of dietary intake and acquired immune deficiency syndrome in HIV-seropositive homosexual men. *J Acquir Immune Defic Syndr.*, Vol. 6, No. 8, pp. 949-58.

Abrescia N, D'Abbraccio M, Figoni M, Busto A, Maddaloni A & De Marco M. (2005). Hepatotoxicity of antiretroviral drugs. *Current Pharmaceutical Design*, Vol. 11, pp. 3697-3710.

Allard JP, Aghdassi E, Chau J, Tam C, Kovacs CM, Salit IE & Walmsley SL. (1998). Effects of vitamin E and C supplementation on oxidative stress and viral load in HIV-infected subjects. *AIDS*, Vol. 12, No. 13, (September 10), pp. 1653-9.

de la Asunción JG, del Olmo ML, Sastre J, Millán A, Pellín A, Pallardó FV & Viña J. (1998). AZT treatment induces molecular and ultrastructural oxidative damage to muscle mitochondria. Prevention by antioxidant vitamins. *J Clin Invest.*, Vol.102, No. 1, (July 1), pp. 4-9.

Bauer A, Harrer T, Peukert M, Jahn G, Kalden JR & Fleckenstein B. (1991). Alpha-lipoic acid is an effective inhibitor of human immuno-deficiency virus (HIV-1) replication. *Klin Wochenscher*, Vol. 69, No. 15, (October 2), pp. 722-724.

Baum MK, Shor-Posner G, Lu Y, Rosner B, Sauberlich HE, Fletcher MA, Szapocznik J, Eisdorfr C, Buring JE & Hennekens CH. (1995). Micronurients and HIV-1 disease progression. *AIDS*, Vol. 9, No. 9, pp. 1051-1056.

Beach RS, Mantero-Atienza E, Shor-Posner G, Javier JJ, Szapocznik J, Morgan R, Sauberlich HE, Cornwell PE, Eisdorfer C & Baum MK. (1992). Specific nutrient abnormalities in asymptomatic HIV-1 infection. *AIDS*, Vol. 6, No. 7, pp. 701-8.

Carr A, Samaras K, Chisholm DJ & Cooper DA. (1998). Pathogenesis of HIV-1-protease inhibitor-associated peripheral lipodystrophy, hyperlipidaemia, and insulin resistance. *Lancet*, Vol. 351, No. 9119, (June 20), pp. 1881-3.

Carr A, Morey A, Mallon P, Williams D & Throburn DR. (2001). Fatal portalhypertension, liver failure, and mitochondrial dysfunction after HIV-1 nucleoside analogue-induced hepatitis and lactic acidaemia. *Lancet*, Vol. 357, No. 9266, (May 5), pp. 1412-4.

Costello C. (1988). Haematological abnormalities in human immunodeficiency virus (HIV) disease. *Journal of clinical pathology*, Vol. 41, pp. 711-715.

Fassina G, Buffa A, Benelli R, Varnier OE, Noonan DM & Albini A. (2002). Polyphenolic antioxidant (-)-epigallocatechin-3-gallate from green tea as a candidate anti-HIV agent. *AIDS*, Vol. 16, No. 6, (April 12), pp. 939-41.

Fawzi WW, Msamanga GI, Spiegelman D, Urassa EJ, McGrath N, Mwakagile D, Antelman G, Mbise R, Herrera G, Kapiga S, Willett W & Hunter DJ. (1998). Randomised trial of effects of vitamin supplements on pregnancy outcomes and T cell counts in HIV-1-infected women in Tanzania. *Lancet*, Vol. 351, No. 9114, (May 16), pp. 1477-82.

Fawzi W, Msamanga G, Antelman G, Xu C, Hertzmark E, Spiegelman D, Hunter D & Anderson D. (2004). Effect of prenatal vitamin supplementation on lower-genital levels of HIV type 1 and interleukin type 1 beta at 36 weeks of gestation. *Clin Infect Dis.*, Vol. 38, No. 5, (Mar 1), pp. 716-22.

Fischl MA, Richman DD, Grieco MH, Gottlieb MS, Volberding PA, Laskin OL, Leedom JM, Groopman JE, Mildvn D, Schooley RT *et al.* (1987). The efficacy of azidothymidine (AZT) in the treatment of patients with AIDS and AIDS-related complex. A double-blind, placebo-controlled trial. *N Engl J Med*, Vol. 317, No. 4, (July 23), pp. 185-91.

Gallo RC, Salahuddin SZ, Popovic M, Shearer GM, Kaplan M, Haynes BF, Palker TJ, Redfield R, Oleske J, Safai B, et al. (1984). Frequent detection and isolation of cytopathic retroviruses (HTLV-III) from patients with AIDS and at risk for AIDS. , Vol. 224, No. 4648, (May 4), pp. 500-3.

Gray RH. (1984). Similarities between AIDS and PCM. *AM J Public Health*, Vol. 73, No. 11, pp. 1332.

Harakeh S, Jariwalla RJ & Pauling L. (1990). Suppression of human immunodeficiency virus replication by ascorbate in chronically and acutely infected cells. *Proc. Natl. Acad. Sci USA*, Vol. 87, No. 18, pp. 7245-49.

Harakeh S & Jariwalla RJ. (1991). Comparative study of the anti-HIV activities of ascorbate and thiol-containing reducing agents in chronically HIV-infected cells. *Am J Clin. Nutr.*, Vol. 54, No. 6S, pp. 1231S-1235S.

Herzenberg LA, De Rosa SC, Dubs JG, Roederer M, Anderson MT, Ela SW & Deresinski SC. (1997). Glutathione deficiency is associated with impaired survival in HIV disease. *Proc Natl Acad Sci U S A*, Vol. 94, No. 5, (March 4), pp. 1967-72.

Hogg RS, Yip B, Chan KJ, Wood E, Craib KJ, O'Shaughnessy MV & Montaner JS. (2001). Rates of disease progression by baseline CD4 cell count and viral load after initiating triple-drug therapy. *JAMA*, Vol. 286, No. 20, (November 28), pp. 2568-77.

Jariwalla RJ. (1995). Micronutrient imbalance in HIV infection and AIDS: Relevance to pathogenesis and therapy. *J Nutr Environ Med*, Vol. 5, pp. 297-306.

Jariwalla RJ, Niedzwiecki A, & Rath M. (2008a). Micronutrients and nutrient synergy in immunodeficiency and infectious disease. In: *Botanical Medicine in Clinical Practice* (R. R. Watson & V. R. Preedy, Eds), pp 203-12. CAB International, London, UK.

Jariwalla RJ, Lalezari J, Cenko D, Mansour SE, Kumar A, Gangapurkar B & Nakamura D. (2008b). Restoration of blood total glutathione status and lymphocyte function following alpha-lipoic acid supplementation in patients with HIV infection. *J Altern Complement Med.*, Vol. 14, No. 2, pp. 139-46.

Jariwalla RJ, Niedzwiecki A, & Rath M. (2009). The essentiality of nutritional supplementation in HIV infection and AIDS: Review of clinical Studies and results from a community helath micronutrient program. In: Bioactive Foods in Promoting Health: Fruits and Vegetables (R. R. Watson & V. R. Preedy, Eds), pp 323-342. Oxford: Academic Press, ISBN: 978-0-12-374628-3.

Jariwalla RJ, Gangapurkar B, Pandit A, Kalinovsky T, Niedzwiecki A & Rath M. (2010). Micronutrient cooperation in the suppression of HIV production in chronically and latently infected cells. *Mol Med Report,* Vol. 3, No. 3, pp. 377-85.

Jiamton S, Pepin J, Suttent R, Filteau S, Mahakkanukrauh B, Hanshaoworakul W, Chaisilwattana P, Suthipinittharm P, Shetty P & Jaffar S. (2003). A randomized trial of the impact of multiple micronutrient supplementation on mortality among HIV-infected individuals living in Bangkok. *AIDS*, Vol. 17, No. 17, (November 21), pp. 2461-9.

Kaiser JD, Campa AM, Ondercin JP, Leoung GS, Pless RF & Baum MK. (2006). Micronutrient supplementation increases CD4 count in HIV-infected individuals on highly active antiretroviral therapy: a prospective, double-blinded, placebo-controlled trial. *J Acquir Immune Defic Syndr.*, Vol. 42, No. 5, (August 15), pp. 523-8.

Kalebic T, Kinter A, Poli G, Anderson ME, Meister A & Fauci AS. (1991). Suppression of human immunodeficiency virus expression in chronically infected monocytic cells by glutathione, glutathione ester, and N-acetylcysteine. *Proc Natl Acad Sci USA*, Vol. 88, No. 3, (February 1), pp. 986-90.

Mahmood N, Pizza C, Aquino R, De Tommasi N, Piacente S, Colman S, Burke A & Hay AJ. (1993). Inhibition of HIV infection by flavonoids. *Antiviral Res.*, Vol. 22, No. 2-3, pp. 189-99.

Mihm S, Ennen J, Pessara U, Kurth R & Droge W. (1991). Inhibition of HIV-1 replication and NF-κB by cysteine and cysteine derivatives. *AIDS*, Vol. 5, No. 5, pp. 497-503.

Morgan D, Mahe C, Mayanja B, Okongo, Lubega R & Whitworth JA. (2002). HIV-1 infection in rural Africa: Is there a difference in median time to AIDS & survival compared with that in industrialized countries. *AIDS*, Vol. 16, No. 4, (March 8), pp. 597-603.

Müller F, Svardal AM, Nordoy I, Berge RK, Aukrust P & Frøland SS. (2000).Virological and immunological effects of antioxidant treatment in patients with HIV infection. *Eur J Clin Invest.*, Vol. 30, No. 10, pp. 905-14.

Namulemia E, Sparling J & Foster HD. (2007). Nutritional supplements can delay the progression of AIDS in HIV-infected patients: results from a double-blinded, clinical trial at Mengo hospital, Kampala, Uganda. *Journal of orthomolecular Medicine,* Vol. 22, pp. 129-136.

Nobelprize.org (1929-1964). The nobel prize and the discovery of vitamins (by K.J. Carpenter), Retrieved from http://nobelprize.org/nobel_prizes/medicine/articles/carpenter

Pakker NG, Notermans DW, de Boer RJ, Roos MT, de Wolf F, Hill A, Leonard JM, Danner SA, Miedema F & Schellekens PT. (1998). Biphasic kinetics of peripheral blood T cells after triple combination therapy in HIV-1 infection: a composite of redistribution and proliferation. *Nat Med.*, Vol. 4, No. 2, pp. 208-14.

Paton NI, Sangeetha S, Earnest A & Bellamy R. (2006). The impact of malnutrition on survival and the CD4 count response in HIV-infected patients starting antiretroviral therapy. *HIV Med.*, Vol. 7, No. 5, pp. 323-30.

Patton GC, Coffey C, Sawyer SM, Viner RM, Haller DM, Bose K, Vos T,Ferguson J & Mathers CD. (2009). Global patterns of mortality in young people: a systematic analysis of population health data. *Lancet*, Vol. 374, No. 9693, (September 12), pp. 881-92.

Popovic M, Sarngadharan MG, Read E & Gallo RC. (1984). Detection, isolation, and continuous production of cytopathic retroviruses (HTLV-III) from patients with AIDS and pre-AIDS. *Science*, Vol. 224, No. 4648, (May 4), pp. 497-500.

Rath M & Niedzwiecki A. (1996). Nutritional supplement program halts progression of early coronary atherosclerosis documented by ultrafast computed tomography. *Journal of Applied Nutrition*, Vol. 48, pp. 67-78.

Rath M, Kalinovsky T & Niedzwiecki A. (2005). Reduction in the frequency of arrhythmic episodes in patients with paroxysmal atrial arrhythmia with a vitamin/essential nutrient program. *JANA*, Vol. 8, pp. 21-25.

Richman DD, Fischl MA, Grieco MH, Gottlieb MS, Volberding PA, Laskin OL, Leedom JM, Groopman JE, Mildvan D, Hirsch MS, Jackson GG, Durack DT & Nusinoff-Lehrman S. The AZT collaborative working group. (1987). The toxicity of azidothymidine (AZT) in the treatment of patients with AIDS and AIDS related complex. A double-blind, placebo-controlled trial. *New England Journal of Medicine*, Vol. 317, pp. 192-197.

Roederer M. (1998). Getting to the HAART of T cell dynamics. *Nat Med.*, Vol. 4, pp. 145-6.

Roederer M, Staal FJ, Raju PA, Ela SW & Herzenberg LA. (1990). Cytokine-stimulated human immunodeficiency virus replication is inhibited by N-acetyl-L-cysteine. *Proc. Natl. Sci USA*, Vol. 87, No. 12, pp. 4884-8.

Sappey C, Legrand-Poels S, Best Belpomme M, Favier A, Rentier B & Piette J. (1994). Stimulation of glutathione peroxidase activity decreases HIV type 1 activation after oxidative stress. *AIDS Res. Hum. Retroviruses*, Vol. 10, No. 11, pp. 1451-61.

Scrimshaw NS. (2003). Historical concepts of interactions, synergism and antagonism between nutrition and infection. *Journal of Nutrition*, Vol. 133, No. 1, pp. 316S-321S.

Sleaseman JW and Goodenow MM. (2003). HIV-1 infection. *J Allergy Clin Immunol.*, Vol. 111, No. 2 suppl, pp. S582-S592.

Suzuki YJ & Packer L. (1993). Inhibition of NF-κB activation by vitamin E derivatives. *Biochem. Biophys. Res. Commun.*, Vol. 193, No. 1, (May 28), pp. 277-83.

Tang AM, Graham NM, Kirby AJ, McCall LD, Willett WC & Saah AJ. (1993). Dietary micronutrient intake and risk of progression to acquired immunodeficiency syndrome (AIDS) in human immunodeficiency virus type 1 (HIV-1)-infected homosexual men. *Am J Epidemiol.*, Vol. 138, No. 11, (December 1), pp. 937-51.

Turchenko LV, Voloshchuk EO, Ivanov V, Kalinovsky T, Niedzwiecki A & Rath M. (2008). Clinical improvement of active tuberculosis patients with complex treatment and nutritional supplementation. *The Open Natural Products Journal*, Vol. 1, pp. 20-26.

UNAIDS (2010). UNAIDS Report on the Global AIDS Epidemic, Retrieved from http://www.unaids.org/globalreport/

Webb AL & Villamor E. (2007). Update: effects of antioxidant and non-antioxidant vitamin supplementation on immune function. *Nutr Rev.*, Vol. 65, No. 5, pp. 181-217.

12

The Pertinence of Applying Qualitative Investigation Strategies in the Design and Evaluation of HIV Prevention Policies

Carmen Rodríguez, Teresa Blasco, Antonio Vargas and Agustín Benito
National Centre for Tropical Medicine, Health Institute Carlos III
Spain

1. Introduction

"We think that there still exists a vast sector of science in which we are no further than in taylorian stages of intellectual work rationalization and which can do nothing but contribute to scientific rigor. Rigor when reasoning is more important that rigor when calculating. Questions is more important than rigor than questionnaires."
Edgar Morin [1]

In the last decade, the incidence of HIV has globally diminished by 19% (Joint United Nations Programme on HIV/Aids, [Unaids], 2010). Likewise, new cases of children infected by HIV have diminished due to the spread of vertical mother-child prevention among pregnant women. The percentage of people who received anti-retroviral treatment increased by 30% due to improvements in the accessibility of therapeutic treatment. Also, the annual percentage of death caused by Aids has decreased (Unaids, 2010). Nevertheless, in spite of this progress, HIV/Aids pandemic continues to be one of the main threats to global health. On a world scale, pandemic epidemiological data shows alarming numbers: there are more than 33 million people around the world living with HIV. Approximately, 7,000 new cases of infection arise every day. Every year, an average of 1,800,000 people die as a consequence of Aids. It is estimated that 12 million children have been orphaned (Unaids, 2010).

However, such numbers are distributed in unequal proportions throughout the world. Thus, since not every country presents the same level of prevalence, big differences can be found. Currently, most of the countries suffering from HIV pandemic are developing countries. Also, these countries show low or medium levels of human development. The Table 1 shows the relation between Human Development Index in some countries with a higher pandemic level.

As seen on table 1, the distribution of the pandemic tendency throughout these countries reveals a clear correlation: The less socio-economically developed a country is, the higher the HIV prevalence is. This being so, it is hardly surprising that sub-Saharan African or Asian countries present widespread epidemic HIV levels. On a world scale, these countries hold the highest Multidimensional Poverty Index (United Nations Development Programme, [Unpd], 2010). For instance, the worst Human Development Index in the world belongs to

---

[1] Morin, Eder. (2006). *The method* (ed. Cátedra).

Countries	2009 HIV estimates in Adults and children	HDI 2010
Nigeria	3,300,000	0.432
India	2,400,0000	0.59
United Republic Of Tanzania	140,000	0.398
Zimbawe	120,000	0.140
Uganda	120,000	0.422
Malawi	920,000	0.385
Zambia	98,000	0.395

Table 1. Relation between HIV and HDI prevalence
Self-made

belongs to Zimbabwe (0.291) and, at the same time, the highest levels of HIV prevalence can be found there – around 20% and 25%-, (UNPD, 2010). With the one before, in countries like Sweden, where the Human Development Index is very high, (0.773) such prevalence varies between 1% and 5% (UNPD, 2010).

Therefore, the highest number of cases are to be found in lesser developed countries, bearing almost 90% of the whole HIV prevalence worldwide. In these countries, the HIV epidemic is one of the largest National Health problems faced by their Governments. As a consequence, strategic plans of prevention, together with the provision of welfare coverage in the treatment of HIV, are given top priority by the National policies. Nonetheless, HIV epidemic does not only mean a challenge at political level, it also entails a menace to entails a menace to democracy and governability in these countries' political systems. Regarding this last statement, the South African Institute for Democracy has published a report highlighting the negative effect of HIV/Aids in the electoral processes of these countries.

HIV epidemic in these countries does not only mean a medical and sanitary problem, it also constitutes one of the main obstacles for their socio-economic development. Given the huge percentage of adults who die as a consequence of Aids, these countries lose their young people, those who could help with their economic development to a higher degree. In addition, economic productivity also decreases due to the fact that the number of people infected by Aids or those who take care of them must quit their jobs. Besides, their educational systems are affected due to the percentage of teachers who die as a consequence of Aids. This situation brings about an important loss of highly educated inhabitants. Likewise, medical expenses generated out of the provision of health services to people who live with HIV (PLHIV) and Aids, involve budgetary restrictions in the investment of public expenses in other sectors, with the aim of promoting the economic and social development of these countries. In connection with this, the UNPD estimates that in Bostwana the State Revenue dropped by 20% in 2010 as a direct result of HIV/Aids (PNUD, 2010).

Regarding families, the consequences of this epidemic in the domestic economy of these countries are also devastating. When they lose the "head of the family" –the one who has to meet the economic needs of the family– they lose their income, their nutrition worsens, agricultural production falls, medical expenses increase, savings turn into debts, funeral expenses multiply, children leave schools, people's health deteriorates, and so on. In fact, a survey carried out in Zambia shows that two thirds of urban homes which have lost the head of the family as a consequence of Aids have seen their income drop by 80%. The same survey revealed that 61% of these families moved to cheaper places to live, 39% lost their access to drinking water and also 21% of girls and 17% of boys gave up their school studies (PUND, 2001).

Finally, the spread of the epidemic in these countries is increasing, deepening existing poverty and social inequality, and reversing the trend towards their level of human development. Hence, HIV/Aids epidemic has become one of the main key aspects in national policies of Poverty Reduction Strategies (PRS) (PNUD, 2002) Such strategies are becoming the main national planning instrument in many countries. That is why HIV/Aids plays a central role in the processes of national development planning and in the budgetary allocation of these States. This contributes to the creation of adequate policies and providing the necessary resources, in order to give a wide multisectorial response to the HIV problem.

Generally, a higher prevalence of the pandemic in countries with low human development index increases social injustice and emphasizes the north-south divide. So that the fight against HIV/Aids together with the fight poverty has become two parts of the same parts of the same battle. Therefore, regarding poverty in certain countries, there will be no possibility to achieve the Millenium Development Goals (MDGs) unless HIV/Aids is efficiently treated. That is why the fight against HIV/Aids has been chosen as the sixth MDG (United Nations, [Nu], 2000).

2. The importance of prevention in the response to the epidemic

After three decades fighting against the epidemic, in the field of public health there is no doubt that the intervention from prevention policies is the most efficient weapon in order to eliminate and combat the epidemic (World Health Organization, [Who], 2010). In this sense, competent international organizations struggle more and more to make governments and other institutions aware of the importance of implementing efficient actions in order to prevent HIV. So, the last UNAIDS world report has included measurement indexes for different aspects of prevention processes carried out in different countries as evaluative indicators of the current state of the epidemic (Unaids, 2010).

All over the world, the high number of new cases of HIV in 2010 corroborate the pressing need for intervention in order to stop the development of the epidemic. There again, a higher incidence of HIV cases in developing countries has established prevention as a priority in the national policies of these countries. In connection with this, it is worth knowing that 97% of the new infections produced every day are to be found in people who live in countries with medium or low human development index (Unaids, 2010). Specifically, it is in the African context where the cases of incidence occur more frequently.

As for the development of HIV prevention policies, experience reveals that there are no universal formulae for success that might be applied to all countries. Therefore, certain strategies of prevention proved to be successful in a given country may not constitute any guarantee in another, due to the multiple factors that interfere in the development of the different policies. For instance, each context presents a set of specific needs which must be taken into account for the design and implementation of such policies. Among other things, exclusive qualities of the social and cultural elements also play a part when defining the context in which the intervention is going to take place. That is why it is advised to take into account all of these aspects and adapt the design of HIV prevention policies to the context in which they will be implemented.

Currently, there is a big concern about how to adapt prevention policies to African countries. On the one hand, it is due to the urgent need to change the development of the epidemic considering its magnitude and, on the other hand, to the ineffectiveness shown by prevention policies to date, considering the high rates of incidence. As a consequence, the epidemic stabilization has not yet been reached in some countries.

2.1 Prevention policies in the African context

HIV prevention actions developed in Africa are key to slow down the great development of this disease. Besides, prevention actions have an added value since either they must be linked to or they must incorporate values, such as justice, fairness and the promotion of dignity. At the same time, it constitutes basic principles which help to improve the African context.

Now, some of the international recommendations on public health as well as some of the existing evidence on HIV prevention in the African context to date are described.

Prevention actions must be aware of the main HIV routes of transmission in the continent. In Africa, the HIV epidemic spreads mainly through sexual intercourse. The percentage of people who became infected by this disease through routes other than the sexual intercourse is low. Nevertheless, mother-to-child transmission and hemoderivatives transfusion are the other two relevant aspects when assessing prevention measures in countries where, like in the African context, the investment in public health is not enough.

It is advisable to develop HIV prevention policies that interact with the different levels of prevention. According to the World Organization of Family Doctors (Wonca), there are four grades of prevention. Primary prevention is the one that involves action before the disease appears and, among these actions are the ones in charge of promoting health, those focused on environmental hygiene or those like vaccination or chemical prophylaxis. Secondary prevention deals with actions aimed at identifying ill patients within the population, implementing strategies of population sifting, enabling the early detection of diseases. Through implemented actions, tertiary prevention involves easing or avoiding the effects of the disease once it has been contracted. Finally, in 1986 Marc Jamoulle defined quaternary prevention as *"those actions designed to restrict unnecessary damage produced as a consequence of health-care activity"*.

Within the current priority of international recommendations on health-HIV, five guidelines for intervention have been developed. These guidelines are especially relevant in countries with higher prevalence, as in most of the African countries (Who, 2009). They mainly include preventive actions in the three first levels:

1. Strengthening actions in primary prevention of the disease from the health sector.
2. Making it possible for the population to know its serological status.
3. Accelerating the spread of the treatment as well as the HIV/Aids care.
4. Strengthening health systems capacities.
5. Increasing knowledge in order to improve response.

In general, as a maxim of intervention in public health, the development of HIV-related actions, including all actions and not only preventive ones, should be adapted to each and every context in three determining factors. Firstly, they should adapt to the specific characteristics of the epidemic in question, like the particular context of each country as well as that of its community. Secondly, they should pay attention to the cultural context and, thirdly, to the level of provision of services and resources set aside for health. Related to this last aspect and in order to strengthen the adaptation of international frameworks at local level, actions developed to prevent HIV are considered to be complex interventions as gards their evaluation processes (Campbell et al., 2000). In order to do so, it is advisable to ke into account the adaptation of the process to the local circumstances before being nplemented once it has been completely standardized. Therefore, for an optimal nplementation, it is currently considered as necessary to have the adequate knowledge to rientate this process of adaptability of the standard theoretical framework.

the African context, a low specific applicability of these criteria can be found. That is why a w level of key targets for prevention has been achieved. It is worth mentioning that only 32% of e African population knows their serological status. Likewise, only 45% of pregnant women ceive proper care in order to prevent their children from contracting the disease. (Who, 2010).

s regards the type of epidemic, actions carried out in the African context must have plenty characteristics unique to the generalized epidemic. This is the most common ridemiological situation in most countries of the continent. The fact of presenting nieralized epidemic levels determines the monitoring of intervention priorities within the revention area:

Using strategies that would cover all risk behaviour of contracting the disease. Besides, these strategies must be as accessible as possible to the population in need of help.

Decentralizing the provision of services by incorporating primary care actions as well as community actions.

Integrating prevention services together with treatment and care services into primary care services.

Giving priority to actions aimed at tertiary prevention making it possible to interrupt the epidemiological chain of the disease, diminishing the appearance of new cases.

Recommending the diagnostic sifting of every person who makes use of health care services and to all pregnant women or those in a lactation period.

he existence of a whole multiplicity of cultural components characteristic of every area and nique to every social group is something that, for the time being, has not been sufficiently flected in the adaptation of the general frameworks to each context. The recommendation at second generation epidemiological vigilance (Grulich & Kaldor, 2002) (Who, 2000) iould be integrated into the tracking and monitoring processes of the disease makes it rssible to count on a broader knowledge of people's attitudes and practices. Moreover, laptation to strategies has improved. The use of qualitative methodologies in order to nerate this knowledge is still very recent and, in some contexts, almost nonexistent. This is iown as a tool that supplies key elements, having a deeper impact on health when lapting actions to contexts.

eakness in health systems which implement actions and policies is a very common factor around Africa. Such weakness does not always derive from the low budget allocated to i development. In the last years, poor systems and limited resources, together with iportant obstacles that eliminate the possibility to improve these systems, demand the ied to search for evidence-based knowledge in order to determine which actions are the ost cost-effective in HIV. This knowledge would help to establish criteria that could iprove the management of the intervention.

ut of all this generated knowledge, taking into account the target context of the chapter as ell as efficiency criteria previously mentioned, we wanted to pay special attention to the ilue of implementing associated measures of secondary and tertiary prevention, like agnosis and treatment, respectively.

he initial intervention model in the fight against HIV implemented only tertiary prevention easures, in spite of its low efficiency when trying to reduce the progression of the disease.

The target was to reduce the high rate of mortality caused by this disease at that time Nowadays, the antiretroviral treatment has evolved and it is considered to be highly activ (HAART). Cohort studies in serodiscordant couples and pregnant women living with HIV have proved that patients who receive good treatment and have an undetectable viral load are less likely to transmit the disease (Quinn et al., 2000). This ART has proved to be a ver good method to reduce the transmission of this disease and that is the reason why currently, on a global scale, all countries are advised to reach universal coverage (Granich e al, 2009) of the treatment. The reason is not only that the rate of mortality decreases but als its effect on the transmission chain.

There is a great variability when it comes to value the cost-effectiveness of HIV strategie depending, above all, on the country where the action is implemented (Andrew, 2002) Following this criteria, actions of prevention that cause a deeper impact and those enjoying better cost-effectiveness criteria are meant to limit mother-to-child transmission of the disease. Regarding the diagnosis of the disease in the population, the HIV strategies meet th requirements defined by Frame and Carslon (Frame & Carslon, 1975) in order to be able t carry out actions of secondary prevention and, therefore, make quite an impact both on th health of the patient and on the health of the whole population. The necessary criteria fo this applicability are the following:

1. The disease must be an important health problem, having a clear effect on the quality o life and life expectancy.
2. The disease must develop through an asymptomatic initial stage and its natural histor must be known.
3. There must be an effective treatment accepted by the population in the case that th disease is detected in its initial state.
4. There must be a sifting test which has to be quick, safe, easy-to-do, highly sensitive, highl specific, of high positive predictive value and well accepted by doctors and patients.
5. The sifting test must keep a good cost-effectiveness balance.
6. The early detection of the disease and its treatment during the asymptomatic perio must diminish morbidity as well as global or each of them separately.

In the last years, the scientific community issued an appeal for the innovation of develope prevention strategies (Piot,2008). Current recommendations in order to cause a greate impact on health in the African context suggest that actions of secondary prevention, such a diagnosis, and actions of tertiary prevention, such as ARV treatment, are joined (Dooc 2010). It is important to bear in mind that without diagnosis there is no treatment and, a seen before, preventing this disease from being transmitted becomes a limited task.

3. Application of qualitative methodologies in HIV prevention

"Aids has proved that epidemics take place at different levels: biological event, social perceptior collective response and individual phenomenon, both existential and moral [...].Each disease, as soci phenomenon, is a unique configuration of events and responses both in the biological sphere and i the social sphere"(Mariano Bronfman[2]

In the scientific field, HIV epidemic has traditionally been investigated by clinica epidemiology. For this reason, the predominant theoretical development has been th

---

[2] Mariano Bronfman: Social Sciences and Aids. Magazine of Public Health and Mexico 1999;Vol.41(2):8 84.

biomedical model. Concerning this subject, most of the investigations to be found on scientific literature are prevalence and/or ecological studies. In this sense and in general terms, knowledge based on data that mainly describe the way this epidemic is distributed throughout the population according to certain factors predominate (Caitlin et al., 2010). However, the relevance and significance that HIV epidemic has gained in the social sphere nowadays constitute evidence. This fact can be clearly seen, for instance, when paying attention to the social stigma generated around HIV (Skinner & Mfecane, 2004). That is why most of the interventions being carried out in the field of HIV take into account the social dimension of the problem. In this sense, epidemic research beyond simple observation of how it is distributed throughout a given population is required.

Currently, the HIV epidemic represents a social phenomenon that mainly affects the area of public health. The HIV epidemic as a social phenomenon acquires different meanings depending on the kind of society in which it is found, since cultural and social contexts play an important role in all countries. For example, although HIV is seen as a cronical disease in the collective unconscious of most developed countries, this virus is considered to be fatal and lethal in the developing countries (Conde, 1997). There again, as HIV is meddled in social constructs like life, health, dead and disease, it is also steeped in specific connotations that every culture attributes to these social values.

So that HIV acquires meanings, representations, perceptions, values and erelated to social and cultural contexts. Such contexts give meaning and guide people's behaviour and actions to confront HIV. These distinctive values, meanings and so forth, will have an effect on preventive actions that are being taken in order to face the HIV phenomenon. As can be seen, qualitative aspects that are also important to know in order to prevent and eliminate the epidemic mark the HIV phenomenon.

By applying the methodologies which have developed the traditional approaches to HIV study, the knowledge of HIV qualitative aspects is difficult to achieve. Nowadays, with the aim of setting out a deeper and more holistic HIV knowledge, other perspectives and theoretic approaches belonging to disciplines other than health are applied. For instance, approaches to the epidemic phenomenon have been carried out by different sciences -like hermeneutics, phenomenology or ethnography- in which their theoretical frameworks from disciplines like Anthropology or Sociology (Arachu & Pau, 2003). The efforts made by UNESCO in order to develop and promote a cultural approach to the HIV epidemic are especially worthy of notice (United Nations Educational, Scientific and Cultural Organozation, [Unicef], 2003).

Theoretical approaches in the field of social sciences have incorporated HIV study methodologies different from the quantitative, which is traditionally applied by clinic epidemiology. Among these methodologies, the use of qualitative methodology prevails. Therefore, qualitative methodology is no longer a method exclusively used in disciplines connected to the social sphere. In this sense, it appears more and more frequently in health related studies, whose scientific expansion displays as much on publications and seminars as on medicine and public health related conferences.

On an international level, different authors have placed particular emphasis on the necessity and in the advantages of using this methodology in the field of public health (Bryman, 1984). Also, its relevance to social epidemiology has been highlighted. For instance, it has been pointed out its importance when used in order to evaluate peoples' health care from a more dynamic and comprehensive perspective. It has also been stated the necessity to know both the adaptation of qualitative methodology for its study and the socio-cultural background together with people's values as health determining factors.

As compared to other diseases or to other health related subjects, qualitative methodology has been widely used in the study of the HIV. However, qualitative investigations performed in this field are still few. But there are still fewer qualitative research aimed at putting into practice the necessary knowledge in order to evaluate and design HIV prevention policies.

Nevertheless, the results of the studies carried out show the adaptation and benefits of this methodology to the understanding and comprehension of the different factors that intervene in the HIV epidemic phenomenon. So that the adaptation of qualitative strategies to the study of the HIV phenomenon constitutes a potential instrument of support to design effective preventive strategies and, therefore, carry out effective and efficient policies in the intervention of this epidemic.

4. Application of a case: Equatorial Guinea

4.1 Epidemiological context

The HIV/Aids epidemic is also severely affecting Guinean people's health. On the basis of parameters established by the WHO, Equatorial Guinea suffers from generalized epidemic (Unaids, 2010 b). The HIV prevalence among people between 15 and 49 years of age is 3.2% (IC 95% 2.0 -4.4%). Likewise, Aids represents the main cause of individual mortality (Who, 2008).

In a context of generalized epidemic, competent international organizations warn of the urgent need for these countries to set appropriate measures in motion in order to reverse the epidemic curve. They also emphasize the importance of carrying out prevention policies with the aim of diminishing and eliminating the magnitude of the epidemic. At the same time, they urge the governments of these countries to establish and coordinate effective strategic plans for the prevention of the HIV. In this regard, one of the preventive measures recommended by the WHO is to spread the HIV diagnosis tests throughout the whole population, regardless whether there is clinical suspicion or not, and suggests having the test done at least once a year (Who, 2007) given the positive results that this action would carry with it in both individual level and community level. On an individual level: it initiates and holds preventive behaviour towards the HIV acquisition and transmission, immediate access to care, treatment and support of people living with HIV, major efficacy on interventions in order to prevent mother-to-child transmission, better planning to improve the future life. On community level: it diminishes denial, stigma and discrimination associated to the HIV and demands aid for an adequate answer. However, evidence suggests that, in terms of cost-effectiveness, everyone having the test done becomes profitable on the long term, regardless whether they take part in high risk behaviour or not. (Patiel, 2005).

As for HIV preventive measures carried out by the Guinean population, there is almost no information that describes and explains this aspect due to the lack of research in this field of study. Nevertheless, there is some data extracted from a transversal study conducted by ISCIII in collaboration with MINSABS. In this study, people aged between 15 and 50 were given a questionnaire – the CAP survey[3] – about different aspects concerning sexual life and

---

[3] "Knowledge, attitudes and practices about nuptiality, sexual activity, HIV/Aids and STD"

HIV/Aids. Results related to the execution of HIV diagnosis show that almost ¾ of the people who participated in the survey had never had the tests done (Ministry of Health and Social Welfare of Malabo, 2006). The fact that an important percentage of the population is not aware of their serological status aggravates the magnitude of the epidemic due to the existing risk of exponential growth, as a consequence of HIV transmission through people unaware of their seropositive status. Likewise, this study also stresses the vulnerability of this society towards the epidemic, since evidence shows that being aware of one's serological status is the first step to be taken in order to prevent and treat the disease.

Regarding the use of male condoms among the Guinean population, the CAP survey produced alarming results. Sexual intercourse is the main HIV transmission route in Equatorial Guinea. That is why, in this country, different social agents competent in HIV prevention have made tremendous efforts to extend and promote the use of male condoms when having sex in order to control this transmission route. In spite of the efforts made, the results of the CAP survey show that the use of the male condom has not been one of the prevention methods used by a vast majority of the Guinean population. Although 73% of those polled point out that they do know how to use male condoms as an HIV preventive measure, almost seven out of ten declared that they had not used them in the last twelve months when having occasional sex with different partners. The male condom was not used by 73% of those men who had sex with prostitutes either.

Generally, CAP results reveal that the Guinean population has taken few measures regarding HIV prevention.

4.2 Justification for the study

No sociological investigation considering HIV as a social phenomenon had been previously carried out in Equatorial Guinea. That is why there was no holistic or hermeneutic knowledge about the epidemic phenomenon in the country.

Until the completion of the ESEVIGUE study, there was no qualitative data about the epidemic. In this sense, the qualitative aspects of the epidemic constitute key elements to take into account when designing HIV prevention policies. For instance, there was no information about the meaning or possible meanings that the epidemic had acquired in society. Moreover, there was no information about the elements –whatever their nature: cultural, social, political, economic…-that could be interfering with the results of the implemented prevention strategies, acting like barriers and/or facilitators. In general, explanatory information about people's practices and behaviours related to the implemented prevention strategies was non-existent.

Given the absence of these data, the possibility to carry out an investigation in order to announce this situation arises. In the last analysis, the reasons why the preventive measures developed in the country got such results will be evaluated and explained. In this context, the ESEVIGUE comes into being with the general aim of: "understanding and generating knowledge about the epidemic phenomenon in Equatorial Guinea".

This study targeted the use of generated knowledge as support in order to direct the decision taking process, regarding the different strategies and measures to be implemented in the area of HIV prevention.

This research started in Bata in August 2009 and has been led jointly by MINSABBS, in Malabo, and the National Centre for Tropical Medicine of the Carlos III Health Institute, (Referential Centre for the Control of Endemic Diseases [CRCE], 2009) in Spain. This investigation has been carried out by a research team made up of professionals belonging to both institutions.

4.3 The basis of the methodological design

Although epidemiological methods have been traditionally regarded as the standard reference for the study of public health, these methodologies are based on a reductionist view of the world in which simple causality standards are established through statistical processes (Baum, 1997). Health and disease are the result of a complex interrelation of social, economical, political and environmental factors. Interpretative methods based on qualitative techniques are generally well prepared for the analysis of complex situations and contribute to a large extent to the study of public health (Baum, 1997).

The aim of the research was to observe the epidemic as a social phenomenon so that, considering biological investigative or medical approaches, a social perspective of the HIV study was adopted. The design of the investigation has been a qualitative one. The decision of carrying out a qualitative methological design was backed up by the adaptation that qualitative strategies have shown in order to generate holistic, deep and comprehensive knowledge of the real situation under study. Nowadays, in the area of public health, the effective use of qualitative techniques for the understanding and comprehension of factors and processes affecting health and disease is also sufficiently verified. To be more specific, many examples of qualitative methodology applied to the study of the HIV and its context can be found in scientific literature (Medicus Mundi, 2007). In this respect, it is worth mentioning that, confronting epidemiological and quantitative HIV medical study, this type of investigations have proliferated over the last decades.

The sample used in the investigation was a structural one. As in quantitative investigations, the sample design consitutes one of the first methodological aspects to be defined. However, its theoretical basis differs from the sample design in quantitative research. Whereas sample design in quantitative research is based on the concept of statistic representation, in qualitative research it is based on the social signification criteria of the individuals (Valles, 1997). In this sense, sample validity is not given by the number of individuals that make up the sample but by the pertinence of selected individuals in connection with the aims of the study.

Regarding the object of the study, a first general criterion of sample inclusion was established: Individuals aged between 13 and 60. Defining this section of age span became relevant due to the fact that the main HIV route of transmission is sexual intercourse. Therefore, in view of prevention, getting to know the meaning of the HIV epidemic phenomenon and other related aspects within the sexually active population in Guinea was considered to be pertinent.

In the second place, the sample was segmented according to certain variables of interest: being infected by HIV or not, sex, age, education level and place of residence. This segmentation was aimed at identifying and gathering different perceptions and experiences of the HIV. For instance, the initial hypothesis was that, in general terms, there would be differences between PLWHIV and those who do not, as regards perceptions, meanings and practices. Likewise, it was also considered to be pertinent to pay attention to the thoughts of different social groups so as to know the various conceptions of HIV that there may be throughout the whole variety of social groups that form the Guinean society. The objective was to adequate prevention strategies to the specific needs of each social group. For the purpose of this research, the sex and the gender of the individuals, their education level, etc. was taken into account.

Information gathering techniques applied in order to produce and collect information were: semi-structured individual interview and discussion group. These techniques are generically named qualitative techniques. In order to develop both techniques, the script item was outlined. The script item is a gathering information tool that contains qualitative techniques. This script item was drawn up through open questions that explored analytical dimensions related to the object of study. Now, in table 2, some of the analytical dimensions are shown:

ANALYTICAL DIMENSION	CATEGORIES AND QUESTIONS
Health meaning and value	What are the important things in your life? What does health mean to you?
Social Perception of the HIV	What do you think about the HIV? What do people say about the HIV?
Knowledge about the HIV	What is the HIV? Are the HIV and Aids the same disease? How can a person become infected by the HIV?

Table 2. Analytical Dimensions of the ESEVIGUE research

Before the fieldwork was performed, the script item was tested following preliminary interviews. The aim of testing this instrument was to check the validity of its technical design as regards the content of the questions, the format and the language.

4.3.1 The reasons why semi-structured interviews are applied

Semi-structured interviews were done to people living with the HIV. The application of this technique, in opposition to other group qualitative techniques like discussion groups, has the advantage of preserving anonymity and confidentiality about the serological status of the interviewee.

Semi-structured interview is performed on the basis of a face-to-face conversation between the interviewer and the interviewee. That involves immediate and personal norms of verbal interaction generating, therefore, a subjective knowledge of the observed reality (Alonso, 1994). The interview is a communicative tool that sets out to grasp meanings that are influenced by the constructions made by the individuals themselves according to their experience:

> "Personal interview results very productive to the study of extreme or typical cases in which the attitudes of certain people embody, in every sense, the ideal model of a certain attitude much less crystallized in the average of the group of reference (Ortí, 1986)".

So that this technique was carried out with the aim of getting to know the experiences and meanings felt by people living with the HIV. Therefore, its application in the ESEVIGUE resulted in the knowledge of the subjective aspect of suffering HIV. Also, this technique provided information about the phenomenon of the epidemic from the point of view of the people living with the HIV.

4.3.2 The reason why the discussion group is applied to the study

The discussion group was performed among the population segment of participants who did not know if they were seropositive and/or those whose blood tests results were negative. Since it is a group technique, it has the advantage of confronting and gathering discourse from the different social groups in one session. At the same time, in economical terms, this technique becomes more profitable

The different points of view of the studied reality regarding the position occupied by the individual in the social framework can be known through the application of discussion groups (ref.). This used to be a key aspect of the technical selection since it allowed the gathering of different HIV related discourses in order to produce and adapt prevention strategies to the specificities of each social group. Therefore, the application of such technique created diverse knowledge about the different social aspects regarding the HIV.

4.3.3 Fieldwork

Finally, fieldwork based on qualitative methodological strategies was done with the aim of generating knowledge about the HIV phenomenon. Prior to the phase of gathering information, the research team applied the non-participant observation technique. It was aimed at validating different aspects of the study protocol such as sample design or instruments to collect information. It was also aimed at later development of fieldwork.

Geographically, this research took place in Bata between January and April 2010 and it was carried out by a multidisciplinary working group made up of sociologists, doctors, nurses and lab assistants.

5. Conclusions

In terms of results achieved, the application of qualitative methodology has turned out to be very adequate and valid in order to generate holistic and comprehensive information of the HIV epidemic phenomenon in Equatorial Guiena. So that data has been generated in order to allow both evaluating some of the prevention strategies in the country and showing some of the key aspects to take into account in decision-making processes in the strategy to be implemented.

For instance, results show the inadequacy of massive HIV/Aids information and prevention campaigns carried out in Equatorial Guinea. The association established between the HIV, Aids and death has caused much alarm and fear among the population. Nowadays, it constitutes one of the main barriers for the population to have diagnostic tests done of their own free will. The conducted campaigns played a decisive role in the HIV social construction, which does not favour the integration of people living with Aids into society. Such social construction about people living with the HIV having abandoned the services of the HIV treatment and diagnosis, influenced the reasons given in order to explain why they decided to give up their treatment.

Results have also revealed the importance and necessity of implementing and carrying out prevention strategies considering already existing specificities and needs among different social groups. In this sense, interviewed women's and men's different ways of understanding health and facing the disease are shown. These aspects must be taken into account when designing prevention strategies in order to achieve maximal efficiency and effectiveness in results.

Nevertheless, the development of the methodology has not been exempt from difficulties and inconveniences. The first drawback was brought about by the application of this type of methodology in a context of low involvement of the population in social movements and slender culture of social discussion forums. In spite of counting on the collaboration and participation of MINSABS, occasionally people did not want to participate in group sessions for fear of attending politically oriented meetings. Likewise, this fear was also revealed through some of the participants' concerns regarding the confidentiality of the provided information related to personal assessment and opinions about the country.

Difficulties were also revealed due to the lack of tradition in qualitative research in the country. That is why human resources educated and/or qualified in this methodology can scarcely be found. As a consequence, identifying and integrating Guinean personnel into the research team was quite difficult.

To sum up, the HIV epidemic is a complex social phenomenon in the Guinean society. In this sense, the HIV epidemic phenomenon has acquired particular connotations that require specific interventions in this field. Moreover, it also reveals that working frameworks and multidisciplinary action is required in order to prevent and treat the epidemic.

6. Acknowledgment

To the people who took part in interviews and discussion groups, for sharing their time and HIV experiences with the research team. To Jesús Nzang for the generosity that he showed during the development of fieldwork. His dedication and collaboration made it possible to overcome the problems found during the data collection. To Catalina Mangue, Gaspar Nkoni and Luis Mbonio from the CRCE in Equatorial Guinea, for the support they gave me during the recruitment of participants. To Doctor Nemesio Abeso, Director of the MINSABS National Plan of Fight against Aids in Malabo, and Pilar Aparicio, for his support and confidence in the study for his support and confidence in the study. To Jose Luís Cenal, Leticia Díaz and Alberto Hedo from the Foundation for International Health and Cooperation of the National Health System of Spain, for his assistance in the logistic management of the project. And To the Spanish Agency for International Development Cooperation, for financing the study. The study was co-funded by the Instituto de Salud Carlos III, Spanish Research Network of Tropical Diseases (RICET;RD06/0021/0000), Ministry of Science and Innovation of Spain.

It has been possible to write these pages thanks to the contributions made by all these people and institutions.

7. References

Alonso, LE. (1994). Subject and Discourse: The place of the open interview in the practices of qualitative sociology. In: *The Qualitative look on sociology*, Síntesis, pp. 144-53, Madrid

Arachu & Pau. (2003). Aids and structural violence: The blaming of the victim. *Notebooks on Social Anthropology*, Vol.14, pp.29-47

Baum, F. (1997). Public health research: The debate about qualitative and quantitative methodologies. *Public health reviews*, Vol.5, pp.175-193

Bryman, A. (1984). The debate about quantitative and qualitative research: a question of method or epistemology?. *Br J Sociol*, Vol 35, pp. 33- 77

Caitlin, E.; Amy, K.; Medly, M.; Sweat, M. & Reilly, K. (2010). Behavioural Interventions for the prevention of HIV in developed countries: systematic revision and meta-analysis. *WHO bulletin*, Vol. 88, pp. 561-640

Campbell, M. ; Fitzpatrick, R. ; Haines, A.; Kinmonth, A. ; Sandecork, P. ; Spiegelhalter, D.; & Tyrer, P. (2000). Framework for the design and evaluation of complex interventions to improve health. *BMJ*, Vol.321, pp. 694–96

Centre of Reference for the Endemic disease Control. (2009) Presentation of the ESEVIGUE study in the MINSABS. Date of access, 1/4/2010. Available from: http://www.crceguinea.org/index.php?option=com_content&task=view&id=118 &Itemid=86

Conde, F. (1997). HIV/Aids future scenarios: from the disease «event» to the diffuse chronicity. From the moral stigma to the central areas of social vulnerability. *Public health magazine*, Vol.71, No.1, pp.1-7

Creese, A.; Floyd, K.; Alban, A.; & Guinness, L. (2002). Cost-effectiveness of HIV/Aids interventions in Africa: a systematic review of the evidence. *Lancet*, Vol.359, pp. 1635-42

Dodd, P.; Garnett, G. & Hallett, T. (2010). Examining the promise of HIV elimination by 'test and treat' in hyper-endemic settings. *AIDS*, Vol.24, pp. 729–35

Frame & Carlson. (1975). A critical review of periodic health screening using specific screening criteria. Part 4: selected miscellaneous diseases. *J Fam Pract.* Vol.2, No.4, pp.283-9

Granich, M.; Gilks, F.; Dye, C.; De Cock, M. & Williams, G. (2009). Universal voluntary HIV testing with immediate antiretroviral therapy as a strategy for elimination of HIV transmission: a mathematical model. *Lancet, Vol.* 373, pp. 48–57

Grulich & Kaldor. (2002). Evidence of success in HIV prevention in Africa. *The Lancet*, Vol. 360, pp.41-6

Quinn, C.; Wawer, J.; Sewankambo, N.; Serwadda, D.; Li, C.; Wabwire, F. & Meehan, M. (2000). Viral load and heterosexual transmission of human immunodeficiency virus type 1. *N Engl J Med*, Vol. 342, pp.921–29

Idasa. (2004).HIV/Aids and Democratic Governance in South Africa http://www.aceproject.org/ace-es/focus/fo_aids/onePage Consulted: 23/3/2011

Medicus Mundi. (2007). *Women, Aids and access to health in Sub-saharan Africa: Approach from Social Sciences*, (Medicus Mundi Barcelona), B-9865-2007, Spain

Salinero, J., García-Inés, M., Sánchez, I., Sidro, I. (2006). *Survey on knowledge, attitudes and practices about nuptiality, sexual activity, HIV/Aids and STD among the sexually active population in Equatorial Guinea.* (MINSABS). Malabo, Guinea Ecuatorial

Paltiel, A.; Weinstein, M.; Kimmel, A.; Seage, G.; Losina, E. & Zhang, H. (2005). Expanded screening for HIV in the United States. An analysis of cost-effectiveness. *N Engl J Med.* Vol.352, pp.586-95

Piot, P.; Bartos, M. & Larson, H. (2008). Coming to terms with complexity: a call to action for HIV prevention. *Lancet,* Vol.372, pp.845-59

Skinner & Mfecane.(2004). Stigma, discrimination and the implications for people living with HIV/Aids in South Africa. *Sahara J,* Vol.1.N3, pp.157-64

Unaids. (2010 a). Report on the global Aids epidemia. Available in: http://www.unaids.org/documents/20101123_GlobalReport_em.pdf   Consulted: 29/11/2010

Unaids. (2010 b). National report on progresses made in the performance of UNGAS. Available in: http://www.unaids.org/en/dataanalysis/monitoringcountryprogress/2010progre ssreportssubmittedbycountries/equatorialguinea_2010_country_progress_report_e s.pdf Consulted: 29/11/2010

Unpd. (2011). Human Devolopment Report 2010. Avaible in: http://hdr.undp.org/en/reports/global/hdr2011/ Consulted: 4/2/2011

Unpd. (2002). HIV/Aids and strategies for poverty reduction. Diponible en: http://www.pnud.cl/areas/4.asp Consulted: 4/3/2011

UN. (2000). Millenium Goals Declaration. Resolution 58/291. General Assembly. Available in: http://www.un.org/es/comun/docs/?symbol=A/RES/55/2.   Consulted 29/11/2010 Consulted: 8/3/2011

Unesco.(2003). A cultural approach to HIV/Aids prevention and attention. Collection of methodological manuals N° 1

Ortí, A. (1986). The opening and the qualitative or structural approach: The semi-managerial open interview and the discussion group, In: *The analysis of social reality: methods and techniques of social investigation,* M. García, J. Ibañez & F. Alvira (comps.), pp. 171-203, Madrid

Valles, M. (1997). Qualitative techniques of social investigation: methodological reflexion and professional practice. Síntesis, Madrid

Who.(2010). Towards universal access: scaling up priority HIV/Aids interventions in the health sector. Progress report 2010. Available in: http://www.who.int/hiv/pub/2010progressreport/report/en/index.html Consulted: 23/3/2011

Who. (2009). Prioritary HIV/Aids interventions, prevention, treatment and care in the health sector. Available in : http://www.aidslex.org/site_documents/HP-0062F.pdf Consulted: 15/3/2011

Who. (2008). Epidemiological Country Profile on HIV and Aids. Available in: http://www.unaids.org/es/resources/unaidspublications/2008/ Consulted:12/02/2011

Who. (2007). Mortality country fact sheet 2006. Available in: http://www.unaids.org/es/resources/unaidspublications/2007/ Consulted:15/3/2011

Who. (2000). Guidelines for Second Generation Surveillance of HIV Infection. Geneva: Who and Joint United Nations Programme on HIV/Aids Available in:

http://www.unaids.org/es/resources/unaidspublications/2000/
Consulted:14/2/2011
Who.(1998). Public health approach for STD control. Available in:
http://www.who.int/hiv/pub/sti/en/stdcontrol_sp.pdf Consulted: 15/2/2011

Permissions

The contributors of this book come from diverse backgrounds, making this book a truly international effort. This book will bring forth new frontiers with its revolutionizing research information and detailed analysis of the nascent developments around the world.

We would like to thank Yi-Wei Tang, MD, PhD, for lending his expertise to make the book truly unique. He has played a crucial role in the development of this book. Without his invaluable contribution this book wouldn't have been possible. He has made vital efforts to compile up to date information on the varied aspects of this subject to make this book a valuable addition to the collection of many professionals and students.

This book was conceptualized with the vision of imparting up-to-date information and advanced data in this field. To ensure the same, a matchless editorial board was set up. Every individual on the board went through rigorous rounds of assessment to prove their worth. After which they invested a large part of their time researching and compiling the most relevant data for our readers. Conferences and sessions were held from time to time between the editorial board and the contributing authors to present the data in the most comprehensible form. The editorial team has worked tirelessly to provide valuable and valid information to help people across the globe.

Every chapter published in this book has been scrutinized by our experts. Their significance has been extensively debated. The topics covered herein carry significant findings which will fuel the growth of the discipline. They may even be implemented as practical applications or may be referred to as a beginning point for another development. Chapters in this book were first published by InTech; hereby published with permission under the Creative Commons Attribution License or equivalent.

The editorial board has been involved in producing this book since its inception. They have spent rigorous hours researching and exploring the diverse topics which have resulted in the successful publishing of this book. They have passed on their knowledge of decades through this book. To expedite this challenging task, the publisher supported the team at every step. A small team of assistant editors was also appointed to further simplify the editing procedure and attain best results for the readers.

Our editorial team has been hand-picked from every corner of the world. Their multi-ethnicity adds dynamic inputs to the discussions which result in innovative outcomes. These outcomes are then further discussed with the researchers and contributors who give their valuable feedback and opinion regarding the same. The feedback is then collaborated with the researches and they are edited in a comprehensive manner to aid the understanding of the subject.

Apart from the editorial board, the designing team has also invested a significant amount of their time in understanding the subject and creating the most relevant covers. They scrutinized every image to scout for the most suitable representation of the subject and create an appropriate cover for the book.

The publishing team has been involved in this book since its early stages. They were actively engaged in every process, be it collecting the data, connecting with the contributors or procuring relevant information. The team has been an ardent support to the editorial, designing and production team. Their endless efforts to recruit the best for this project, has resulted in the accomplishment of this book. They are a veteran in the field of academics and their pool of knowledge is as vast as their experience in printing. Their expertise and guidance has proved useful at every step. Their uncompromising quality standards have made this book an exceptional effort. Their encouragement from time to time has been an inspiration for everyone.

The publisher and the editorial board hope that this book will prove to be a valuable piece of knowledge for researchers, students, practitioners and scholars across the globe.

List of Contributors

Gail Reid and Richard M. Novak
University of Illinois, Chicago, U.S.A.

Chi Dola, Sean Kim and Juliet Tran
Department of Obstetrics and Gynecology, Tulane University School of Medicine, New Orleans, Louisiana, USA

Gerrit Schreij
Maastricht University Medical Centre, Maastricht, The Netherlands

Rob Janknegt
Orbis Medical Centre, Sittard-Geleen, The Netherlands

Scott Ledger
The Faculty of Medicine, The University of New South Wales, Sydney, Australia

Borislav Savkovic
The School of Mathematics and Statistics, The University of New South Wales, Sydney, Australia

Michelle Millington, Helen Impey and Maureen Boyd
Calimmune Australia, 405 Liverpool St Darlinghurst, NSW, Australia

John M. Murray
The School of Mathematics and Statistics, The University of New South, Australia
The Kirby Institute, The University of New South Wales, Sydney NSW, Australia
St Vincent's Institute for Applied Medical Research, 405 Liverpool St Darlinghurst, NSW, Australia

Geoff Symonds
Calimmune Australia, 405 Liverpool St Darlinghurst, NSW, Australia
St Vincent's Institute for Applied Medical Research, 405 Liverpool St Darlinghurst, NSW, Australia

Lisa Egerer, Dorothee von Laer and Janine Kimpel
Innsbruck Medical University, Department of Hygiene, Microbiology and Social Medicine, Division of Virology, Innsbruck, Austria

Ramesh B. Batchu
Laboratory of Surgical Oncology & Developmental Therapeutics, Department of Surgery, Wayne State University, Detroit, MI
John D. Dingell VA Medical Center, Detroit, MI, USA

Oksana V. Gruzdyn
Laboratory of Surgical Oncology & Developmental Therapeutics, Department of Surgery, Wayne State
University, Detroit, MI, USA

Aamer M. Qazi
Laboratory of Surgical Oncology & Developmental Therapeutics, Department of Surgery, Wayne State University, Detroit, MI, USA
John D. Dingell VA Medical Center, Detroit, MI, USA

Assaad Y. Semaan, Shelly M. Seward, Christopher P. Steffes, David L. Bouwman and Donald W. Weaver
Laboratory of Surgical Oncology & Developmental Therapeutics, Department of Surgery, Wayne State University, Detroit, MI, USA

Scott A. Gruber
John D. Dingell VA Medical Center, Detroit, MI, USA

María José Abad, Luis Miguel Bedoya and Paulina Bermejo
Department of Pharmacology, Faculty of Pharmacy, University Complutense, Ciudad Universitaria s/n, 28040, Madrid, Spain

Alexandre de Almeida, Telma Miyuki Oshiro, Alessandra Pontillo and Alberto José da Silva Duarte
University of São Paulo, Brazil

Maja A. Sommerfelt
Bionor Pharma ASA, Norway

Thomas F Kresina, Robert Lubran and Laura W. Cheever
Centre for Substance Abuse Treatment, Substance Abuse and Mental Health Services, Administration and HIV/AIDS Bureau, Health Resources and Services Administration, USA

Raxit J. Jariwalla, Aleksandra Niedzwiecki and Matthias Rath
Dr. Rath Research Institute, Santa Clara, CA, USA

Carmen Rodríguez, Teresa Blasco, Antonio Vargas and Agustín Benito
National Centre for Tropical Medicine, Health Institute Carlos III, Spain

Printed in the USA
CPSIA information can be obtained
at www.ICGtesting.com
JSHW011434221024
72173JS00004B/793

9 781632 410276